MW01038060

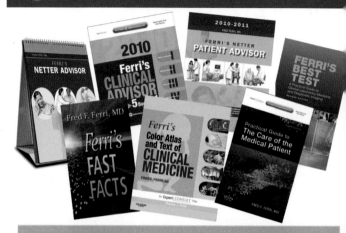

Ferri's Fast Facts in Dermatology

Ferri's Fast Facts in Dermatology
A Practical Guide to Skin Diseases and Disorders

EDITOR

Fred F. Ferri, MD, FACP
Clinical Professor
Warren Alpert Medical School
Brown University
Providence, Rhode Island

ASSOCIATE EDITORS

James S. Studdiford, MD, FACP
Associate Professor
Department of Family and Community Medicine
Jefferson Medical College
Thomas Jefferson University
Philadelphia, Pennsylvania

Amber Tully, MD
Assistant Professor of Family Medicine
Jefferson Medical College
Thomas Jefferson University
Philadelphia, Pennsylvania

SAUNDERS
ELSEVIER

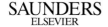

1600 John F. Kennedy Blvd.
Ste 1800
Philadelphia, PA 19103-2899

FERRI'S FAST FACTS IN DERMATOLOGY   ISBN: 978-1-4377-0847-9
A Practical Guide to Skin Diseases and Disorders

Notice

Knowledge and best practice in this field are constantly changing. As new research and experience broaden our
understanding, changes in research methods, professional practices, or medical treatment may become necessary.
Practitioners and researchers must always rely on their own experience and knowledge in evaluating and using any
information, methods, compounds, or experiments described herein. In using such information or methods they
should be mindful of their own safety and the safety of others, including parties for whom they have a professional responsibility. With respect to any drug or pharmaceutical products identified, readers are advised to check
the most current information provided (i) on procedures featured or (ii) by the manufacturer of each product to
be administered, to verify the recommended dose or formula, the method and duration of administration, and
contraindications. It is the responsibility of practitioners, relying on their own experience and knowledge of their
patients, to make diagnoses, to determine dosages and the best treatment for each individual patient, and to take
all appropriate safety precautions. To the fullest extent of the law, neither the Publisher nor the authors, contributors, or editors, assume any liability for any injury and/or damage to persons or property as a matter of products
liability, negligence or otherwise, or from any use or operation of any methods, products, instructions, or ideas
contained in the material herein.

The Publisher

Library of Congress Cataloging-in-Publication Data

Ferri, Fred F.
  Ferri's fast facts in dermatology : a practical guide to skin diseases and disorders / Fred F. Ferri ; associate editors,
James S. Studdiford, Amber Tully.—1st ed.
    p. ; cm.
  ISBN 978-1-4377-0847-9
  Includes index.
  1. Skin—Diseases—Handbooks, manuals, etc. 2. Skin—Diseases—Atlases. I. Studdiford, James S. II. Tully,
Amber. III. Title. IV. Title: Fast facts in dermatology.
  [DNLM: 1. Skin Diseases—Handbooks. WR 39 F388f 2011]
  RL74.F47 2011
  616.5—dc22   2009025859

The patient images without a credit line were taken from the following collections:
1) The Honickman Collection of Medical Images in memory of Elaine Garfinkel
2) The Jefferson Clinical Images Collection (through the generosity of JMB, AKR, LKB, and DA)

Acquisitions Editor: Jim Merritt
Developmental Editor: Nicole DiCicco
Project Manager: Bryan Hayward
Design Direction: Steven Stave

Printed in China

Last digit is the print number: 9   8   7   6   5   4   3   2   1

CONTENTS

CHAPTER 3 DISEASES AND DISORDERS 41

APPENDICES

INDEX

PREFACE

This manual is meant to be a "portable, visual, peripheral brain" for medical students, residents, practicing physicians, and allied health professionals in dealing with the diagnosis and treatment of disorders of the skin. It is not meant to serve as a replacement for the many voluminous dermatology textbooks currently available to those specializing in dermatology.

Every attempt has been made to incorporate practical information in a standard format and to provide pearls of wisdom accumulated in clinical training. The book is subdivided into three main sections. The first section deals primarily with a basic initial approach to skin lesions. The second section provides a practical dermatologic differential diagnosis. The final section covers 164 specific disorders, most of them primary skin diseases, others being systemic diseases with skin manifestations. Each topic is subdivided into five major sections: General Comments (definition, etiology), Keys to Diagnosis (clinical manifestations, physical examination, diagnostic tests), Differential Diagnosis, Treatment, and Clinical Pearls. I hope that this standardized approach will facilitate the rapid diagnosis and treatment of dermatologic disorders commonly encountered in the daily practice of medicine.

Fred F. Ferri, MD, FACP
Clinical Professor
Alpert Medical School
Brown University
Providence, Rhode Island

ACKNOWLEDGMENTS

I gratefully acknowledge the generosity of the many colleagues listed below who have lent text material to this book. A special thank you to James S. Studdiford, MD, FACP, and Amber Tully, MD, both at Family and Community Medicine at Jefferson Medical College of Thomas Jefferson University, for providing me with most of the fine illustrations used in this manual. If I have left anyone out, it is not out of immodesty or unintended claims of original material but simply an oversight given the myriad of sources involved in this project:

Purva Agarwal, MD
Tanya Ali, MD
George O. Alonso, MD
Ruben Alvero, MD
Srivdya Anandan, MD
Mel L. Anderson, MD, FACP
Michelle Stozek Anvar, MD
Kelly Bossenbrok, MD
Maria A. Corigliano, MD, FACOG
George T. Danakas, MD, FACOG
Rami Eltibi, MD
Mark J Fagan, MD
Gil M. Farkash, MD
Staci A. Fisher, MD, FACP
Glenn G. Fort, MD, MPH
Joseph Grillo, MD
Mohammed Hajjiri, MD
Sajeev Handa, MD
Christine Hartley, MD

Jennifer Jeremiah, MD
Michael P. Johnson, MD
Joseph Masci, MD
Lonnie R. Mercier, MD
Dennis Mickolich, MD, FACP, FCCP
James J. Ng, MD
Gail M. O'Brien, MD
Steven M. Opal, MD
Pranav M. Patel, MD
Eleni Patrozou, MD
Peter Petropoulos, MD, FACC
Arundathi G. Prasad, MD
Deborah L. Shapiro, MD
Jennifer Souther, MD
Dominick Tammaro, MD
Iris Tong, MD
Tom Wachtel, MD
Marie Elizabeth Wong, MD

I also extend a special thanks to the authors and contributors of the following texts who have lent illustrations and text material to this book:

Goldstein BG, Goldstein AO: *Practical Dermatology,* ed 2, St. Louis, 1997, Mosby.
Lebwohl MG, Heymann WR, Berth-Jones J, Coulson I [eds]: *Treatment of Skin Disease,* St. Louis, 2002, Mosby.
McKee PH, Calonje E, Granter SR [eds]: *Pathology of the Skin with Clinical Correlations,* ed 3, St. Louis, 2005, Mosby.
Swartz MH: *Textbook of Physical Diagnosis,* ed 5, Philadelphia, 2006, Saunders.
White GM, Cox NH [eds]: *Diseases of the Skin, a Color Atlas and Text,* ed 2, St. Louis, 2006, Mosby.

Fred F. Ferri, MD, FACP
Clinical Professor
Alpert Medical School
Brown University
Providence, Rhode Island

CHAPTER 1

EVALUATION OF SKIN DISORDERS

A. HISTORY AND PHYSICAL EXAMINATION

- The initial step in the dermatologic evaluation involves obtaining a detailed dermatologic history. **Box 1-1** describes pertinent questions.
- When examining the patient it is essential to detail the skin lesions, their distribution, and their characteristics.
- Classically skin lesions have been classified as primary or secondary:
  - Primary lesions represent the initial basic lesion.
  - Secondary lesions may result from evolution of the primary lesions or may be created by scratching or infection.
- The proper terminology in describing these lesions is described in **Box 1-2** and **Box 1-3**.
- For diagnostic purposes it is also important to note the distribution of the skin lesions. **Table 1-1** describes vascular and miscellaneous skin dermatoses.

BOX 1-1 Dermatologic History

A. Initial Questions
 1. When did the rash start?
 2. What did it look like when it first started, and how has it changed?
 3. Where did it start, and where is it located now?
 4. What treatments, especially over-the-counter medications or self-remedies, has the patient tried? What was the effect of each of these treatments?
 5. Are there symptoms (e.g., itching, pain)?
 6. What is the patient's main concern about the rash (e.g., itching, pain, cancer)?
 7. How is the rash affecting the patient's life?
 8. Are other family members concerned or affected?
 9. Has the patient ever had this rash before? If so, what treatment worked?
 10. What does the patient think caused the rash?

B. Follow-up Questions
 1. Does the patient have a history of chronic medical problems?
 2. What is the patient's social history, including occupation (chemical exposures), hobbies, alcohol and tobacco use, and any underlying interpersonal or family stress?
 3. What medications is the patient taking, acutely or chronically, including birth control pills and over-the-counter medications?
 4. Does the patient have any underlying allergies?
 5. Is there a family history of hereditary or similar skin diseases?
 6. Will the patient's education or financial status influence treatment considerations?

From Goldstein BG, Goldstein AO: Practical Dermatology, ed 2, St. Louis, 1997, Mosby.

BOX 1-2 Primary Skin Lesions

Macule: Small spot, different in color from surrounding skin, that is neither elevated nor depressed below the skin's surface

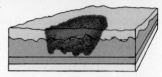

Papule: Small (≤5 mm diameter) circumscribed solid elevation on the skin

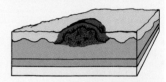

Plaque: Large (≥5 mm) superficial flat lesion, often formed by a confluence of papules

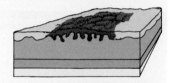

Nodule: Large (5-20 mm) circumscribed solid skin elevation

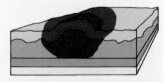

Pustule: Small circumscribed skin elevation containing purulent material

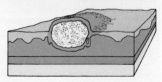

BOX 1-2 Primary Skin Lesions—cont'd

Vesicle: Small (<5 mm) circumscribed skin blister containing serum

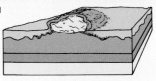

Wheal: Irregular elevated edematous skin area, which often changes in size and shape

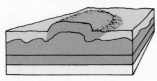

Bulla: Large (>5 mm) vesicle containing free fluid
Cyst: Enclosed cavity with a membranous lining, which contains liquid or semisolid matter
Tumor: Large nodule, which may be neoplastic
Telangiectasia: Dilated superficial blood vessel

From Goldstein BG, Goldstein AO: Practical Dermatology, ed 2, St. Louis, 1997, Mosby.

BOX 1-3 Secondary Skin Lesions

Scale: Superficial epidermal cells that are dead and cast off from the skin

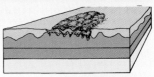

Erosion: Superficial, focal loss of part of the epidermis; lesions usually heal without scarring

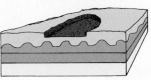

(Continued)

BOX 1-3 Secondary Skin Lesions—cont'd

Ulcer: Focal loss of the epidermis extending into the dermis; lesions may heal with scarring

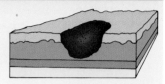

Fissure: Deep skin split extending into the dermis

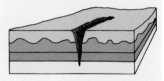

Crust: Dried exudate, a "scab"

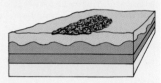

Erythema: Skin redness
Excoriation: Superficial, often linear, skin erosion caused by scratching
Atrophy: Decreased skin thickness due to skin thinning
Scar: Abnormal fibrous tissue that replaces normal tissue after skin injury
Edema: Swelling due to accumulation of water in tissue
Hyperpigmentation: Increased skin pigment
Hypopigmentation: Decreased skin pigment
Depigmentation: Total loss of skin pigment
Lichenification: Increased skin markings and thickening with induration secondary to chronic inflammation caused by scratching or other irritation
Hyperkeratosis: Abnormal skin thickening of the superficial layer of the epidermis

From Goldstein BG, Goldstein AO: Practical Dermatology, ed 2, St. Louis, 1997, Mosby.

TABLE 1-1

Vascular Skin Lesions

Lesion	Characteristics	Examples
Erythema	Pink or red blanchable discoloration of the skin secondary to dilatation of blood vessels	
Petechiae	Reddish-purple; nonblanching; smaller than 0.5 cm	Intravascular defects
Purpura	Reddish-purple; nonblanching; greater than 0.5 cm	Intravascular defects
Ecchymosis	Reddish-purple; nonblanching; variable size	Trauma, vasculitis
Telangiectasia	Fine, irregular dilated blood vessels	Dilatation of capillaries
Spider Angioma	Central red body with radiating spider-like arms that blanch with pressure to the central area	Liver disease, estrogens

Miscellaneous Skin Lesions

Lesion	Characteristics	Examples
Scar	Replacement of destroyed dermis by fibrous tissue; may be atrophic or hyperplastic	Healed wound
Keloid	Elevated, enlarging scar growing beyond boundaries of wound	Burn scars
Lichenification	Roughening and thickening of epidermis; accentuated skin markings	Atopic dermatitis

From Swartz MH: Textbook of Physical Diagnosis: History and Examination, ed 6, Philadelphia, 2010, Saunders.

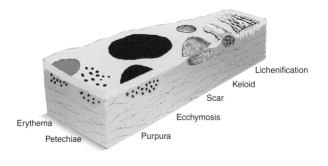

B. DERMATOSES BY REGION

1. *SCALP*

Papules/Plaques

- Actinic keratosis
- Appendageal tumor
- Cyst
- Hemangioma
- Lichen planopilaris
- Lupus erythematosus
- Melanoma
- Nevus
- Seborrheic keratosis

Nodules

- Actinic keratosis
- Appendageal tumor
- Basal cell carcinoma
- Cyst
- Hemangioma
- Kerion
- Metastatic carcinoma
- Nevus
- Prurigo nodularis
- Seborrheic keratosis

Eruptions

- Contact dermatitis
- Dissecting cellulitis
- Eczema
- Folliculitis
- Herpes zoster
- Pediculosis capitis
- Psoriasis
- Seborrheic dermatitis
- Tinea capitis

Alopecias

- Alopecia areata
- Anagen effluvium
- Androgenetic alopecia

- Discoid lupus erythematosus
- Hypervitaminosis A
- Lichen planopilaris
- Syphilis
- Systemic disease
- Telogen effluvium
- Tinea capitis
- Traction/chemical alopecia
- Trichotillomania

2. *FACE*

Isolated Papules

- Acrochordon
- Actinic keratosis
- Angioma
- Appendageal tumors
- Basal cell carcinoma
- Cyst
- Dermatosis papulosa nigra
- Hemangioma
- Keratoacanthoma
- Lentigo maligna
- Milia
- Nevus
- Sebaceous hyperplasia
- Seborrheic keratosis
- Solar lentigo
- Squamous cell carcinoma
- Telangiectasia
- Venous lake
- Xanthelasma

Eruptions

- Acne rosacea
- Acne vulgaris
- Adenoma sebaceum
- Dermatomyositis
- Eczema, including contact dermatitis
- Erysipelas
- Favre-Racouchot (comedones in actinically damaged skin)
- Fifth disease
- Herpes simplex/zoster

- Impetigo
- Lupus erythematosus
- Lymphocytoma cutis
- Melasma
- Pemphigoid/pemphigus
- Perioral dermatitis
- Photodrug eruption
- Pityriasis alba
- Postinflammatory hypopigmentation
- Psoriasis
- Sarcoidosis
- Scleroderma
- Seborrheic dermatitis
- Steroid rosacea
- Syphilis
- Tinea corporis
- Urticaria, angioedema
- Warts, especially flat or molluscum

3. ORAL MUCOSA

Oral Mucosa (See also Erosions and Ulcers)

- Kaposi's sarcoma
- Leukoplakia
- Melanoma
- Mucous cysts
- Oral hairy leukoplakia
- Oral melanotic macule
- Pyogenic granuloma
- Verruca

4. AXILLA

- Acanthosis nigricans
- Acrochordon
- Axillary freckling in neurofibromatosis
- Bullous pemphigoid
- Contact dermatitis
- Epidermal inclusion cyst
- Erythrasma
- Fox-Fordyce disease
- Fungal or yeast infection
- Hailey-Hailey disease
- Hidradenitis suppurativa

- Intertrigo
- Pediculosis corporis
- Pseudoxanthoma elasticum
- Scabies
- Striae distensae
- Trichomycosis axillaris

5. *HANDS AND FEET*

Isolated Papules

- Actinic keratosis
- Arsenical keratosis
- Basal cell carcinoma
- Callus/clavus
- Keratoacanthoma
- Melanoma
- Nevus
- Painful fat herniations
- Phelon
- Pyogenic granuloma
- Solar lentigo
- Squamous cell carcinoma
- Warts

Eruptions

- Acute or chronic paronychia
- Cutaneous larva migrans (feet)
- Dermatomyositis
- Drug eruption
- Eczema, including contact dermatitis
- Emboli
- Epidermolysis bullosa
- Erythema multiforme
- Granuloma annulare
- Hand-foot-and-mouth disease
- Herpetic whitlow
- Hyperhidrosis
- Juvenile plantar dermatosis
- Keratolysis exfoliativa
- Lichen planus (wrists, ankles)
- Lupus erythematosus
- Pitted keratolysis (feet)
- Pityriasis rubra pilaris

- Porphyria cutanea tarda
- Psoriasis
- Reiter's syndrome
- Rocky Mountain spotted fever
- Scabies
- Scleroderma
- Syphilis
- Tinea pedis, manus
- Viral exanthems
- Vitiligo

6. GENITALIA/INGUINAL

- Acrochrodons
- Accrodermatitis enteropathica
- Angiokeratoma
- Balanitis
- Bowen's disease
- Candidiasis
- Chancroid
- Condyloma acuminata
- Contact dermatitis
- Diaper dermatitis
- Erythema multiforme
- Erythrasma
- Fixed drug eruption
- Folliculitits
- Furunculosis
- Herpes simplex/zoster
- Hidradenitis suppurativa
- Intertrigo
- Kawasaki syndrome
- Lichen planus
- Lichen sclerosus
- Lichen simplex chronicus
- Lymphogranuloma venereum
- Molluscum contagiosum
- Paget's disease, extramammary
- Pearly penile papules
- Pediculosis pubis
- Perianal streptococcal cellulitis
- Pinworm
- Pityriasis rubra pilaris
- Psoriasis
- Reiter's syndrome

- Scabies
- Seborrheic dermatitis
- Squamous cell carcinoma
- Syphilis
- Tinea cruris

7. *PHOTODISTRIBUTED*

- Dermatomyositis
- Lupus erythematosus
- Pellagra
- Photodrug eruption
- Polymorphous light eruption
- Porphyria cutanea tarda

C. DERMATOSES BY MORPHOLOGY

1. *MACULES*

Hypopigmented

- Halo nevus
- Leprosy
- Postinflammatory
- Sarcoidosis
- Tinea versicolor
- Tuberous sclerosis
- Vitiligo

Hyperpigmented

- Café au lait spot
- Drug eruption
- Ephelis (freckle)
- Lentigo
- Mastocytosis
- Melanoma
- Melasma
- Mongolian spot
- Nevus
- Ochronosis
- Postinflammatory
- Purpura
- Stasis dermatitis

Erythematous

- Drug eruption
- Rheumatic fever
- Secondary syphilis
- Viral exanthem

2. PAPULES

Isolated Papules

- Acrochordon
- Actinic keratosis
- Angiofibroma
- Angioma
- Appendageal tumors (benign or malignant)
- Baciliary angiomatosis
- Basal cell carcinoma
- Chondrodermatitis nodularis helicis
- Dermatofibroma
- Fungal infections, early
- Hemangioma
- Keratoacanthoma
- Melanoma
- Milia
- Molluscum contagiosum
- Neurofibroma
- Nevus
- Pyogenic granuloma
- Sebaceous hyperplasia
- Seborrheic keratosis
- Squamous cell carcinoma
- Warts

Papular Eruptions

- Acne rosacea
- Acne vulgaris
- Appendageal tumors (usually benign)
- Arthropod bite
- Bacillary angiomatosis
- Dermatomyositis
- Drug eruption
- Eczematous dermatitis
- Flat warts

- Folliculitis
- Granuloma annulare
- Keratosis pilaris
- Lichen nitidus
- Lichen planus
- Lichen sclerosus
- Lupus erythematosus
- Lymphoma
- Miliaria
- Molluscum contagiosum
- Neurofibromatosis
- Pediculosis corporis
- Perioral dermatitis
- Pityriasis rosea
- Polymorphous light eruption
- Pruritic urticarial papules, plaques of pregnancy
- Psoriasis
- Sarcoidosis
- Sarcoma (Kaposi's other)
- Scabies
- Syphilis
- Urticaria
- Vasculitis
- Venous lake
- Viral exanthem
- Xanthoma

3. *PUSTULES*

- Acne rosacea/perioral dermatitis
- Acne vulgaris
- Arthropod bite (fire ants)
- Drug eruption
- Eosinophilic folliculitis
- Erythema toxicum neonatorum
- Folliculitis
- Fungal or yeast infections, especially tinea capitis and Majocchi's granuloma
- Furunculosis
- Gonorrhea, disseminated
- Herpes simplex/zoster
- Impetigo
- Keratosis pilarus
- Neonatal pustulosis
- Pseudofolliculitis barbae
- Pustular psoriasis

- Pyoderma gangrenosum
- Syphilis
- Varicella

4. *PLAQUES*

- Acanthosis nigricans
- Candidiasis
- Cellulitis
- Deep fungal infections
- Dermatomyositis
- Diaper dermatitis
- Eczematous dermatitis, including lichen simplex chronicus
- Erythrasma
- Fungal infections (e.g., tinea corporis, pedis, cruris, manus)
- Granuloma annulare
- Ichthyosis
- Lichen planus
- Lichen sclerosis
- Lupus erythematosus
- Lyme disease
- Lymphoma, cutaneous T-cell
- Morphea
- Myxedema
- Necrobiosis lipoidica diabeticorum
- Paget's disease, mammary/extramammary
- Pityriasis rosea
- Psoriasis
- Sarcoidosis
- Seborrheic dermatitis
- Sweet's syndrome
- Syphilis
- Tinea veriscolor
- Vasculitis
- Xanthelasma

5. *NODULES AND TUMORS*

- Acrochordon
- Angioma
- Appendageal tumors
- Basal cell carcinoma
- Callus/calvus
- Chondrodermatitis nodularis helicis
- Erythema nodosum

- Hidradenitis suppurativa
- Histiocytosis
- Inclusion cyst
- Kaposi's sarcoma
- Keloid
- Lipoma
- Lymphoma cutaneous
- Melanoma
- Metastatic carcinoma
- Neurofibroma
- Nevus
- Prurigo nodularis
- Pyogenic granuloma
- Seborreheic keratosis
- Squamous cell carcinoma
- Syphilis
- Tuberous sclerosis
- Venous lake
- Warts
- Xanthoma

6. *VESICLES AND BULLAE*

- Bullous disease in diabetes
- Bullous pemphigoid
- Burn
- Cellulitis
- Congenital syphilis
- Contact dermatitis
- Dermatitis herpetiformis
- Eczema, especially of the hand or foot
- Epidermolysis bullosa
- Erythema multiforme
- Fixed drug eruption
- Fungal infection, especially of tinea pedis
- Herpes gestationis
- Herpes simplex
- Herpes zoster
- Id reaction
- Impetigo
- Insect bite reaction
- Lichen planus
- Lupus erythematosus bullous
- Pemphigus vulgaris/foliaceus
- Porphyria cutanea tarda

- Scabies
- Staphylococcal scaled skin syndrome
- Streptococcal toxic shock like–syndrome
- Toxic epidermal necrolysis
- Varicella
- Vasculitis

7. EROSIONS AND ULCERS

Mouth

- Aphthae
- Avitaminosis
- Bullous pemphigoid
- Burn
- Candidiasis
- Epidermolysis bullosa
- Erythema multiforme
- Hand-foot-mouth disease
- Herpangina
- Herpes simplex
- Lichen planus
- Lupus erythematosus
- Pemphigus bulgaris
- Perleche
- Toxic epidermal necrolysis

Genital

- Balanitis
- Candidiasis
- Chancroid
- Diaper dermatitis, severe
- Erythema multiforme
- Fixed drug eruption
- Fungal infections, tinea cruris
- Herpes simplex
- Intertrigo
- Lichen planus
- Lichen sclerosus
- Lymphogranuloma venereum
- Squamous cell carcinoma
- Syphilis

Other

- Basal cell carcinoma
- Bullous pemphigoid
- Echthyma
- Erythema multiforme
- Ischemia
- Necrobiosis lipoidica
- Pemphigus vulgaris
- Porphyria cutanea tarda
- Pyoderma gangrenosum
- Spider bite
- Squamous cell carcinoma
- Stasis ulcer
- Toxic epidermal necrosis

8. DESQUAMATION

- Exfoliative dermatitis
- Kawasaki syndrome
- Keratolysis exfoliativa (hands and feet)
- Scarlet fever
- Scarletiniform eruption
- Staphylococcal scalded skin syndrome
- Toxic shock syndrome, late

D. DERMATOSES IN THE YOUNG

1. NEWBORN INFANTS WITH VESICOPUSTULES

- Congenital cutaneous candidiasis
- Congenital herpes simplex
- Erythema toxicum neonatorum
- Genodermatosis
- Impetigo
- Miliaria
- Scabies
- Syphilis
- Transient neonatal pustulosis

2. CHILDREN WITH PRURITIC RASHES

- Atopic dermatitis
- Contact dermatitis
- Diaper dermatitis

- Eczema, especially xerotic
- Histiocytosis
- Impetigo
- Insect bite
- Dermatosis pilaris
- Pediculosis, especially capitis
- Pityriasis rosea
- Scabies
- Seborrheic dermatitis
- Tinea corporis and tinea capitis

3. *FEBRILE CHILDREN WITH RASH*

- Bacteremia
- Dermatomyositis
- Drug exanthem, including serum sickness
- Erysipelas
- Henoch-Schönlein purpura
- Kawasaki syndrome
- Lupus erythematosus
- Lyme disease
- Rocky Mountain spotted fever
- Scarlet fever
- Staphylococcal scalded skin syndrome
- Still's disease
- Urticaria
- Viral exanthem

CHAPTER 2

DIFFERENTIAL DIAGNOSIS

1. ALOPECIA, NONSCARRING

- Androgenetic alopecia
- Cosmetic treatment
- Tinea capitis
- Trichotillomania (hair pulling)
- Anagen arrest
- Telogen arrest
- Alopecia areata
- Structural hair shaft disease

2. ALOPECIA, SCARRING

- Trauma
- Tinea capitis with inflammation (kerion)
- Bacterial folliculitis
- Discoid lupus erythematosus
- Congenital (aplasia cutis)
- Lichen planopilaris
- Folliculitis decalvans
- Neoplasm

3. ANHYDROSIS

- Drugs (anticholinergics)
- Dehydration
- Hysteria
- Obstruction of sweat ducts (e.g., inflammation, miliaria)
- Local radiant heat or pressure
- Central nervous system (CNS) lesions (medulla, hypothalamus, pons)
- Spinal cord lesions
- Lesions of sympathetic nerves
- Congenital sweat gland disturbances

4. ARTHRITIS, FEVER, AND RASH

- Lyme borreliosis
- Rocky Mountain spotted fever
- Parvovirus B-19
- Gonococcemia
- Meningococcemia
- Secondary syphilis

- Acute rheumatic fever
- Still's disease
- Kawasaki syndrome
- Vasculitic urticaria
- Acute sarcoidosis
- Rubella
- Familial Mediterranean fever
- Hyperimmunoglobulinemia D and periodic fever syndrome

5. BLISTERS, SUBEPIDERMAL

- Burns
- Porphyria cutanea tarda
- Bullous pemphigoid
- Bullous drug reaction
- Arthropod bite reaction
- Toxic epidermal necrosis
- Dermatitis herpetiformis
- Polymorphous light eruption
- Variegate porphyria
- Lupus erythematosus
- Epidermolysis bullosa
- Pseudoporphyria
- Acute graft-versus-host reaction
- Linear IgA disease
- Leukocytoclastic vasculitis
- Pressure necrosis
- Urticaria pigmentosa
- Amyloidosis

6. BULLOUS DISEASES

- Bullous pemphigoid
- Pemphigus vulgaris
- Pemphigus foliaceus
- Paraneoplastic pemphigus
- Cicatricial pemphigoid
- Erythema multiforme
- Dermatitis herpetiformis
- Herpes gestationis
- Impetigo
- Erosive lichen planus
- Linear IgA bullous dermatosis
- Epidermolysis bullosa acquisita

7. CUTANEOUS COLOR CHANGES

Blue

- Cardiovascular disease
- Pulmonary diseases
- Raynaud's disease

Brown

- Liver disease
- Pituitary disease
- Andrenocorticotropic hormone (ACTH)–producing tumor (e.g., oat cell lung carcinoma)
- Localized: nevi, neurofibromatosis

White

- Vitiligo
- Albinism
- Raynaud's disease

Red (Erythema)

- Anxiety reaction
- Fever
- Polycythemia
- Viral exanthems
- Generalized urticaria
- Localized: inflammation, infection, Raynaud's disease

Yellow

- Hepatitis, liver disease
- Chronic renal failure
- Anemia
- Hypothyroidism
- Increased intake of vegetables containing carotene
- Localized: resolving hematoma, infection, peripheral vascular insufficiency

8. CUTANEOUS INFECTIONS, ATHLETES

- Tinea pedis
- Tinea cruris
- Molluscum contagiosum

- Herpes simplex
- Verrucal vulgaris
- Folliculitis
- Impetigo
- Furuncles
- Otitis externa
- Erythrasma

9. EXANTHEMS

- Enterovirus
- Adenovirus
- Erythema infectiosum (fifth disease)
- Scarlet fever
- Measles
- Rubella
- Roseola exanthema
- Varicella
- Epstein-Barr virus
- Kawasaki syndrome
- Staphylococcal scalded skin
- Meningococcemia
- Rocky Mountain spotted fever

10. FEVER AND RASH

- Drug hypersensitivity: penicillin, sulfonamides, thiazides, anticonvulsants, allopurinol
- Viral infection: measles, rubella, varicella, erythema infectiosum, roseola, enterovirus infection, viral hepatitis, infectious mononucleosis, acute human immunodeficiency virus (HIV)
- Other infections: meningococcemia, staphylococcemia, scarlet fever, typhoid fever, *Pseudomonas* bacteremia, Rocky Mountain spotted fever, Lyme disease, secondary syphilis, bacterial endocarditis, babesiosis, brucellosis, listeriosis
- Serum sickness
- Erythema multiforme
- Erythema marginatum
- Erythema nodosum
- Systemic lupus erythematosis (SLE)
- Dermatomyositis
- Allergic vasculitis
- Pityriasis rosea
- Herpes zoster

11. FINGER LESIONS, INFLAMMATORY

- Paronychia
- Herpes simplex type 1 (herpetic whitlow)
- Dyshidrotic eczema (pompholyx)
- Herpes zoster
- Bacterial endocarditis (Osler's nodes)
- Psoriatic arthritis

12. FLUSHING

- Anxiety
- Menopause
- Ingestion of hot drink
- Monosodium glutamate ingestion
- Ingestion of hot peppers
- Ingestion of alcoholic beverages
- Drugs: nicotinic acid, diltiazem, nifedipine, levodopa, bromocriptine, vancomycin, amyl nitrate
- Carcinoid syndrome
- Polycythemia, systemic mastocytosis
- Renal cell carcinoma
- Chronic myelogenous leukemia (CML)
- Vipoma
- Agnogenic flushing

13. FOOT DERMATITIS

- Tinea pedis
- Dyshidrotic eczema
- Tylosis (mechanically induced hyperkeratosis, fissuring, and dryness)
- Allergic contact dermatitis
- Psoriasis
- Peripheral vascular insufficiency
- Neuropathic foot ulcers (diabetes mellitus [DM], poorly fitting shoes)
- Acquired plantar keratoderma
- Sézary syndrome

14. FOOT LESIONS, ULCERATING

- Cellulitis
- Plantar wart
- Squamous cell carcinoma
- Actinomycosis (Madura foot)

- Plantar fibromatosis
- Pseudoepitheliomatous hyperplasia

15. GENITAL SORES

- Trauma
- Herpes genitalis
- Syphilis
- Condyloma acuminatum
- Neoplastic lesion
- Chancroid
- Lymphogranuloma venereum
- Granuloma inguinale

16. GRANULOMATOUS DERMATITIDES

- Granuloma annulare
- Sarcoidosis
- Necrobiosis lipoidica diabeticorum
- Cutaneous Crohn's disease
- Rheumatoid nodules
- Annular elastolytic giant cell granuloma (actinic granuloma)
- Foreign body granuloma

17. HIV INFECTION, CUTANEOUS MANIFESTATIONS

Viral Infection

- Herpes simplex
- Herpes zoster
- HIV
- Human papillomavirus
- Kaposi's sarcoma (herpesvirus)
- Molluscum contagiosum

Bacterial Infection

- Bacillary angiomatosis
- *Staphylococcus aureus*
- Syphilis

Fungal Infection

- Candidiasis
- Cryptococcoses
- Seborrheic dermatitis

Arthropod Infestations

- Scabies

Noninfectious

- Drug reactions
- Psoriasis
- Vasculitis
- Nutritional deficiencies

18. HYPERPIGMENTATION

- Pregnancy
- Drug induced (e.g., antimalarials, some cytotoxic agents)
- Addison's disease*
- ACTH- or MSH-producing tumors (e.g., oat cell carcinoma of the lung)*
- Hemochromatosis
- Malabsorption syndrome (Whipple's disease and celiac sprue)
- Melanoma
- Pheochromocytoma
- Porphyrias (porphyria cutanea tarda and variegate porphyria)
- Progressive systemic sclerosis and related conditions
- Psoralen and UVA (PUVA) therapy for psoriasis and vitiligo*
- Melanotropic hormone injection*
- Arsenic ingestion

19. HYPERTRICHOSIS

Systemic Illness

- Anorexia nervosa
- Hypothyroidism
- Malnutrition
- Porphyria
- Dermatomyositis

Drugs

- Minoxidil
- Dilantin
- Cyclosporine
- Hexachlorobenzene
- Penicillamine

---

*Accentuation on sun-exposed surfaces.

20. HYPOPIGMENTATION

- Vitiligo
- Tinea versicolor
- Atopic dermatitis
- Chemical leukoderma
- Idiopathic hypomelanosis
- Sarcoidosis
- SLE
- Scleroderma
- Oculocutaneous albinism
- Phenylketonuria
- Nevoid hypopigmentation

21. LEG ULCERS

Trauma

- Insect bites
- Burns
- Cold injury
- Radiation dermatitis
- Factitial
- Excessive pressure

Vascular

- Superficial varicosities
- Arteriovenous (AV) malformation
- Arteriosclerosis
- Thromboangiitis obliterans
- Lymphatic abnormalities
- Incompetent perforators
- Cholesterol emboli
- Deep venous thrombosis (DVT)

Vasculitis/Hematologic

- Sickle cell anemia
- Lupus anticoagulant, antiphospholipid syndrome
- Cold agglutinin disease
- Polycythemia vera
- Leukemia
- Macroglobulinemia
- Protein C and protein S deficiency

- Cryoglobulinemia
- Thalassemia

Infectious

- Furuncle
- Septic emboli
- Coccidioidomycosis
- Blastomycosis
- Histoplasmosis
- Sporotrichosis
- Ecthyma
- Leishmaniasis

Metabolic

- Necrobiosis lipoidica diabeticorum
- Gout
- Localized bullous pemphigoid
- Calcinosis cutis
- Gaucher's disease

Tumors

- Basal cell carcinoma
- Squamous cell carcinoma
- Melanoma
- Mycosis fungoides
- Kaposi's sarcoma
- Metastatic neoplasms

Neuropathic

- Diabetic ulcers
- Tabes dorsalis
- Syringomyelia

Drugs

- Warfarin
- Intravenous (IV) colchicine extravasation
- Hydroxyurea
- Methotrexate
- Halogens
- Ergotism

Panniculitis

- Pancreatic fat necrosis
- Alpha-antitrypsinase deficiency
- Weber-Christian disease

22. LIVEDO RETICULITIS

- Emboli (subacute bacterial endocarditis [SBE], left atrial myxoma, cholesterol emboli)
- Thrombocythemia or polycythemia
- Antiphospholipid antibody syndrome
- Cryoglobulinemia, cryofibrinogenemia
- Leukocytoclastic vasculitis
- SLE, rheumatoid arthritis, dermatomyositis
- Pancreatitis
- Drugs (quinine, quinidine, amantadine, catecholamines)
- Physiologic (cutis marmorata)
- Congenital

23. MELANONYCHIA

- Pregnancy
- Trauma
- Medications (e.g., AZT, 5-fluorouracil, doxorubicin, psoralens)
- Nail matrix nevus
- HIV infection
- Onychomycosis
- Melanocyte hyperplasia
- Verrucae
- Pustular psoriasis
- Lichen planus
- Basal cell carcinoma
- Nail matrix melanoma
- Subungual keratosis
- Addison's disease
- Bowen's disease

24. NAIL CLUBBING

- Chronic obstructive pulmonary disease (COPD)
- Pulmonary malignancy
- Cirrhosis
- Inflammatory bowel disease
- Chronic bronchitis

- Congenital heart disease
- Endocarditis
- AV malformations
- Asbestosis
- Trauma
- Idiopathic

25. NAIL, HORIZONTAL WHITE LINES (BEAU'S LINES)

- Malnutrition
- Idiopathic
- Trauma
- Prolonged systemic illnesses
- Pemphigus
- Raynaud's disease

26. NAIL KOILONYCHIA

- Trauma
- Iron deficiency
- SLE
- Hemochromatosis
- Raynaud's disease
- Nail-patella syndrome
- Idiopathic

27. NAIL ONYCHOLYSIS

- Infection
- Trauma
- Psoriasis
- Connective tissue disorders
- Sarcoidosis
- Hyperthyroidism
- Amyloidosis
- Nutritional deficiencies

28. NAIL PITTING

- Psoriasis
- Alopecia areata
- Reiter's syndrome
- Trauma
- Idiopathic

29. NAIL SPLINTER HEMORRHAGE

- SBE
- Trauma
- Malignancies
- Oral contraceptives
- Pregnancy
- SLE
- Antiphospholipid syndrome
- Psoriasis
- Rheumatoid arthritis
- Peptic ulcer disease

30. NAIL STRIATIONS

- Psoriasis
- Alopecia areata
- Trauma
- Atopic dermatitis
- Vitiligo

31. NAIL TELANGIECTASIA

- Rheumatoid arthritis
- Scleroderma
- Trauma
- SLE
- Dermatomyositis

32. NAIL WHITENING (TERRY'S NAILS)

- Malnutrition
- Trauma
- Liver disease (cirrhosis, hepatic failure)
- Diabetes mellitus
- Hyperthyroidism
- Idiopathic

33. NAIL YELLOWING

- Tobacco abuse
- Nephrotic syndrome
- Chronic infections (tuberculosis [TB], sinusitis)
- Bronchiectasis

- Lymphedema
- Raynaud's disease
- Rheumatoid arthritis
- Pleural effusions
- Thyroiditis
- Immunodeficiency

34. NIPPLE LESIONS

- Contact dermatitis
- Trauma
- Paget's disease
- Sebaceous hyperplasia
- Neurofibroma
- Accessory nipple
- Papillary adenoma
- Nevoid hyperkeratosis
- Cellulitis

35. NODULAR LESIONS, SKIN

- Lipoma
- Cherry angioma
- Angiokeratoma
- Hemangioma
- Classic Kaposi's sarcoma
- Nodular melanoma
- Pyogenic granuloma
- Angiosarcoma
- Eccrine poroma

36. NODULES, PAINFUL

- Arthropod bite or sting
- Erythema nodosum
- Glomus tumor
- Neuroma
- Leiomyoma
- Angiolipoma
- Dermatofibroma
- Osler's node
- Blue rubber bleb nevus
- Vasculitis
- Sweet's syndrome

37. ORAL MUCOSA, ERYTHEMATOUS LESIONS

- Burn from hot beverage
- Viral infection
- Allergy
- Erythroplakia
- Candidiasis
- Pemphigus vulgaris
- Geographic tongue
- Stomatitis areata migrans
- Plasma cell gingivitis
- Pemphigus vulgaris

38. ORAL MUCOSA, PIGMENTED LESIONS

- Smoker's melanosis
- Chloasma
- Racial pigmentation
- Oral melanotic macule
- Peutz-Jeghers syndrome
- Neurofibromatosis
- Melanoma
- Addison's disease
- Drug reaction: quinacrine, Minocin, chlorpromazine, Myleran
- Amalgam tattoo
- Nevi
- Lead line
- Albright's syndrome

39. ORAL MUCOSA, PUNCTATE LESIONS

- Aphthous stomatitis
- Herpes simplex
- Coxsackievirus (A, B, A16)
- Drug reaction
- Neutropenia
- Inflammatory bowel disease
- Contact allergy
- Sutton's disease (giant aphthae)
- Behçet's syndrome
- Reiter's syndrome
- Acute necrotizing ulcerative gingivostomatitis (ANUG)
- Herpes zoster

40. ORAL MUCOSA, WHITE LESIONS

- Candidiasis
- Leukoplakia
- Stomatitis nicotinica
- Allergy
- White, hairy leukoplakia
- Squamous cell carcinoma
- Lichen planus
- Benign intraepithelial dyskeratosis
- White spongy nevus
- Leukoedema
- Darier-White disease
- Pachyonychia congenital
- SLE

41. ORAL VESICLES AND ULCERS

- Aphthous stomatitis
- Primary herpes simplex infection
- Coxsackievirus A (herpangina)
- Vincent's stomatitis
- Syphilis
- Behçet's syndrome
- SLE
- Reiter's syndrome
- Crohn's disease
- Erythema multiforme
- Pemphigus
- Pemphigoid
- Fungi (histoplasmosis)

42. PAPULOSQUAMOUS DISEASES

- Psoriasis
- Lichen planus
- Pityriasis rubra pilaris
- Pityriasis rosea
- Tinea versicolor
- Secondary syphilis
- Lichen nitidus
- Pityriasis lichenoides
- Parapsoriasis
- Mycosis fungoides
- Dermatophytosis

43. PENILE RASH

- Herpes simplex 2
- Balanitis *(Candida)*
- Condyloma acuminata
- Molluscum contagiosum
- Scabies
- Pediculosis pubis
- Pearly penile papules
- Lichen nitidus
- Fox-Fordyce disease (follicular papules)

44. PHOTODERMATOSES

- Polymorphous light eruption
- Phototoxicity and photoallergy
- Chronic actinic dermatitis
- Solar urticaria
- Porphyrias

45. PHOTOSENSITIVITY

- Solar urticaria
- Photoallergic reaction
- Phototoxic reaction
- Polymorphous light eruption
- Porphyria cutanea tarda
- SLE
- Drug induced (e.g., tetracyclines)

46. PREMATURE GRAYING, SCALP HAIR

- Chemical exposure (e.g., phenol/catechol derivatives, sulfhydryls, arsenic)
- Physical agents (e.g., ionizing radiation, lasers)
- Hyperthyroidism
- Vitamin B_{12} deficiency
- Down syndrome
- Chronic and severe protein deficiency
- Vitiligo
- Idiopathic
- Myotonic dystrophy
- Ataxia telangiectasia
- Progeria
- Wermer's syndrome

47. PRURITUS

- Dry skin
- Drug-induced eruption, fiberglass exposure
- Scabies
- Skin diseases
- Myeloproliferative disorders: mycosis fungoides, Hodgkin's lymphoma, multiple myeloma, polycythemia vera
- Cholestatic liver disease
- Endocrine disorders: diabetes mellitus, thyroid disease, carcinoid, pregnancy
- Carcinoma: breast, lung, gastric
- Chronic renal failure
- Iron deficiency
- Acquired immunodeficiency syndrome (AIDS)
- Neurosis
- Sjögren's syndrome

48. PRURITUS ANI

- Poor hygiene
- Pinworms
- Hemorrhoids
- Scabies
- Bacterial infection, viral infection
- Spicy foods, citrus foods
- Anesthetic agents, topical corticosteroids, perfumed soap
- Psoriasis, seborrhea, lichen simplex or sclerosus
- Polycythemia vera, Hodgkin's disease
- Fissure, fistula
- Skin tags, perianal clefts
- Syphilis
- Herpes simplex virus
- Human papillomavirus
- Chronic renal failure
- Thyroid disorders
- Polycythemia vera
- Hodgkin's disease

49. PURPURA

- Trauma
- Septic emboli, atheromatous emboli
- Disseminated intravascular coagulation (DIC)
- Thrombocytopenia
- Meningococcemia

- Rocky Mountain spotted fever
- Hemolytic-uremic syndrome
- Viral infection: echovirus, coxsackievirus
- Scurvy
- Other: left atrial myxoma, cryoglobulinemia, vasculitis, hyperglobulinemic purpura

50. SEXUALLY TRANSMITTED DISEASES, ANORECTAL REGION

Nonulcerative

- Condyloma acuminatum
- Gonorrhea
- Syphilis
- Chlamydia *(Chlamydia trachomitis)*

Ulcerative

- Herpes simplex virus
- Early (primary) syphilis
- Idiopathic (usually HIV positive)
- Lymphogranuloma venereum
- Chancroid *(Haemophilus ducreyi)*
- Cytomegalovirus (CMV)

51. STOMATITIS, BULLOUS

- Erythema multiforme
- Erosive lichen planus
- Bullous pemphigoid
- SLE
- Pemphigus vulgaris
- Mucous membrane pemphigoid

52. TELANGIECTASIA

- Oral contraceptive agents
- Pregnancy
- Rosacea
- Varicose veins
- Trauma
- Drug induced (corticosteroids, systemic or topical)
- Spider telangiectases
- Hepatic cirrhosis
- Mastocytosis
- SLE, dermatomyositis, systemic sclerosis

53. TICK-RELATED INFECTIONS

- Lyme disease
- Rocky Mountain spotted fever
- Babesiosis
- Tularemia
- Q fever
- Colorado tick fever
- Ehrlichiosis
- Relapsing fever

54. VASCULITIS, DISEASES THAT MIMIC VASCULITIS

- Drug effects (vasoconstrictors, anticoagulants)
- Atherosclerosis
- DIC
- Protein C and S deficiencies, factor V/Leiden mutation
- Antiphospholipid syndrome
- Radiation
- Infectious or marantic endocarditis
- Cardiac mural thrombus
- Atrial myxoma
- Cholesterol embolization syndrome
- Arterial fibromuscular dysplasia
- Radiation
- Genetic disease (neurofibromatosis, Ehlers-Danlos syndrome)
- Amyloidosis
- Intravascular malignant lymphoma
- Thrombotic thrombocytopenic purpura
- Hemolytic-uremic syndrome

55. VASCULITIS, CLASSIFICATION

Large Vessel Disease

- Giant cell arteritis
- Arteritis associated with Reiter's syndrome, ankylosing spondylitis
- Takayasu's arteritis

Medium and Small Vessel Disease

- Polyarteritis nodosa
- Wegener's granulomatosis
- Behçet's disease
- Primary (idiopathic)

- Associated with viruses (Hepatitis B or C, CMV, HIV, herpes zoster)
- Associated with malignancy (hairy cell leukemia)
- Kawasaki syndrome (mucocutaneous lymph node syndrome)
- Familial Mediterranean fever
- Granulomatous vasculitis
- Lymphomatoid granulomatosis

Predominantly Small Vessel Disease

- Vasculitis associated with connective tissue diseases (SLE, Sjögren's syndrome)
- Erythema nodosum
- Hypersensitivity vasculitis (leukocytoclastic vasculitis)
- Henoch-Schönlein purpura
- Mixed cryoglobulinemia
- Serum sickness
- Vasculitis associated with specific syndromes:
  - Primary biliary cirrhosis
  - Lyme disease
  - Chronic active hepatitis
  - Drug-induced vasculitis
  - Churg-Strauss syndrome
  - Goodpasture's syndrome
- Panniculitis
- Buerger's disease (thrombophlebitis obliterans)

56. VERRUCOUS LESIONS

- Warts
- Seborrheic keratosis
- Lichen simplex
- Acanthosis nigricans
- Scabies (Norwegian, crusted)
- Verrucous carcinoma
- Nevus sebaceous
- Deep fungal infection

57. VESICULOBULLOUS DISEASES

- Impetigo
- Bullous pemphigoid
- Dermatitis herpetiformis
- Herpes gestationis
- Mucous membrane pemphigoid
- Epidermolysis bullosa acquisita
- Diabetic blisters

- Pemphigus (vulgaris, foliaceus, paraneoplastic)
- Erythema multiforme minor
- Erythema multiforme major (Stevens-Johnson syndrome)
- Toxic epidermal necrolysis
- Porphyria cutanea tarda
- Pseudoporphyria
- Epidermolysis bullosa
- Staphylococcal scalded skin syndrome
- Herpes simplex
- Varicella
- Herpes zoster

58. VULVAR LESIONS

Red Lesion

Infection/Infestation
- *Candida*
- Tinea cruris
- Intertrigo
- Folliculitis: *Staphylococcus aureus*
- Hidradenitis suppurativa
- Pityriasis versicolor
- Granuloma inguinale: *Calymmatobacterium granulomatis*
- Behçet's syndrome
- *Sarcoptes scabiei*
- Erythrasma: *Corynebacterium minutissimum*

Inflammation
- Mechanical trauma: scratching (psoriasis, seborrheic dermatitis)
- Chemical irritation (lubricants, spermicide, hygiene sprays)
- Medications (topical 5-fluorouracil, podophyllum)
- Irritation from semen, saliva
- Essential vulvodynia

Neoplasm
- Vulvar intraepithelial neoplasia (VIN)
- Squamous cell carcinoma, melanoma, Paget's disease, Bowen's disease

White Lesion
- Lichen sclerosus
- Vitiligo
- Intertrigo
- Radiation treatment
- Partial albinism

Dark Lesion

- Melanoma
- Lentigo
- Nevi (mole)
- Reactive hyperpigmentation
- Seborrheic keratosis
- Pubic lice

Ulcerative Lesion

- Herpes simplex
- *Treponema pallidum*
- Condyloma acuminatum
- Molluscum contagiosum
- Hidradenitis suppurativa
- Basal cell carcinoma
- Squamous cell carcinoma
- Neurofibroma
- Acrochordon
- Bartholin cyst or abscess
- Behçet's disease
- Crohn's disease
- Pemphigus
- Pemphigoid
- Lymphogranuloma venereum
- Granuloma inguinale

DISEASES AND DISORDERS

1. ACANTHOSIS NIGRICANS (AN)

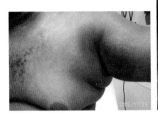

FIGURE 03-001. Velvety thickening of skin in flexural areas such as the axilla with brown-black hyperpigmentation. Because of excess chafing, skin tags appear occasionally, as seen in this obese patient.

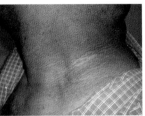

FIGURE 03-002. Darkened, "dirty" appearing thick skin with prominent lighter-colored deep skin lines. Several overlying warty or papillomatous growths are common in this condition.

General Comments

Definition
■ *Acanthosis nigricans* refers to the presence of symmetrical brown velvety or verrucous plaques with a predilection for intertriginous sites as the back of the neck, groin, and axillae (**Fig. 03-001**).

Etiology
■ It is most commonly seen in obese individuals with insulin resistance or an internal malignancy and in those taking certain medications (nicotinic acid, glucocorticoids, contraceptives, and diethylstilbestrol).

Keys to Diagnosis

Clinical Manifestation(s)
■ Asymptomatic. The axilla and neck are the most commonly involved. In obese females who are hyperandrogenic, the vulva is the most commonly affected site.

Physical Examination
■ Symmetrical hyperpigmented velvety plaques of the major flexures (axilla, groin), neck (**Fig. 03-002**), nipples, and vulva.

Diagnostic Tests
- Laboratory evaluation often reveals elevated glucose levels. Additional useful laboratory tests are thyroid-stimulating hormone (TSH) and follicle-stimulating hormone (FSH)/luteinizing hormone (LH).

Differential Diagnosis
- Seborrheic keratosis
- Hyperpigmented nevus (Becker nevus), linear epidermal nevus
- Pemphigus vegetans
- Lichen simplex chronicus
- Confluent and reticulated papillomatosis

℞ Treatment

First Line
- Therapy for underlying cause (weight loss in obese, discontinuation of offending drugs, treatment of malignancy if present)

Second Line
- Topical tretinoin, dermabrasion, ammonium lactate, carbon dioxide laser

Third Line
- Oral contraceptives, cyproheptadine, oral isotretinoin

😮 Clinical Pearl(s)
- The sudden onset of acanthosis nigricans should be followed by investigation for internal malignancy (e.g., upper endoscopy to rule out gastric cancer and computed tomography [CT] of abdomen and pelvis).
- Skin changes precede the malignancy diagnosis (usually neoplasm of abdominal cavity) in one third of cases.
- Consider drug use as a cause and review new medications (e.g., nicotinic acid, contraceptives, glucocorticoids).

2. ACNE KELOIDALIS

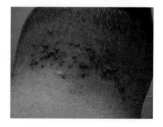

FIGURE 03-003. A papular, pustular eruption found on the nape of the neck and often associated with keloidal scarring. A typical finding as seen here is the emergence of hair follicles from the center of the lesion.

General Comments

Definition
- Acne keloidalis is an idiopathic chronic inflammatory eruption of the nape of the neck occurring most commonly in dark-skinned men. Also known as acne keloidalis nuchae, acne keloid, and folliculitis keloidalis. These are misnomers because there is no family history of keloids, no presence of keloids at other sites, and no development of keloid formation following excision. Despite the name, acne vulgaris also is not associated.

Etiology
- Unknown. Close shaving of the hair, picking by patients, and chronic rubbing by collars have been suggested as possible contributing factors.

 Keys to Diagnosis

Clinical Manifestation(s)
- Onset is usually after puberty and before age 50.
- Clinical presentation consists of a follicular pustular eruption on the nape of the neck (**Fig. 03-003**).

Physical Examination
- Hard papules with hair emerging from the center are seen on the nape of neck and occipital scalp. Comedomes are not seen.
- Papules coalesce into sclerotic plaques.
- Pustules, crusting, and drainage may occur with secondary infections.

Diagnostic Tests
- Pustule swab
- Deep biopsy

DDx Differential Diagnosis
- Folliculitis
- Simple ingrowing hairs (pili incurvatorum)
- Nevus sebaceous
- Traumatic causes of keloid
- Acne vulgaris
- Pseudofolliculitis
- Pediculosis capitis

R Treatment

First Line
- Dissuade close cutting. Allow hair to grow long in affected areas.
- Limit mechanical irritation by a tight collar.

- Encourage patient not to pick or squeeze lesions.
- Administer topical antibiotics (clindamycin or erythromycin).

Second Line
- Oral doxycycline, tetracycline, or minocycline

Third Line
- Intralesional triamcinolone alone or following use of CO_2 laser vaporization
- Oral isotretinoin
- Surgery: punch biopsy for small papular lesions, surgical debulking for larger lesions. Any excision must be carried out to the subfollicular depth. If any of the hair follicle is left, recurrence is common.

🪱 Clinical Pearl(s)

- Most cultures are sterile, but when a bacterium is found it is usually *Staphylococcus aureus*

3. ACNE VULGARIS

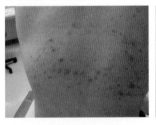

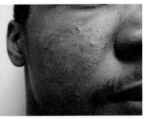

FIGURE 03-004. Erythematous nodulocystic acne vulgaris found on the back, often resulting in scarring.

FIGURE 03-005. Acne vulgaris consisting of open comedones ("blackheads") and closed comedones ("whiteheads").

📋 General Comments

Definition
- Acne vulgaris is a chronic disorder of the pilosebaceous apparatus caused by abnormal desquamation of follicular epithelium leading to obstruction of the pilosebaceous canal, resulting in inflammation and subsequent formation of papules, pustules, nodules, comedones, and scarring (**Fig. 03-004**). Acne can be classified by the type of lesion (comedonal, papulopustular, and nodulocystic). The American Academy of Dermatology classification scheme for acne denotes the following three levels:
  1. Mild acne: characterized by the presence of comedomes (noninflammatory lesions), few papules and pustules (generally <10), but no nodules.

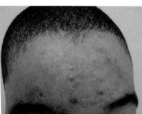

FIGURE 03-006. Acne vulgaris is often found on the face. Other common areas include the chest and the back.

FIGURE 03-007. Presence of scars and comedones.

2. Moderate acne: presence of several to many papules and pustules (10-40) along with comedomes (10-40). The presence of more than 40 papules and pustules along with larger, deeper nodular inflamed lesions (up to 5) denotes moderately severe acne.
3. Severe acne: presence of numerous or extensive papules and pustules as well as many nodular lesions.

Etiology

- Overactivity of the sebaceous glands and blockage in the ducts result in acne vulgaris. The obstruction leads to the formation of comedones, which can become inflamed because of overgrowth of *Propionibacterium acnes.*
- The condition is exacerbated by environmental factors (hot, humid, tropical climate), medications (e.g., iodine in cough mixtures, hair greases), and industrial exposure to halogenated hydrocarbons.

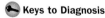 Keys to Diagnosis

Clinical Manifestation(s)

- Various stages of development and severity may be present concomitantly.
- Common distribution of acne is on the face, back, and upper chest.

Physical Examination
- Open comedones (blackheads), closed comedones (whiteheads) (**Fig. 03-005**)
- Greasiness (oily skin) (**Fig. 03-006**)
- Presence of scars from prior acne cysts (**Fig. 03-007**)
- Inflammatory papules, pustules, and ectatic pores

Diagnostic Tests
- Laboratory evaluation is generally not helpful.
- Patients who are candidates for therapy with isotretinoin (Accutane) should have baseline liver enzymes, cholesterol, and triglycerides checked, because this medication may result in elevation of lipids and liver enzymes.
- A negative serum pregnancy test or two negative urine pregnancy tests should also be obtained in female patients 1 week before initiation of isotretinoin; it is also imperative to maintain effective contraception during and 1 month after therapy with isotretinoin ends because of its teratogenic effects. Pregnancy status should be rechecked at monthly visits.
- In female patients, if hyperandrogenism is suspected, levels of dehydroepiandrosterone sulfate (DHEAS), testosterone (total and free), and androstenedione should be measured. Generally for women with regular menstrual cycles, serum androgen measurements are not necessary.

DDx Differential Diagnosis
- Gram-negative folliculitis
- Staphylococcal pyoderma
- Acne rosacea
- Drug eruption
- Sebaceous hyperplasia
- Angiofibromas, basal cell carcinomas, osteoma cutis
- Occupational exposures to oils or grease
- Steroid acne
- Flat warts

R Treatment

First Line
Treatment generally varies with the type of lesions (comedones, papules, pustules, cystic lesions) and the severity of acne.
- Comedones (noninflammatory acne) can be treated with retinoids or retinoid analogs. Topical retinoids are comedolytic and work by normalizing follicular keratinization. Commonly available agents are adapalene (0.1% gel or cream, applied once or twice daily), tazarotene (0.1% cream or gel applied daily), tretinoin (0.1% cream or 0.025% gel applied once nightly), tretinoin microsphere (0.1% gel, applied at bedtime). Tretinoin is inactivated by UV light and

oxydized by benzoyl peroxide; therefore, it should only be applied at night and not used concomitantly with benzoyl peroxide.

- Tretinoin is pregnancy category C; tazarotene is pregnancy category X. Salicylic acid preparations (e.g., 2% wash) have keratolytic and antiinflammatory properties and are also useful in the treatment of comedones. Large open comedones (blackheads) should be expressed.

- Patients should be reevaluated after 4 to 6 weeks. Benzoyl peroxide gel (2.5% or 5%) may be added if the comedones become inflamed or form pustules. The most common adverse effects are dryness, erythema, and peeling. Topical antibiotics (erythromycin, clindamycin lotions or pads) can also be used in patients with significant inflammation. They reduce *P. acnes* in the pilosebaceous follicle and have some antiinflammatory effects. The combinations of 5% benzoyl peroxide and 3% erythromycin or 1% clindamycin with 5% benzoyl peroxide are highly effective in patients who have a mixture of comedonal and inflammatory acne lesions.

- Pustular acne can be treated with tretinoin and benzoyl peroxide gel applied on alternate evenings; drying agents (e.g., sulfacetamide/sulfur lotions) are also effective when used in combination with benzoyl peroxide.

- Azelaic acid, a bacteriostatic dicarboxylic acid, is used to normalize keratinization and reduce inflammation.

Second Line

- Oral antibiotics (doxycycline 100 mg QD or erythromycin 1 g QD in 2-3 divided doses) are effective in patients with moderate to severe pustular acne; patients not responding well to these antibiotics can be switched to minocycline 50 to 100 mg BID; however, this medication is more expensive.

- Patients with nodular cystic acne can be treated with systemic agents: antibiotics (erythromycin, tetracycline, doxycycline, minocycline), isotretinoin, or oral contraceptives. Periodic intralesional triamcinolone injections are also effective. The possibility of endocrinopathy should be considered in patients responding poorly to therapy.

- Oral contraceptives reduce androgen levels and therefore sebum production. They represent a useful adjunctive therapy for all types of acne in women and adolescent girls. Commonly used agents are norgestimate/ethinyl estradiol and drospirenone/ethinyl estradiol.

- Spironolactone 100 to 200 mg/day can be administered to women only.

- Blue light can be used for treatment of moderate inflammatory acne vulgaris. Light in the violet/blue range can cause bacterial death by a photoreaction in which porphyrins react with oxygen to generate reactive oxygen species, which damage the cell membranes of *P. acnes*. Treatment usually consists of 15-minutes of exposure twice weekly for 4 weeks.

Third Line

- Isotretinoin is indicated for acne resistant to antibiotic therapy and severe acne; dosage is 0.5 to 1 mg/kg/day in 2 divided doses (maximum of 2 mg/kg/day); duration of therapy is generally 20 weeks for a cumulative dose 120 mg/kg or more for severe cystic acne; before using this medication, patients should undergo baseline laboratory evaluation. This drug is absolutely contraindicated during pregnancy because of its teratogenicity. It should be used with caution in patients with a history of depression. In order to prescribe this drug, physicians must be registered members of the manufacturer's System to Manage Accutane-Related Teratogenicity (SMART) program.

Clinical Pearl(s)

- Gram-negative folliculitis should be suspected if inflammatory acne worsens after several months of oral antibiotic therapy.
- Acne may worsen during the first 3 to 4 weeks of retinoid therapy before improving.
- Indications for systemic therapy of acne are painful deep papules or nodules, extensive lesions, active acne with severe scarring or hyperpigmentation, and patient's morale.
- Erythromycin has a high incidence of early drug resistance.
- Doxycycline has a high incidence of sun sensitivity.
- Benzoyl peroxide will cause bleaching of clothes.
- Spironolactone can produce menstrual irregularity.
- Tetracyclines are contraindicated in children and pregnant women.
- Isotretinoin is contraindicated in patients with depression.

4. ACROCHORDON

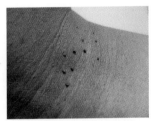

FIGURE 03-008. Acrochordons are soft, flesh-colored, pedunculated papules that are commonly located on the neck and axilla.

General Comments

Definition

- Acrochordons are benign outgrowths of the skin, also known as skin tags or fibroepithelial polyps.

Etiology

■ Unknown. They are more prevalent in obese individuals and in women. Acrochordon may be associated with pregnancy and acanthosis nigricans.

 Keys to Diagnosis

Clinical Manifestation(s)

■ This condition is asymptomatic unless irritated by clothing, jewelry, or friction. It is most common in middle-aged and elderly persons.

Physical Examination

■ Skin-colored or brown fleshy outgrowths (**Fig. 03-008**) are usually seen on the side of the neck and around the axillae and groin.

Diagnostic Tests

■ None necessary. A shave/snip biopsy can be done when diagnosis is unclear.

DDx Differential Diagnosis

■ Wart
■ Seborrheic keratosis
■ Melanocytic nevus
■ Dermatosis papulosa nigra
■ Neurofibroma
■ Melanoma

 Treatment

First Line

■ No treatment is needed.
■ Scissor excision with or without local anesthesia may be done for cosmetic reasons or when the skin tag is irritated.

Second Line

■ Electrodessication

Third Line

■ Liquid nitrogen cryosurgery

Clinical Pearl(s)

■ Skin tags in periorbital area are often confused with neoplastic skin lesions.
■ Freezing of a skin tag in dark-skinned patients may result in a white spot.

5. ACTINIC KERATOSIS

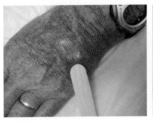

FIGURE 03-009. Several scaly, adherent, yellow-brown lesions on the sun-exposed dorsum of the hand.

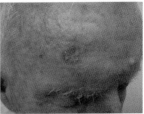

FIGURE 03-010. An actinic keratosis located on this patient's forehead is often best appreciated by its rough, tactile quality, similar to that of sandpaper.

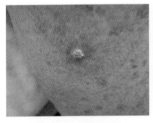

FIGURE 03-011. Scaly, raised lesion on sun-exposed back. Pain was elicited when scraping this lesion.

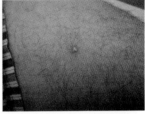

FIGURE 03-012. Raised, rough, gritty actinic keratosis on the anterior thigh of an outdoorsman.

General Comments

Definition
■ Actinic keratosis is a common skin lesion usually presenting as multiple, erythematous or yellow-brown, dry, scaly lesions in the middle aged or elderly. It is also known as solar keratosis or senile keratosis.

Etiology
■ Sun exposure, ionizing radiation

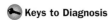 Keys to Diagnosis

Clinical Manifestation(s)

- Typical lesions occur on sun-damaged skin usually on the face and neck and the dorsal aspects of hands (**Fig. 03-009**) and forearms.
- Actinic keratosis is more common in males than females, especially in those with fair complexions who burn rather than tan following sun exposure.

Physical Examination

- Advanced lesions are characterized by a hard spiky scale (**Fig. 03-010**) and usually measure 1 cm in diameter or less. Early lesions manifest with redness and minimal scale. With progression scales become thicker and yellow (**Fig. 03-011**) and may resemble a small squamous cell carcinoma. On examinations lesions are rough and gritty (**Fig. 03-012**)
- The surrounding skin often shows additional features of sun damage, including atrophy, pigmentary changes, and telengiectasia.

Diagnostic Tests

- Skin biopsy can be performed for recurrent lesions or when diagnosis is unclear to rule out squamous cell or basal cell carcinoma.

Differential Diagnosis

- Lentigo maligna (heavily pigmented variants may be clinically mistaken for this condition)
- Basal cell or squamous cell carcinoma
- Seborrheic keratosis
- Eczema
- Bowen's disease (intraepithelial carcinoma)
- Wart
- Lichenoid keratosis
- Cutaneous lupus

℞ Treatment

First Line

- Avoidance of sun exposure, use of sunscreens
- Cryosurgery with liquid nitrogen

Second Line

- Topical 5-fluorouracil BID for 3 to 6 weeks
- Topical diclofenac
- Carbon dioxide laser
- Dermabrasion
- Curettage

Third Line

- Excision
- Photodynamic therapy with aminolevulinic acid and blue light
- Imiquimod 5% cream BID for 3 to 4 months
- Oral retinoids

 Clinical Pearl(s)

- Actinic keratoses are of particular importance because they are a sensitive indicator of exposure to ultraviolet (UV) light and strongly predict the likelihood of developing cutaneous squamous cell carcinoma.
- The cumulative probability of development of invasive squamous cell carcinoma in patients with 10 or more actinic keratoses has been estimated at 14% in a 5-year period.
- It is estimated that up to 10% of actinic keratoses tend to progress to invasive carcinoma.

6. ALOPECIA AREATA

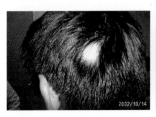 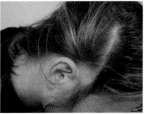

FIGURE 03-013. Round, well-demarcated area of hair loss is characteristic of alopecia areata.

FIGURE 03-014. Alopecia areata presenting as an annular band of hair loss anterior to the right ear in this case with no erythema or scarring.

 General Comments

Definition

- Alopecia areata is a variant of alopecia in which large numbers of hair follicles undergo progression into catagen and telogen while smaller numbers enter an abnormal anagen stage. Alopecia areata is also known as autoimmune alopecia.
- Alopecia areata affects up to 1% of the population and is more common between 15 and 40 years of age.

Etiology

- Alopecia areata is basically a disease driven by cellular immunity with autoantibody production representing a secondary phenomenon.
- The increased frequency of this disorder in genetically related individuals suggests that there is a genetic link to the disease.
- Histologically, alopecia areata is characterized by normal numbers of follicular units and hair follicles, an increase in the number of catagen and telogen follicles, and a lymphocytic infiltrate affecting the bulbs of the anagen.

Keys to Diagnosis

Clinical Manifestation(s)

- Typically patients present with an abrupt development of patches of nonscarring alopecia in different patterns: circumscribed (**Fig. 03-013**), bandlike (**Fig. 03-014**), and reticular. The degree of involvement is highly variable and can range from very mild disease to diffuse hair loss that may affect the entire scalp (alopecia totalis).

Physical Examination

- Examination of the involved scalp generally reveals that except for the absence of hair, the skin appears normal.

Diagnostic Tests

- Laboratory evaluation is generally not helpful.
- Antinuclear antibody (ANA), TSH, complete blood cell count (CBC), and B_{12} level should be considered in patients with a family history of the disease or other manifestations of autoimmune diseases.
- VDRL can be performed in selected patients.

Differential Diagnosis

- Androgenic alopecia
- Trichotillomania
- Secondary syphilis
- Telogen effluvium
- Tinea capitis

R Treatment

First Line

- Intralesional corticosteroids (triamcinolone acetonide, 5 to 10 mg/mL, raising a small bleb within the affected patch)

Second Line

- Topical corticosteroids such as clobetasol 0.05% cream BID, cycled (2 weeks on, 1 week off)
- Topical minoxidil

- Topical sensitizing agent or irritants (dithranol, diphencyprone)
- Phototherapy (ultraviolet radiation or psoralen with ultraviolet A [PUVA])

Third Line
- Systemic immune modulators (e.g., cyclosporine)
- Oral minoxidil

Clinical Pearl(s)

- Fifty percent of cases resolve spontaneously without treatment within 1 year.
- Ten percent evolve to chronic disease.

7. AMALGAM TATTOO

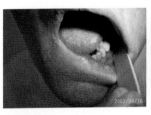

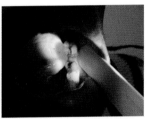

FIGURE 03-015. Amalgam tattoo is a benign hyperpigmented area of the gingival mucosa adjacent to teeth with amalgam fillings.

FIGURE 03-016. Amalgam tattoo, occasionally mistaken for melanoma, results from the local absorption of amalgam particles (mercury, silver, or copper) used to fill carious teeth.

General Comments

Definition
- Amalgam tattoo is characterized by painless gray, bluish, black, or slate-colored macules that generally occur on the gingival/alveolar ridge or buccal mucosa.

Etiology
- Particles of amalgam restorations may be traumatically implanted into the mucosa by the dentist during placement or removal of a restoration, by the patient from bite injury, from leakage and disintegration of a restoration (or root canal filling material), or from a restoration falling into a tooth socket after extraction.

Keys to Diagnosis

Clinical Manifestation(s)
- This condition is asymptomatic, generally noted by dentist during routine dental examination.

Physical Examination
- Gray, bluish, black or slate-colored macules can be seen on the gingival/alveolar ridge or buccal mucosa (**Fig. 03-015**).

Diagnostic Tests
- None necessary. Biopsy only when diagnosis is uncertain and neoplasm is being considered.

DDx Differential Diagnosis
- Melanoma or mucosal melanosis
- Nevus
- Peutz-Jeghers
- Hemangioma or venous lake

R Treatment
- No treatment is necessary.

Clinical Pearl(s)
- The only significance of this lesion is that its appearance can be mistaken for melanoma (**Fig. 03-016**).

8. ANAGEN EFFLUVIUM

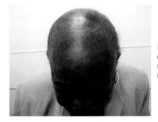

FIGURE 03-017. Generalized hair loss, thinning of hair shafts, and normal appearing scalp secondary to chemotherapy for breast cancer in this patient.

General Comments
Definition
- Anagen effluvium is nonscarring hair loss of the scalp following a toxic insult to growing hair (in anagen phase).

Etiology
- Cancer chemotherapy (e.g., cyclophosphamide, nitrosoureas, doxorubicin) is the most common cause.

Keys to Diagnosis

Clinical Manifestation(s)
- Hair loss occurs usually within 2 weeks of cancer chemotherapy.

Physical Examination
- Hair loss may be slight but is often extensive.
- Alopecia is noninflammatory and nonscarring (**Fig. 03-017**).

Diagnostic Tests
- None necessary.

DDx Differential Diagnosis

- Iron deficiency
- Malnutrition
- Androgenic alopecia
- Telogen effluvium
- Trichotillomania
- Traction alopecia

R Treatment

- No treatment is necessary; the disorder is self-limited.

Clinical Pearl(s)

- Be sympathetic, even if hair loss seems trivial to you. Reassure patient that hair loss is only temporary.

9. ANDROGENIC ALOPECIA

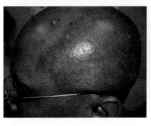

FIGURE 03-018. Frontal recession of hairline typical of early androgenic alopecia.

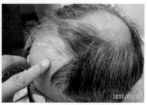

FIGURE 03-019. Progressive androgenic alopecia with loss of hair extending from frontal to vertex regions.

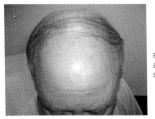

FIGURE 03-020. The loss of hair in advanced androgenic alopecia leaves the scalp smooth, shiny, and devoid of hair follicles.

 General Comments

Definition

- Androgenic alopecia is characterized by progressive patterned hair loss of the scalp due to androgens in genetically susceptible men.

Etiology

- Androgens are the main regulators of hair growth. After puberty, they promote transformation of vellus hair follicles, resulting in production of either tiny, nonpigmented hairs or large pigmented terminal hairs. However, androgens may also reverse this process, resulting in the gradual replacement of terminal hairs with vellus hairs and the onset of androgenetic alopecia. This phenomenon is the direct result of 5-alpha-reductase activity, which is mainly found on the external root sheath and the hair bulb papilla. The enzyme converts testosterone into dihydrotestosterone, which has a great affinity for the androgen receptors in the hair follicle.

Keys to Diagnosis

Clinical Manifestation(s)

- In males the condition usually starts early after puberty, mainly affecting the crown, vertex, frontal (**Fig. 03-018**), central, and temporal areas of the scalp *(Hamilton's male pattern).* There is usually no involvement of the occipital and lower parietal regions.
- In females the hair loss is patterned and characterized by progressive thinning over the frontal/parietal scalp, retention of the frontal hairline *(Ludwig's female pattern),* and the presence of miniaturized hairs. The hair loss often starts around the onset of menopause.

Physical Examination

- Noninflammatory, nonscarring alopecia is seen in defined patterns often resulting in a smooth, shiny scalp devoid of hair follicles (**Fig. 03-019**, **Fig. 03-020**).

Diagnostic Tests
- Ferritin and iron studies, TSH, serum testosterone and dihydrotestosterone levels, ANA
- Scalp biopsy if diagnosis is unclear

DDx Differential Diagnosis
- Iron deficiency
- Malnutrition
- Hypothyroidism
- Telogen effluvium
- Trichotillomania
- Traction alopecia
- Alopecia areata
- Anagen effluvium
- Tinea capitis

R Treatment

First Line
- Topical minoxidil 5% applied BID
- Finasteride 1 mg PO QD (men only)

Second Line
- Hair transplant from occipital scalp
- Hair weaves, wigs

Third Line
- Spironolactone 100 mg BID (women only)

Clinical Pearl(s)
- Androgenetic alopecia affects more than 50% of males over age 50 and 40% of females by age 70. There is usually a familial history of baldness.
- Patients with low iron and alopecia are rarely anemic (the hair is sacrificed before the blood).
- At least 6 months are needed to assess a response to minoxidil and nearly 12 months for finasteride.

10. ANGIOEDEMA

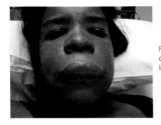

FIGURE 03-021. Angioedema is a hivelike swelling of the mucosa that can involve the tongue, lips, or larynx and at times can encroach on the airway.

General Comments

Definition

■ Mucocutaneous swelling caused by the release of vasoactive mediators. The hivelike swelling involves the deep layers of the dermis and the subcutaneous tissue.

■ Angioedema is classified as acquired (allergic or idiopathic) or hereditary.

Etiology

■ Angioedema is primarily due to mast cell activation and degranulation with release of vasoactive mediators (e.g., histamine, serotonin, bradykinins) resulting in postcapillary venule inflammation, vascular leakage, and edema in the deep layers of the dermis and subcutaneous tissue.

■ Hereditary angioedema is an autosomal dominant disease caused by a deficiency of C1 esterase inhibitor (C1-INH). C1-INH is a protease inhibitor that is normally present in high concentrations in the plasma.

■ Other causes of angioedema include infection (e.g., herpes simplex, hepatitis B, and coxsackie A and B viruses; *Streptococcus, Candida, Ascaris,* and *Strongyloides* bacteria), insect bites and stings, stress, physical factors (e.g., cold, exercise, pressure, and vibration), connective tissue diseases (e.g., systemic lupus erythematosis (SLE), Henoch-Schönlein purpura), and idiopathic causes. Angiotensin-converting enzyme (ACE) inhibitors can increase kinin activity and lead to angioedema.

Keys to Diagnosis

Clinical Manifestation(s)

■ This condition is characterized by poorly demarcated, nonpruritic, burning-like edema, often involving the eyelids, lips (**Fig. 03-021**), tongue, and extremities, which resolves slowly.

■ It can involve the upper airway, causing respiratory distress, and can involve the gastrointestinal (GI) tract, leading to cyclic abdominal pain.

Physical Examination
- Edema of the subcutaneous tissues, often resulting in temporary disfigurement, is seen.

Diagnostic Tests
- A detailed history and physical examination usually establish the diagnosis of angioedema.
- Extensive laboratory testing is of limited value.
- CBC, erythrocyte sedimentation rate (ESR), and urinalysis are sometimes helpful as part of the initial evaluation.
- Stool testing can be done to detect ova and parasites.
- Serology testing can be performed.
- C4 levels are reduced in acquired and hereditary angioedema (occuring without urticaria). If C4 levels are low, C1-INH levels and activity should be obtained.
- Skin and radioallergosorbent (RAST) testing may be done if food allergies are suspected.
- Skin biopsy is usually done in patients with chronic angioedema refractory to corticosteroid treatment.

DDx Differential Diagnosis
- Cellulitis
- Arthropod bite
- Hypothyroidism
- Contact dermatitis
- Atopic dermatitis
- Mastocytosis
- Granulomatous cheilitis
- Bullous pemphigoid
- Urticaria pigmentosa
- Anaphylaxis
- Erythema multiforme
- Epiglottitis
- Peritonsillar abscess

R Treatment

First Line
- Acute life-threatening angioedema involving the larynx is treated with:
  - Epinephrine 0.3 mg in a solution of 1:1000 given SC
  - Diphenhydramine 25 to 50 mg intravenously (IV) or intramuscularly (IM)
  - Cimetidine 300 mg IV or ranitidine 50 mg IV
  - Methylprednisolone 125 mg IV
- Mainstay therapy in angioedema is H1 antihistamines.
- H2 antihistamines can be added to H1 antihistamines.

Second Line

■ Corticosteroids are rarely required for symptomatic relief of acute angioedema and are used more often in chronic angioedema. Prednisone 1 mg/kg/day is generally given for 5 days and then tapered over a period of weeks.

Third Line

■ Tricyclic antidepressants (Doxepin 25-50 mg QD) can be used.
■ Androgens (danazol, stanozolol, oxandrolone, methyltestosterone) are used for the treatment of hereditary angioedema which does not respond to antihistamines or corticosteroids. C1-INH replacement therapy is available in some countries.

🦷 Clinical Pearl(s)

■ ACE inhibitors can cause angioedema months after initiation.
■ Acquired angioedema is usually associated with other diseases, most commonly B-cell lymphoproliferative disorders, but may also result from the formation of autoantibodies directed against C1 inhibitor protein.

11. ANGIOMA (CHERRY ANGIOMA)

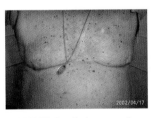

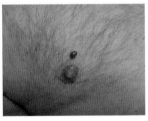

FIGURE 03-022. Example of numerous erythematous to violaceous papules found primarily on the trunk and upper extremities.

FIGURE 03-023. Raised, dark, violaceous angiomas such as this can sometimes be confused with nodular melanomas.

📋 General Comments

Definition

■ Cherry angiomas (also known as Campbell de Morgan spots and senile angiomas) are very common tiny red papules on the trunk (**Fig. 03-022**) and upper limbs of the middle aged and elderly.

Etiology
- Etiology is unknown. Histologically a cherry angioma is a small polypoid lesion with an epidermal collarette and multiple lobules of dilated and congested capillaries in the papillary dermis.

Keys to Diagnosis

Clinical Manifestation(s)
- Asymptomatic lesions appear most often in middle age and increase in size and number with age.

Physical Examination
- Smooth, cherry-red lesions with shape variable from dome to polypoid papules (**Fig. 03-023**).

Diagnostic Tests
- None necessary. Skin biopsy is done only when the diagnosis is unclear.

DDx Differential Diagnosis

- Petechiae
- Telengiectasia
- Bacillary angiomatosis
- Melanoma
- Benign pigmented purpura
- Insect bite
- Pyogenic granuloma
- Angiokeratoma

R Treatment

First Line
- None necessary

Second Line
- Electrodesiccation and curettage

Third Line
- Liquid nitrogen therapy
- Laser surgery

Clinical Pearl(s)

- There is no known association with malignancy.

12. ANGULAR CHEILITIS (PERLECHE)

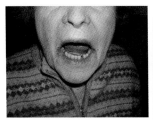

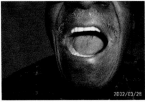

FIGURE 03-024. Angular cheilitis in the elderly is characterized by moist, overlapping skin at the angles of the mouth, which often becomes inflamed and fissured as a result of nocturnal drooling of saliva.

FIGURE 03-025. Chronic inflammation at the corners of the mouth caused by angular cheilitis, which predisposes the skin to secondary bacterial and yeast infections.

 General Comments

Definition
■ Chronic inflammation of the commissures of the lips, also commonly known as perleche.

Etiology
■ Most unilateral lesions are due to trauma (mechanical irritation from dental flossing, excessive salivation, lip licking, mouth breathing, braces, tongue studs). Bilateral lesions are often due to infection (most often *Candida albicans* or *S. aureus*) or nutritional deficiencies (iron deficiency, riboflavin deficiency).

 Keys to Diagnosis

Clinical Manifestation(s)
■ Burning and discomfort are felt at the corners of the mouth.
■ Symptoms made worse by attempts of patients to moisten the area by licking it.

Physical Examination
■ Erythema, fissures (**Fig. 13-024**), scales, and crust may be present at the angles of the mouth (**Fig. 13-025**).
■ Area of fissure may be surrounded by papules and pustules.

Diagnostic Tests
■ Culture for candidiasis and bacteria, potassium hydroxide preparation (KOH) preparation
■ Human immunodeficiency virus (HIV) testing in patients with risk factors

Differential Diagnosis

- Impetigo
- Contact dermatitis (lip balms, mouthwash, toothpaste)
- Lip smacking dermatitis

Ⓡ Treatment

First Line

- Elimination of risk factors (e.g., poorly fitting dentures, repeated attempts by patients to lick and moisten area)
- Topical miconazole or nystatin cream after meals and at bedtime

Second Line

- Topical mupirocin if microbiology swabs reveal *Staphylococcus* colonization
- Protective lip balms or ointments at bedtime

Third Line

- Injection of collagen in the commisures when mechanical factors are causative

🦷 Clinical Pearl(s)

- Angular cheilitis is often present in HIV-positive patients (>10% may have localized candidiasis).

13. ANTIPHOSPHOLIPID SYNDROME

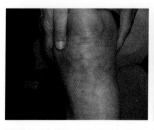

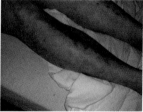

FIGURE 03-026. Bluish, netlike reticular pattern of discoloration involving the lower extremities associated with circulating antiphospholipid antibodies in this patient.

FIGURE 03-027. Lacelike appearance of the skin with blue mottling in this patient with evidence of superficial dermal scarring from prior thrombus formation and infarction.

General Comments

Definition

Antiphospholipid antibody syndrome (APS) is characterized by arterial or venous thrombosis and/or pregnancy loss *and* the presence of antiphospholipid antibodies (aPL). aPL are antibodies directed against either phospholipids or proteins bound to anionic phospholipids. Three types of aPL have been characterized:

- Lupus anticoagulants
- Anticardiolipin antibodies
- Anti-b2 glycoprotein 1 antibodies

Etiology

- APS is an autoimmune disorder.

 Keys to Diagnosis

Clinical Manifestation(s)

- The syndrome is referred to as primary APS when it occurs alone and as secondary APS when in association with systemic lupus erythematosus (SLE), other rheumatic disorders, or certain infections or medications. APS can affect all organ systems and includes venous and arterial thrombosis, recurrent fetal losses, and thrombocytopenia.

Physical Examination

- Cutaneous: livedo reticularis (**Fig. 03-026**, **Fig. 03-027**), cutaneous necrosis, skin ulcerations, gangrene of digits

Diagnostic Tests

- Diagnostic criteria for APS include at least one clinical criterion and at least one laboratory criterion.
- Clinical:
  1. Venous, arterial, or small vessel thrombosis *or*
  2. Morbidity with pregnancy, defined as:
     Fetal death at more than 10 weeks gestation *or*
     More than one premature births before 34 weeks gestation secondary to eclampsia, preeclampsia, or severe placental insufficiency *or*
     More than three unexplained consecutive spontaneous abortions at less than 10 weeks gestation
- Laboratory:
  1. IgG and/or IgM anticardiolipin antibody in medium or high titers *or*
  2. Lupus anticoagulant activity found *or*
  3. Anti-b2 glycoprotein-1 IgM or IgG antibodies found on more than two occasions, at least 12 weeks apart

Laboratory Tests

- Abnormal tests include:
  - False-positive test for syphilis (RPR/VDRL)
  - Lupus anticoagulant activity, demonstrated by prolongation of activated partial thromboplastin time (aPTT) that does not correct with 1:1 mixing study
  - Presence of anticardiolipin antibodies (ELISA for anticardiolipin is most sensitive and specific test [>80%])
  - Presence of anti b_2-glycoprotein 1 antibody

DDx Differential Diagnosis

- Other hypercoagulable states (inherited or acquired)
  - Inherited: antithrombin (ATIII) deficiencies, protein C or S deficiencies, factor V Leiden, prothrombin gene mutation
  - Acquired: heparin-induced thrombocytopenia, myeloproliferative syndromes, cancer, hyperviscosity
  - Nephrotic syndrome
- Cholesterol emboli
- Thrombotic thrombocytopenic purpura
- Hyperhomocysteinemia
- Atherosclerotic cardiovascular disease

Rx Treatment

First Line

- For positive aPL and venous thrombosis:
  - Initial anticoagulation with heparin, then lifelong warfarin treatment (international normalized ratio [INR] 2.0-3.0)
- For positive aPL with arterial thrombosis:
  - Cerebral arterial thrombosis: acetylsalicylic acid (ASA) 325 mg daily or warfarin therapy (INR 1.4-2.8)
  - Noncerebral arterial thrombosis: warfarin therapy (INR 2.0-3.0)
- For pregnant women with previously diagnosed APS:
  - Warfarin should be discontinued secondary to its teratogenic effects.
  - ASA, 81 mg, and heparin subcutaneously (SC) should be administered to partial prothromboplastin time PTT of 1.5 to 2 times control value.
  - Intravenous immunoglobulin (IVIG) and prednisone have also been used with success if aspirin and heparin fail.
- For pregnant women with (+) aPL antibodies and a history of fewer than three spontaneous abortions:
  - ASA 81 mg should be taken daily at conception and subcutaneous heparin 5,000 to 10,000 IU q12h at time of documented viable intrauterine pregnancy. (approximately 7 weeks gestation) until 6 weeks postpartum.
  - A mid-interval PTT should be checked and should be normal or similar to baseline before therapy.

- For pregnant women with (+) aPL antibodies without a history of deep vein thrombosis (DVT) or pregnancy loss:
  - Consider low-dose subcutaneous heparin, ASA 81 mg, or surveillance.
- For catastrophic APS:
  - The highest survival rate is achieved with the combination of anticoagulation, corticosteroids, and IVIG or plasma exchange.
  - Case reports describe Rituximab as a successful therapy for patients with life-threatening thrombosis refractory to anticoagulation.

Clinical Pearl(s)

- Laboratory testing of anticardiolipin and LA antibodies indicated in:
  - Patients with underlying SLE or collagen-vascular disease with thrombosis
  - Patients with recurrent, familial, or juvenile DVT or thrombosis in an unusual location (mesenteric or cerebral)
  - Possibly in patients with lupus or lupuslike disorders in high-risk situations (e.g., surgery, prolonged immobilization, pregnancy)

14. APHTHOUS STOMATITIS (CANKER SORES)

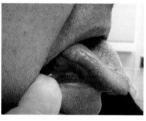

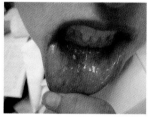

FIGURE 03-028. Aphthous ulcers are most commonly found on the mucous membranes of the oropharynx and appear as shallow, punched-out erosions.

FIGURE 03-029. Painful, gray-based, red-rimmed ulcers are characteristic for aphthous stomatitis.

General Comments

Definition

- Stomatitis is inflammation involving the oral mucous membranes. Aphthous stomatitis is a chronic, painful, relapsing ulcerative condition of the nonkeratinized mucosa (**Fig. 03-028**)

Etiology

- Unknown

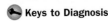 Keys to Diagnosis

Clinical Manifestation(s)

- There are three variants: minor, major, and herpetiform.
- Ulcers of the minor form (the most common variant) are smaller than 1 cm, last 7 to 14 days, and heal without scarring.
- Ulcers of the major form are usually larger than 1 cm, last many weeks, and heal with scarring.
- Ulcers of the herpetiform variety occur in small crops of 10 to 100 ulcers in any one episode.

Physical Examination

- Painful grayish white oval ulcerations with red margins are seen inside the mouth (**Fig. 03-029**).

Diagnostic Tests

- CBC
- Vitamin B_1, B_2, B_6, and B_{12} level; red blood cell (RBC) folate level
- Herpes simplex virus polymerase chain reaction (PCR)

Differential Diagnosis

White Lesions

- Candidiasis (thrush)
- Leukoedema: filmy opalescent-appearing mucosa, can be reverted to normal appearance by stretching; benign condition
- White sponge nevus: thick, white corrugated folds involving buccal mucosa; appears in childhood as an autosomal dominant trait; benign condition
- Darier's disease (keratosis follicularis): white papules on the gingivae, alveolar mucosa, and dorsal tongue; skin lesions also present (erythematous papules); inherited as an autosomal dominant trait
- Chemical injury: white sloughing mucosa
- Nicotine stomatitis: whitened palate with red papules
- Lichen planus: linear, reticular, slightly raised striae on buccal mucosa; skin is involved by pruritic violaceous papules on forearms and inner thighs
- Discoid lupus erythematosus: lesion resembles lichen planus
- Leukoplakia: white lesions that cannot be scraped off; 20% are premalignant epithelial dysplasia or squamous cell carcinoma
- Hairy leukoplakia: shaggy white surface that cannot be wiped off; often seen in HIV infection; caused by Epstein-Barr virus (EBV)

Red Lesions

- Candidiasis: may present with red instead of more frequent white lesion (see "White Lesions"); median rhomboid glossitis is chronic variant

- Benign migratory glossitis (geographic tongue): area of atrophic depapillated mucosa surrounded by a keratotic border; benign lesion, no treatment required
- Hemangiomas
- Histoplasmosis: ill-defined irregular patch with a granulomatous surface, sometimes ulcerated
- Allergy
- Anemia: atrophic reddened glossal mucosa seen with pernicious anemia
- Erythroplakia: red patch usually caused by epithelial dysplasia or squamous cell carcinoma
- Burning tongue (glossopyrosis): normal examination; sometimes associated with denture trauma, anemia, diabetes, vitamin B_{12} deficiency, psychogenic problems

Dark Lesions (Brown, Blue, Black)

- Coated tongue: accumulation of keratin; harmless condition that can be treated by scraping
- Melanotic lesions: freckles, lentigines, lentigo, melanoma, Peutz-Jeghers syndrome, Addison's disease
- Varices
- Kaposi's sarcoma: red or purple macules that enlarge to form tumors; seen in patients with acquired immunodeficiency syndrome (AIDS)

Raised Lesions

- Papilloma
- Verruca vulgaris
- Condyloma acuminatum
- Fibroma
- Epulis
- Pyogenic granuloma
- Mucocele
- Retention cyst

Blisters

- Primary herpetic gingivostomatitis
- Pemphigus and pemphigoid
- Hand-foot-mouth disease: caused by coxsackievirus group A
- Erythema multiforme
- Herpangina: caused by echovirus
- Traumatic ulcer
- Primary syphilis
- Perlèche (or angular cheilitis)
- Recurrent aphthous stomatitis (canker sores)
- Behçet's syndrome (aphthous ulcers, uveitis, genital ulcerations, arthritis, and aseptic meningitis)

- Reiter's syndrome (conjunctivitis, urethritis, and arthritis with occasional oral ulcerations)

Treatment

First Line
- Topical corticosteroids (triamcinolone acetonide 0.1% in Orabase)
- Antimicrobial mouth rinses (tetracycline suspension)
- Intralesional corticosteroids
- 5% anlexanox oral paste (has antiinflammatory and antiallergenic effects)

Second Line
- Oral corticosteroids (prednisone taper)
- Colchicine
- Sucralfate suspension

Third Line
- Pentoxifylline
- Oral acyclovir

Clinical Pearl(s)

- Some conditions often associated with the minor variant include Behçet's syndrome, inflammatory bowel disease, and gluten sensitivity.

15. ATOPIC DERMATITIS (ATOPIC ECZEMA)

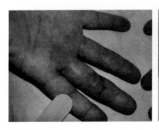 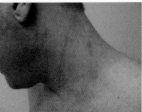

FIGURE 03-030. Dry, erythematous, scaling skin on the palm of this patient during a flare of his atopic dermatitis. Also note fissuring and bleeding secondary to pruritus and scratching.

FIGURE 03-031. Marked erythema, secondary excoriations, and edema of the skin overlying the lateral neck. Skin crease accentuation (hyperlinear creases) is also evident.

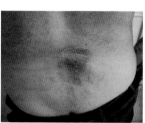

FIGURE 03-032. Thickened, inflamed, scaling skin in the small of the back that was refractory to treatment.

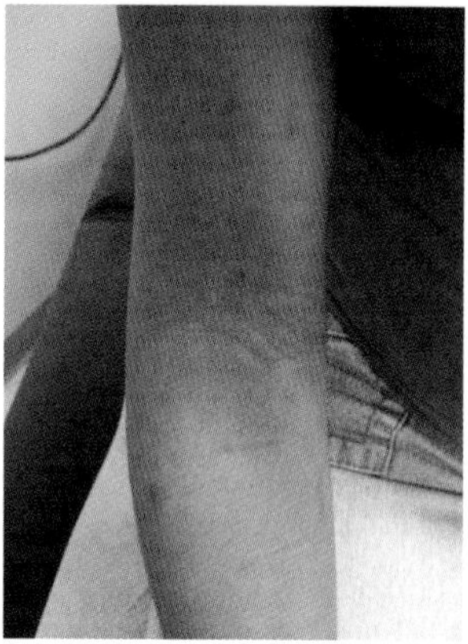

FIGURE 03-033. Chronically inflamed, pruritic, hyperpigmented skin in the antecubital fossa with lichenification and excoriations secondary to excessive scratching.

General Comments

Definition

- Atopic dermatitis is a genetically determined eczematous eruption that is pruritic, symmetric, and associated with personal family history of allergic manifestations (atopy).
- Diagnosis is based on the presence of three of the following major features and three minor features.

Major Features

- Pruritus
- Personal or family history of atopy: asthma, allergic rhinitis, atopic dermatitis
- Facial and extensor involvement in infants and children
- Flexural lichenification in adults

Minor Features

- Elevated IgE
- Eczema-perifollicular accentuation
- Recurrent conjunctivitis
- Ichthyosis
- Nipple dermatitis

- Wool intolerance
- Cutaneous *S. aureus* infections or herpes simplex infections
- Food intolerance
- Hand dermatitis (nonallergic irritant)
- Facial pallor, facial erythema
- Cheilitis
- White dermographism
- Early age of onset (after 2 months of age)

Etiology
- Unknown. Elevated T-lymphocyte activation, defective cell immunity, and B-cell IgE overproduction may play a significant role.

Keys to Diagnosis

Clinical Manifestation(s)
- There are no specific cutaneous signs for atopic dermatitis, and a wide spectrum of presentations are possible, ranging from minimal flexural eczema to erythroderma.
- Inflammation in the flexural areas and lichenified skin is a very common presentation in children.

Physical Examination
- The primary lesions are a result of scratching caused by severe and chronic pruritus. The repeated scratching modifies the skin surface, producing lichenification, dry and scaly skin (**Fig. 03-030**), and redness.
- Lesions are typically found on the neck (**Fig. 03-031**), face, upper trunk, and bends of elbows and knees (symmetric on flexural surfaces of extremities).
- There is dryness, thickening of the involved areas (**Fig. 03-032**), discoloration, blistering, and oozing.
- Papular lesions are frequently found in the antecubital and popliteal fossae.
- In children, red scaling plaques are often confined to the cheeks and the perioral and perinasal areas.
- Constant scratching may result in areas of hypopigmentation or hyperpigmentation (**Fig. 03-033**) (more common in African Americans).
- In adults, redness and scaling in the dorsal aspect of the hands or around the fingers are the most common expression of atopic dermatitis; oozing and crusting may be present.
- Secondary skin infections may be present (*S. aureus*, dermatophytosis, herpes simplex).

Diagnostic Tests
- Skin biopsy can be performed.
- Laboratory tests are generally not helpful.

- Elevated IgE levels are found in 80% to 90% of patients with atopic dermatitis.
- Blood eosinophilia correlates with disease severity.

DDx Differential Diagnosis

- Scabies
- Psoriasis
- Dermatitis herpetiform
- Contact dermatitis
- Photosensitivity
- Seborrheic dermatitis
- Candidiasis
- Lichen simplex chronicus

R Treatment

First Line

- Avoidance of triggering factors:
  - Sudden temperature changes, sweating, low humidity in the winter
  - Contact with irritating substance (e.g., wool, cosmetics, some soaps and detergents, tobacco)
  - Foods that provoke exacerbations (e.g., eggs, peanuts, fish, soy, wheat, milk)
  - Stressful situations
  - Allergens and dust
  - Excessive hand washing
- Clip nails to decrease abrasion of skin.
- Emollients can be used to prevent dryness. Severely affected skin can be optimally hydrated by occlusion in addition to application of emollients.
- Topical corticosteroids may be helpful.

Second Line

- Topical immunomodulators pimecrolimus and tacrolimus are effective steroid-free treatments.
- Oral antihistamines can help with itching.

Third Line

- Oral prednisone, intramuscular triamcinolone, Goeckerman regimen, and PUVA are generally reserved for severe cases.

Clinical Pearl(s)

- The highest incidence is among children (5%-10%). More than 50% of children with generalized atopic dermatitis develop asthma and allergic rhinitis by age 13 years.

16. ATYPICAL MOLE

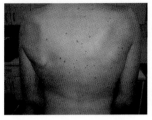 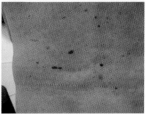

FIGURE 03-034. Atypical nevi located on the back and exhibiting a variety of shapes, sizes (often >6 mm), and borders and colors ranging from brown to black to pink.

FIGURE 03-035. Several 6- to 9-mm brown maculopapular moles, reportedly darkening in color on the back of this patient with a family history of melanoma. He was referred for complete removal and histopathologic examination of the larger nevi.

 General Comments

Definition

- Atypical moles are also commonly known as dysplastic nevi, atypical melanocytic nevi, Clark's nevi, B-K moles, and displastic moles.
- The term refers to nevi that are atypical because of their color, shape, and size.

Etiology

- They can occur sporadically in 5% to 10% of the general population or as a familial syndrome (autosomal dominant trait with incomplete penetrance).

 Keys to Diagnosis

Clinical Manifestation(s)

- Atypical moles may be present on the scalp but are most commonly found on the trunk (**Fig. 03-034**) and upper extremities.
- They may continue appearing into adulthood (unlike acquired melanocytic nevi).

Physical Examination

- Diameter greater than 6 mm
- Irregular edge that can fade into the surrounding skin
- Asymmetrical conformation with variations in pigmentation (**Fig. 03-035**)
- Irregular surface, raised center

Diagnostic Tests
- Diagnostic biopsy if suspecting melanoma
- Ophthalmologic examination (increased risk of intraocular melanoma) and examination of other family members when suspecting familial syndrome

DDx Differential Diagnosis

- Melanoma
- Lentigo maligna
- Compound nevus
- Flat wart
- Seborrheic keratosis

R Treatment

- Periodic follow-up every 6 to 12 months with clinical examination and photographs
- Removal and histopathologic examination of any lesion with documented change

Clinical Pearl(s)

- The risk of melanoma is very high in patients with atypical mole syndrome with a sibling or parent with a history of melanoma.
- The presence of atypically appearing nevi in sun-protected areas in children may be a clue to the presence of the atypical nevus/mole syndrome.

17. BACILLARY ANGIOMATOSIS

General Comments

Definition
- Bacillary angiomatosis is a vasoproliferative lesion that may be readily confused with pyogenic granuloma or Kaposi's sarcoma and is seen predominantly (but not exclusively) in the skin.

Etiology
- The condition may be caused either by *Bartonella henselae* (the organism responsible for cat scratch disease) or, less commonly, by *Bartonella Quintana* (the cause of trench fever).

Keys to Diagnosis

Clinical Manifestation(s)
- Patients may have systemic manifestations, including fever and malaise.
- Lesions have also been described in the bones, soft tissues, liver, lymph nodes, and spleen.

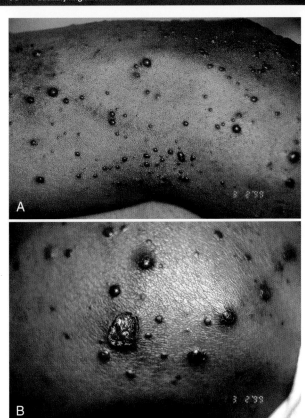

FIGURE 03-036. (A, B) Bacillary angiomatosis: the bright red coloration is characteristic. *(Courtesy N. C. Dlova, MD, Nelson R. Mandela School of Medicine, University of KwaZulu-Natal, South Africa. From McKee PH, Calonje JE, Granter SR: Pathology of the Skin, ed 3, St. Louis, 2005, Mosby, Fig. 17.130.)*

Physical Examination

■ Patients present with widespread, numerous blood-red, smooth, superficial papules and skin-colored or dusky subcutaneous nodules.

■ Hepatosplenomegaly and lymphadenopathy (**Fig. 03-036**) are also seen.

Diagnostic Tests

■ Biopsy and Warthin-Starry stain/electron microscopy, PCR of biopsy material, serology, indirect fluorescence assay (IFA), prolonged culture of blood and biopsy tissue

■ Complete blood cell count (CBC), HIV, alanine aminotransferase (ALT), CD4 lymphocyte count

DDx Differential Diagnosis

■ Pyogenic granuloma
■ Angiokeratoma
■ Kaposi's sarcoma
■ Hemangioma
■ Melanoma
■ Abscess

℞ Treatment

First Line

■ Clarithromycin, azithromycin, or ciprofloxacin

Second Line

■ Erythromycin, doxycycline, rifampin

Third Line

■ Gentamycin
■ Third- and fourth-generation cephalosporins

Clinical Pearl(s)

■ Although bacillary angiomatosis was originally thought to be a disease specific to AIDS, it has also been described in other immunocompromised states and even in apparently normal individuals.

18. BASAL CELL CARCINOMA

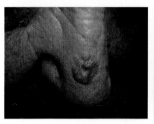

FIGURE 03-037. Nodular basal cell carcinoma presenting as a pearly papule with well-demarcated borders and overlying telangiectasia.

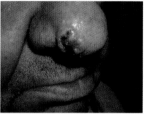

FIGURE 03-038. An ulcerating basal cell carcinoma of the nose (so-called rodent ulcer) with overlying necrosis and dried blood.

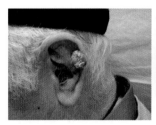

FIGURE 03-039. Nodular basal cell carcinoma of the left ear that has grown irregularly into a multilobular mass with blue-black melanin pigment.

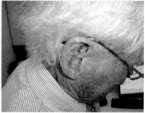

FIGURE 03-040. Brown pigmented basal cell carcinoma embedded in the helix of the right ear.

🗒 General Comments

Definition

■ Basal cell carcinoma (BCC) is a malignant tumor of the skin arising from basal cells of the lower epidermis and adnexal structures. It may be classified as one of six types (nodular, superficial, pigmented, cystic, sclerosing or morpheaform, and nevoid). The most common type is nodular (21%); the least common is morpheaform (1%); a mixed pattern is present in approximately 40% of cases. Basal cell carcinoma advances by direct expansion and destroys normal tissue.

Etiology

■ Risk factors include fair skin, increased sun exposure, use of tanning salons with ultraviolet A or B radiation, history of irradiation (e.g., Hodgkin's disease), personal or family history of skin cancer, and impaired immune system.

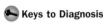 Keys to Diagnosis

Clinical Manifestation(s)

Most common cutaneous neoplasm:

■ 85% appear on the head and neck region
■ Most common site is the nose (30%)
■ Increased incidence with age
■ Increased incidence in men

Physical Examination

Examination varies with the histologic type:

■ Nodular (**Fig. 03-037**): Dome-shaped, painless lesion may become multilobular and frequently ulcerate (rodent ulcer) (**Fig. 03-038**). Prominent telangiectatic vessels are noted on the surface. The border is translucent, elevated, and pearly white. Some nodular basal cell carcinomas may contain pigmentation (**Fig. 03-039**, **Fig. 03-040**), giving an appearance similar to a melanoma.
■ Superficial: Circumscribed scaling black appearance with a thin raised pearly white border is seen. A crust and erosions may be present. These are found most commonly on the trunk and extremities.
■ Morpheaform: Flat or slightly raised and yellowish or white (similar to localized scleroderma), these appear similar to scars. The surface has a waxy consistency.

Diagnostic Tests

■ Biopsy to confirm diagnosis

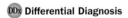 Differential Diagnosis

■ Keratoacanthoma
■ Squamous cell carcinoma
■ Wart
■ Seborrheic keratosis
■ Melanoma (pigmented basal cell carcinoma)
■ Xeroderma pigmentosa
■ Basal cell nevus syndrome
■ Molluscum contagiosum
■ Sebaceous hyperplasia
■ Psoriasis

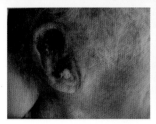 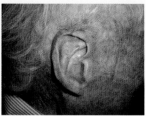

FIGURE 03-041. Same patient from Fig. 03-040 undergoing Mohs' surgery.

FIGURE 03-042. Same patient from Fig. 03-040 with excellent cosmetic result following Mohs' surgery.

℞ Treatment

First Line

Treatment is variable with tumor size, location, and cell type:

- Excision surgery: preferred method for large tumors with well-defined borders on the legs, cheeks, forehead, and trunk.
- Mohs' micrographic surgery (**Fig. 03-041, Fig. 03-042**): preferred for lesions in high-risk areas (e.g., ears, nose, eyelid), very large primary tumors, recurrent basal cell carcinomas, and tumors with poorly defined clinical margins.
- Electrodesiccation and curettage: useful for small (<6 mm) nodular basal cell carcinomas.
- Cryosurgery with liquid nitrogen: useful in basal cell carcinomas of the superficial and nodular types with clearly definable margins; no clear advantages over the other forms of therapy; generally reserved for uncomplicated tumors.

Second Line

- Radiation therapy: generally used for basal cell carcinomas in areas requiring preservation of normal surround tissues for cosmetic reasons (e.g., around lips); also useful in patients who cannot tolerate surgical procedures or for large lesions and surgical failures.

Third Line

- Imiquimod 5% cream can be used for treatment of small, superficial BCCs of the trunk and extremities. Efficacy rate is approximately 80%. Its main advantage is lack of scarring, which must be weighed against higher cure rates with surgical intervention.
- GDC-0449, an orally active small molecule that targets the hedgehog pathway, appears to have antitumor activity in locally advanced or metastatic basal-cell carcinoma.

🩺 Clinical Pearl(s)

- More than 90% of patients are cured; however, periodic evaluation for at least 5 years is necessary because of increased risk of recurrence of another basal cell carcinoma (>40% risk within 5 years of treatment).
- A lesion is considered low risk if it is less than 1.5 cm in diameter, is nodular or cystic, is not in a difficult to treat area (H zone of face), and has not been previously treated.
- Nodular and superficial basal cell carcinomas are the least aggressive.
- Morpheaform lesions have the highest incidence of positive tumor margins (>30%) and the greatest recurrence rate.

19. BECKER'S NEVUS

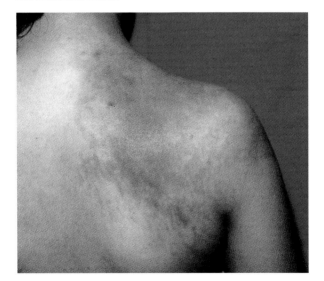

FIGURE 03-043. Becker's nevus. This example shows a characteristic distribution around the shoulder region. (*Courtesy R. A. Marsden, MD, St George's Hospital, London, UK. From McKee PH, Calonje JE, Granter SR: Pathology of the Skin, ed 3, St. Louis, 2005, Mosby, Fig. 23.24.*)

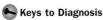 General Comments

Definition

■ Becker's nevus is an androgen-dependent lesion that becomes more prominent after puberty.

Etiology

■ Unknown. It is not a melanocytic nevus.

Keys to Diagnosis

Clinical Manifestation(s)

■ It usually presents in the second decade, initially as an asymptomatic light to dark brown enlarging macular lesion, which subsequently shows hypertrichosis.
■ It most frequently involves the chest, shoulder, or upper arm.
■ Associated abnormalities may include unilateral breast hypoplasia, localized lipoatrophy, vertebral defects, shoulder girdle and pectoralis hypoplasia, accessory mammary tissue, and multiple leiomyomas.

Physical Examination

■ Unilateral irregularly pigmented macular lesions are seen with associated hypertrichosis (**Fig. 03-043**).

Diagnostic Tests

■ Skin biopsy may be performed if diagnosis is uncertain.

DDx Differential Diagnosis

■ Melanoma
■ Congenital melanocytic nevus
■ Postinflammatory pigmentation
■ Nevus spilus
■ Café-au-lait macule

R Treatment

First Line

■ Q-switched ruby laser

Second Line

■ Normal mode ruby laser

Third Line

■ Electrolysis

Clinical Pearl(s)

■ The risk of malignant transformation is very low. Follow-up melanoma screening is unnecessary.

20. BEHÇET'S SYNDROME

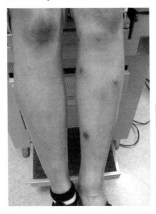

FIGURE 03-044. Erythematous painful nodules on the lower extremity, consistent with erythema nodosum, appeared in this patient with Behçet's syndrome who also had recurrent aphthous ulcers and uveitis.

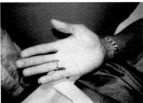

FIGURE 03-045. Patients with Behçet's syndrome may have inflammatory pustules on their hands, in addition to the genital and oral lesions.

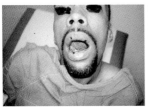

FIGURE 03-046. Recurrent, painful, well-demarcated oral aphthous ulcers are hallmark findings in patients with Behçet's syndrome.

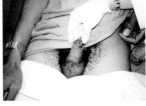

FIGURE 03-047. Punched-out ulcers on the penis, or other areas of the genitalia, in the presence of oral aphthae are consistent with a diagnosis of Behçet's syndrome.

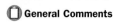 General Comments

Definition

Behçet's syndrome is a chronic, relapsing, inflammatory disorder characterized by the presence of recurrent oral aphthous ulcers, genital ulcers, uveitis, and skin lesions. According to the International Study Group for Behçet's Disease, the diagnosis of Behçet's syndrome is established when recurrent oral ulceration is present along with at least two of the following in the absence of other systemic diseases:

- Recurrent genital ulceration
- Eye lesions
- Skin lesions
- Positive pathergy test (enlarging papules at sterile needle injection sites)

Etiology

- The etiology of Behçet's syndrome is unknown. An immune-related vasculitis is thought to lead to many of the manifestations of Behçet's syndrome. What triggers the immune response and activation is not yet known.

Keys to Diagnosis

Clinical Manifestation(s)

- Behçet's syndrome typically affects individuals in the third to fourth decade of life and primarily presents with painful aphthous oral ulcers. The ulcers occur in crops measuring 2 to 10 mm in size and are found on the mucous membrane of the cheek, gingiva, tongue, pharynx, and soft palate.
- Genital ulcers are similar to the oral ulcers.
- Decreased vision secondary to uveitis, keratitis, or vitreous hemorrhage, or occlusion of the retinal artery or vein, may occur.
- Skin findings include nodular lesions, which are histologically equally divided to erythema nodosum-like lesions (**Fig. 03-044**), superficial thrombophlebitis, and acne lesions; acne lesions are also presented at sites uncommon for ordinary acne (arms and legs).
- Arthritis and arthralgias are common.
- Central nervous system (CNS): meningeal findings, including headache, fever, and stiff neck, can occur. Cerebellar ataxia and pseudobulbar palsy occur with involvement of the brainstem.
- Vasculitis leading to both arterial and venous inflammation or occlusion can result in signs and symptoms of a myocardial infarction, intermittent claudication, deep vein thrombosis, hemoptysis, and aneurysm formation.

Physical Examination

- Papulopustular lesions (**Fig. 03-045**) are the most commonly encountered skin manifestations.
- Recurrent oral ulceration (**Fig. 03-046**) is an invariable feature of this condition.

- The ulcers measure up to 1 cm across and develop anywhere in the oral cavity, pharynx, and even the larynx. They are painful and usually regress spontaneously within 14 days. A yellow, necrotic crust typically covers the ulcer floor.
- Typical of Behçet's syndrome and an important diagnostic clue is the development of sterile pustules at sites of mild skin trauma such as injection sites (pathergy).
- Genital lesions, similar in appearance to those of the oral mucosa, occur on the scrotum, penis (**Fig. 03-047**), vagina, and vulva.

Diagnostic Tests
- The diagnosis of Behçet's syndrome is a clinical diagnosis. Laboratory tests and x-ray imaging may be helpful in working up the complications of Behçet's syndrome or excluding other diseases in the differential.
- There are no diagnostic laboratory tests for Behçet's syndrome.
- Computed tomography (CT) scan, magnetic resonance imaging (MRI), and angiography are useful for detecting CNS and vascular lesions.

DDx Differential Diagnosis

- Ulcerative colitis
- Crohn's disease
- Lichen planus
- Pemphigoid
- Herpes simplex infection
- Benign aphthous stomatitis
- SLE
- Reiter's syndrome
- Ankylosing spondylitis
- AIDS
- Hypereosinophilic syndrome
- Sweet's syndrome

R Treatment

- Oral and genital ulcers:
  - Topical corticosteroids (e.g., triamcinolone acetonide ointment applied TID)
  - Tetracycline tablets 250 mg dissolved in 5 mL water and applied to the ulcer for 2 to 3 minutes
  - Colchicine 0.5 to 1.5 mg/kg/day PO
  - Thalidomide 100 to 300 mg PO daily
  - Dapsone 100 mg PO daily
  - Pentoxifylline 300 mg/day PO
  - Azathioprine 1 to 2.5 mg/kg/day PO
  - Methotrexate 7.5 to 25 mg/wk PO or IV

- Ocular lesions:
  - Anterior uveitis treated by ophthalmologist with topical corticosteroids (e.g., betamethasone 1 to 2 drops TID); topical injection with dexamethasone 1 to 1.5 mg has also been tried
  - Infliximab 5 mg/kg single dose
- CNS disease:
  - Chlorambucil 0.1 mg/kg/day for treatment of posterior uveitis, retinal vasculitis, or CNS disease; patients not responding can be given cyclosporine 5 to 7 mg/kg/day
  - In CNS vasculitis, cyclophosphamide 2 to 3 mg/kg/day; prednisone is an alternative
- Arthritis:
  - Nonsteroidal antiinflammatory drugs (NSAIDs, e.g., ibuprofen 400-800 mg TID PO or indomethacin 50-75 mg/day PO)
  - Alternative treatment: Sulfasalazine 1 to 3 g/day PO
- GI lesions
  - Sulfasalazine 1 to 3 g/day PO
  - Prednisone 40 to 60 mg/day PO
- Vascular lesions
  - Prednisone 40 to 60 mg/day PO
  - Cytotoxic agents as mentioned previously
  - Heparin 5000 to 20,000 U/day followed by oral warfarin

Clinical Pearl(s)

- The aphthous oral ulcers last 1 to 2 weeks, recurring more frequently than genital ulcers.
- Approximately 25% of patients with ocular lesions become blind.

21. BLASTOMYCOSIS

General Comments

Definition

- Blastomycosis is a systemic pyogranulomatous disease caused by a dimorphic fungus, *Blastomyces dermatitidis* (**Fig. 03-048**).

Etiology

- *Blastomyces dermatitidis* exists in warm, moist soil that is rich in organic material. Most patients reside in the southeastern and south central states, especially those bordering the Mississippi and Ohio River valleys, the Midwestern states, and Canadian provinces bordering the Great Lakes. When these microfoci are disturbed, the aerosolized spores or conidia are inhaled into the lungs. Disease at other sites is a result of dissemination from the initial pulmonary infection; the latter may be acute or chronic.

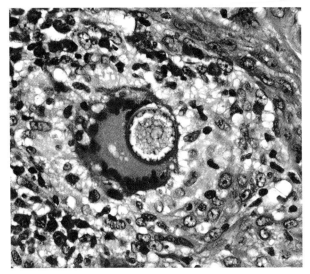

FIGURE 03-048. Coccidioidomycosis: high-power view of spherule. *(Courtesy J. Cohen, MD, Dermatopathology Laboratory, Tucson. From McKee PH, Calonje JE, Granter SR: Pathology of the Skin, ed 3, St. Louis, 2005, Mosby, Fig. 17.319.)*

 Keys to Diagnosis

Clinical Manifestation(s)

- Widely disseminated disease is most common in immunocompromised hosts, especially those with AIDS.
- Initial infections result from inhalation of conidia into the lungs, although primary cutaneous blastomycosis has been reported after dog bites.
- Acute infection: Fewer than 50% of patients are symptomatic. The median incubation period is 30 to 45 days. Symptoms are nonspecific and mimic influenza or bacterial infection with abrupt onset of myalgias, arthralgias, chills, and fever; transient pleuritic pain; and cough that is initially nonproductive. Resolution within 4 weeks is usual.

Physical Examination
- Cutaneous is most common and may occur with or without pulmonary disease. Two different lesions may develop:
  - Verrucous: This begins as a small papulopustular lesion on exposed body areas and may develop into an eschar with peripheral microabscesses.
  - Ulcerative: Subcutaneous nodules (cold abscesses), and rarely cutaneous inoculation blastomycosis, may occur.

Diagnostic Tests
- Presumptive diagnosis can be made by visualizing the distinctive yeast forms in clinical specimens.
- Culture is done on Sabouraud's or more enriched media.
  - Aspirated material from abscesses
  - Skin scrapings
  - Prostatic secretions (urine culture with prostatic massage)
- Direct examination of specimens can be performed.
  - Wet preparation with 10% KOH
  - Histopathology: typically demonstrates pyogranulomas; yeast identification requires special stains

DDx Differential Diagnosis
- Bromoderma
- Pyoderma gangrenosum
- *Mycobacterium marinum* infection
- Squamous cell carcinoma
- Giant keratoacanthoma

R Treatment
First Line
- Itraconazole is the drug of choice except for patients with CNS disease or with fulminant illness who require amphotericin B.
- Amphotericin is recommended in immunocompromised patients, those with life-threatening disease or CNS disease, or those who have failed azole treatment. This is the only drug approved for treating blastomycosis in pregnant women.

Second Line
- Fluconazole 400 to 800 mg/day PO for 6 mo can be given if the patient is unable to tolerate itraconazole or amphotericin.

Third Line
- Ketoconazole 400 mg/day PO × 6 months is an option in mild-to-moderate disease.
- Surgery may be indicated for drainage of large abscesses.

Clinical Pearl(s)

■ Colonization does not occur with blastomycosis as with *Candida* and *Aspergillus* species.

22. BOWEN'S DISEASE

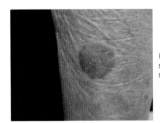

FIGURE 03-049. Bowen's disease, or in situ squamous cell carcinoma, often appears as a scaly, eczematous plaque on the extremities.

 General Comments

Definition

■ Bowen's disease is a type of in situ carcinoma also known as intraepithelial carcinoma, Bowen's carcinoma, or squamous carcinoma in situ or as erythroplasia of Queyrat when involving the glans penis under the foreskin of an uncircumcised penis.

Etiology

■ UV light
■ Human papillomavirus (HPV)
■ Chemicals (arsenic)

Keys to Diagnosis

Clinical Manifestation(s)

■ Insidious onset with slowly enlarging asymptomatic lesion
■ May arise in sun-exposed (head and neck) and sun-protected areas

Physical Examination

■ Scaly patch (**Fig. 03-049**) can be seen that is sharply demarcated and erythematous in appearance.
■ Lesions may be up to several centimeters.
■ Lesions are usually solitary but may be multiple in 20% of cases.

- When involving the penis, there is a red well-demarcated patch often said to be velvety but that may be quite shiny and moist looking. Maceration may at times make it look white and may be mistaken for candidiasis until evaporation brings out the true color.

Diagnostic Tests

- Skin biopsy
- Immunoperoxidase studies for HPV (selected cases)

Differential Diagnosis

- Psoriasis
- Basal cell carcinoma
- Lupus
- Actinic keratosis
- Seborrheic keratosis
- Paget's disease

R Treatment

First Line

- Surgical excision (for well-defined and small lesions) or Moh's micrographic surgery (for ill-defined, large lesions)

Second Line

- 5-Fluorouracil cream 0.5% to 5% applied QD-BID for 8 weeks or topical imiquimod (useful in patients with multiple lesions)
- Electrodessication and curettage
- Liquid nitrogen cryosurgery
- Photodynamic therapy (PDT)

Third Line

- Laser ablation
- Radiation therapy

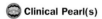 Clinical Pearl(s)

- Erythroplasia of Queyrat is a more aggressive lesion with propensity for invasion and metastases.

23. BULLOUS PEMPHIGOID

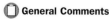 General Comments

Definition

- Bullous pemphigoid refers to an autoimmune, subepidermal blistering disease seen in the elderly. It is the most common of the autoimmune bullous dermatoses.

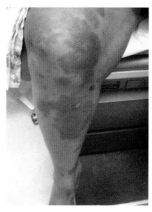

FIGURE 03-050. Urticarial, inflammatory plaques can appear before bulla formation in bullous pemphigoid.

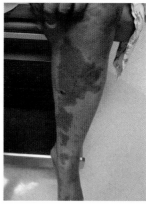

FIGURE 03-051. When bullous pemphigoid affects older adults, erythematous plaques often result.

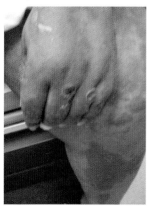

FIGURE 03-052. Bullae may contain serous or hemorrhagic fluid in bullous pemphigoid and may form bleeding erosions when they rupture.

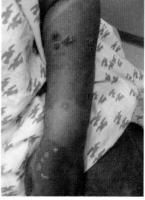

FIGURE 03-053. Bullous pemphigoid appears as round, tense bullae that arise from normal or erythematous skin.

Etiology

- Bullous pemphigoid is an autoimmune disease with IgG and/or C3 complement component reacting with antigens located in the basement membrane zone.
- Drug-induced pemphigoid, although rare, can occur in patients taking penicillamine, furosemide, captopril, penicillin, and sulfasalazine.

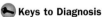 Keys to Diagnosis

Clinical Manifestation(s)

- Bullous pemphigoid typically starts as an eczematous or urticarial rash on the extremities (**Fig. 03-050**). Blisters form between 1 week to several months.
- Anatomic distribution involves the flexor surfaces of the arms, legs (**Fig. 03-051**), groin, axilla, and lower abdomen. The head and neck are generally spared. The lesions are irregularly grouped but sometimes can be serpiginous. Oral lesions can be found occasionally.

Physical Examination

- The typical listering bullae measure from 5 mm to 2 cm in diameter and contain clear or bloody fluid (**Fig. 03-052**). They may arise from normal skin or from an erythematous base (**Fig. 03-053**) and will heal without scarring if denuded.

Diagnostic Tests

- Skin biopsy staining with hematoxylineosin reveals subepidermal blisters.
- Direct and indirect immunofluorescence studies can be done to detect the presence of IgG and C3 immune complexes.
- Immunoelectron microscopy also reveals immune deposits on the basement membrane zone.

DDx Differential Diagnosis

- Cicatricial pemphigoid
- Epidermolysis bullosa acquisita
- Pemphigus
- Pemphigoid nodularis
- Bullous lupus erythematosus
- Herpes gestionalis
- Erythema multiforme

℞ Treatment

First Line

- Treatment of bullous pemphigoid is based on the degree of involvement and rate of disease progression.
- Topical steroids in general have been used in patients with localized bullous pemphigoid

- Systemic corticosteroids are considered the standard treatment for more advanced bullous pemphigoid.

Second Line
- Azathioprine
- Mycophenolate mofetil
- Methotrexate

Third Line
- Cyclophosphamide
- Dapsone
- Plasmapheresis
- IVIG

 Clinical Pearl(s)

- Antibodies to the basement membrane zone are detected in the serum in 70% of patients with bullous pemphigoid.

24. BURNS

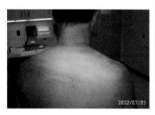

FIGURE 03-054. First-degree burn, confined to the epidermis, with erythema and pain. This patient suffered severe sunburn because of incomplete application of sunscreen.

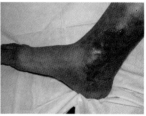

FIGURE 03-055. Severe blistering with distruption of the dermis caused by a second-degree burn from a hot water spill.

 General Comments

Definition
- Burn injuries consist of thermal injuries (sun exposure [**Fig. 03-054**], flames, scalds [**Fig. 03-055**], cigarettes), as well as chemical, electrical, and radiation burns.

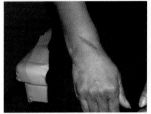

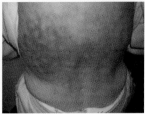

FIGURE 03-056. This linear hyperpigmented lesion represents scarring from a healed oven door burn.

FIGURE 03-057. A white plaque on the trunk of this elderly patient who suffered a first-degree burn from a heating pad, often referred to as erythema ab igne.

Etiology
- Burns can be caused by excessive sun exposure, flames, scalds, and cigarettes, as well as chemical, electrical, and radiation sources.

 Keys to Diagnosis

Clinical Manifestation(s)

Classification of burns is as follows:
- Major burns:
  - Partial-thickness burns covering more than 25% of total body surface area (TBSA) or 20% if younger than 10 or older than 50 years)
  - Full-thickness burns covering more than 10% TBSA
  - Burns crossing major joints or involving the hands, face, feet, or perineum
  - Electrical or chemical burns
  - Burns complicated by inhalation injury or involving high-risk patients (extremes of age/comorbid diseases)
- Moderate burns:
  - Partial-thickness burns covering 15% to 25% TBSA (or 10% in children and older adults)
  - Full-thickness burns covering 2% to 10% TBSA and not involving the specific conditions of major burns
- Minor burns:
  - Partial-thickness burns covering less than 15% TBSA or full-thickness burns covering less than 2% TBSA

Physical Examination
- Burns are defined by size and depth.
- First-degree burns (superficial) involve the epidermis only and appear painful and red.

- Second-degree burns involve the dermis and appear blistered, moist, and red with two-point discrimination intact (superficial partial thickness) or red and blanched white with only sensation of pressure intact (deep partial thickness).
- Third-degree burns (full thickness) extend through the dermis with associated destruction of hair follicles and sweat glands. The skin is charred, pale, painless, and leathery. These burns are caused by flames, immersion scalds, chemicals, and high-voltage injuries.
- The extent of a burn is described as a percentage of the total body surface area.
- Scars (**Fig. 03-056**, **Fig. 03-057**) may develop depending on the depth of the burn.

Diagnostic Tests

- Chest radiographs and bronchoscopy if smoke inhalation suspected
- CBC, electrolytes, blood urea nitrogen (BUN), creatinine, and glucose
- Serial arterial blood gas (ABG) and carboxyhemoglobin if smoke inhalation suspected
- Urinalysis, urine myoglobin, and creatine phosphokinase (CPK) levels if concern for rhabdomyolysis

DDx Differential Diagnosis

- Cellulitis/abscess
- Insect bite (spider bite)
- Bullous erysipelas
- Carbuncle/furuncle
- Anthrax

R Treatment

Minor burns are amenable to outpatient treatment with cool compresses, silver sulfadiazine, nonadherent dressing followed by a sterile gavze wrap. Ruptured blisters should be sharply debrided (except palms and soles). Unruptured blisters should be left intact. Moderate and major burns should be treated in specialized burn care facilities according to the principles described below.

- Establish airway: inspect for inhalation injury and intubate for suspected airway edema (often seen 12 to 24 hr later); administer supplemental O_2.
- Remove jewelry and clothing and place one or two large-bore peripheral intravenous lines (if TBSA affected is >20%).
- Provide fluid resuscitation with Ringer's lactate at 2 to 4 mL/kg/%TBSA/24 hr. with half the calculated fluid given in the first 8 hours.
- Insert Foley catheter and nasogastric (NG) tube (20% of patients develop an ileus).
- Update tetanus if needed.
- Provide medications for pain control.
- Provide stress ulcer prophylaxis in high-risk patients.
- Prophylactic antibiotics are not recommended; however, burn patients should be considered immunosuppressed.

Clinical Pearl(s)

■ High-voltage burn patients should have electrocardiographic (ECG) monitoring because they are at increased risk for arrhythmia.

25. CAFÉ AU LAIT MACULE

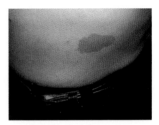

FIGURE 03-058. Isolated 3- by 5-cm light brown macule with irregular borders.

 General Comments

Definition
■ Café au lait spots are well-circumscribed brownish macules caused by an increased number of functionally hyperactive melanocytes.

Etiology
■ They may be found at birth in up to 10% of the population.

Keys to Diagnosis

Clinical Manifestation(s)
■ Asymptomatic
■ Generally no associated abnormalities

Physical Examination
■ Discrete tan-brown macules 2 to 20 mm diameter (**Fig. 03-058**)

Diagnostic Tests
■ None necessary

Differential Diagnosis

■ Seborrheic keratosis
■ Multiple lentigines syndrome
■ Lentigo
■ Nevi

℞ Treatment

First Line
- No treatment necessary

Second Line
- Laser ablation

Third Line
- Hydroquinone 4% cream

🔬 Clinical Pearl(s)

- The presence of more than six macules measuring greater than 5 mm in diameter is suggestive of neurofibromatosis I.

26. CANDIDIASIS

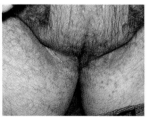

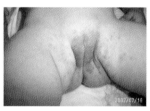

FIGURE 03-059. Erythematous, diffuse eruption occurring in the moist, chafed skin folds of the inner thighs, crural area, and scrotum.

FIGURE 03-060. Candidiasis often occurs in moist areas, such as the diaper area in children.

🗔 General Comments

Definition
- Candidiasis is a cutaneous or mucous membrane infection.

Etiology
- The condition is caused by the yeast *Candida albicans.*

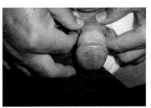 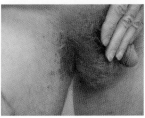

FIGURE 03-061. Candidiasis of the penis appearing as a diffuse, moist, erythematous dermatitis.

FIGURE 03-062. *Candida* intertrigo appearing as a confluent, erythematous dermatitis involving the thighs and scrotum with peripheral satellites typical of such fungal infections.

🔑 Keys to Diagnosis

Clinical Manifestation(s)

- The intertriginous skin folds such as the inner thighs (**Fig. 03-059**) or other moist, occluded sites such as underneath the breasts or in diaper area in infants (**Fig. 03-060**) are most commonly affected.
- The infection may affect the foreskin and glans penis (candidal balanitis [**Fig. 03-061**]) and the scrotum (**Fig. 03-062**).

Physical Examination

- The affected area has a red, glistening surface with an advancing border and cigarette paper–like scaling.

Diagnostic Tests

- Diagnosis is usually made on clinical grounds.
- Presence of pseudohyphae and yeast forms on KOH preparation or other stains confirms the diagnosis.
- Serum glucose and HIV serology can be performed in recurrent cases.

DDx Differential Diagnosis

- Tinea
- Eczema
- Seborrheic dermatitis
- Psoriasis
- Cellulitis

℞ Treatment

First Line
- Affected skin sites that are moist should be dried out with wet-to-dry soaks and exposed to air.
- Topical antifungal products (miconazole, clotrimazole, econazole) are generally effective.

Second Line
- Oral therapy (fluconazole, itraconazole) is reserved for resistant cases.

🦠 Clinical Pearl(s)

- Factors that predispose to infection include diabetes mellitus, obesity, increasing moisture, use of systemic corticosteroids or antibiotics, and immunocompromised status.

27. CELLULITIS

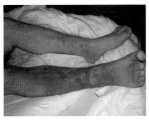

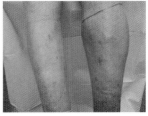

FIGURE 03-063. Erythematous, edematous, tender right leg with recurrent cellulitis. Regression of the cellulitis is evident based on the pre- and post-treatment pen lines.

FIGURE 03-064. Edematous, warm, erythematous left calf present for 3 days. This chronically edematous leg was especially vulnerable to recurrent cellulitis because it had been the site for donor graft vein harvesting several years ago for coronary artery bypass grafting (CABG) surgery.

📋 General Comments

Definition
- Cellulitis is an infection of the subcutaneous tissues.

Etiology
- Group A beta-hemolytic streptococci (may follow a streptococcal infection of the upper respiratory tract)

- Staphylococcal cellulitis
- *Haemophilus influenzae*
- *Vibrio vulnificus*: higher incidence in patients with liver disease (75%) and in immunocompromised hosts (corticosteroid use, diabetes mellitus, leukemia, renal failure)
- *Erysipelothrix rhusiopathiae*: common in people handling poultry, fish, or meat
- *Aeromonas hydrophila*: generally occurring in contaminated open wound in fresh water
- Fungi (*Cryptococcus neoformans*): immunocompromised granulopenic patients
- Gram-negative rods (*Serratia, Enterobacter, Proteus, Pseudomonas* species): immunocompromised or granulopenic patients

Keys to Diagnosis

Clinical Manifestation(s)
- Cellulitis is generally characterized by erythema, warmth, and tenderness of the area involved (**Fig. 03-063**).

Physical Examination
- Erysipelas: A superficial, spreading, warm, erythematous lesion is distinguished by its indurated and elevated margin. Lymphatic involvement and vesicle formation are common.
- Staphylococcal cellulitis: The area involved is erythematous, hot, and swollen; it can be differentiated from erysipelas by nonelevated, poorly demarcated margins. Local tenderness and regional adenopathy are common. Up to 85% of cases occur on the legs (**Fig. 03-064**) and feet.
- *H. influenzae* cellulitis: The area involved is a blue-red/purple-red. It occurs mainly in children and generally involves the face in children and the neck or upper chest in adults.
- *Vibrio vulnificus*: This is characterized by larger hemorrhagic bullae, cellulitis, lymphadenitis, and myositis. It is often found in critically ill patients in septic shock.

Diagnostic Tests
- Gram's stain and culture (aerobic and anaerobic)
- Skin scrapings for mycology
- Blood cultures in hospitalized patients, in patients who have cellulitis superimposed on lymphedema, in patients with buccal or periorbital cellulitis, and in patients suspected of having a salt-water or fresh-water source of infection

DDx Differential Diagnosis

- Erythrasma
- Septic arthritis
- DVT
- Peripheral vascular insufficiency

- Paget's disease of the breast
- Thrombophlebitis
- Acute gout
- Psoriasis
- *Candida* intertrigo
- Pseudogout
- Osteomyelitis
- Insect bite
- Lymphedema

Treatment

- Immobilization and elevation of the involved limb; cool sterile saline dressings to remove purulence from any open lesion
- Erysipelas: dicloxacillin PO or nafcillin or cefazolin IV
- *Staphylococcus* cellulitis: dicloxacillin PO or nafcillin or cefazolin IV
- *H. influenzae* cellulitis: dicloxacillin PO or nafcillin or cefazolin IV
- *V. vulnificus*: doxyxycline or third-generation cephalosporin
- *Erysipelothrix*: penicillin
- *Aeromonas hydrophila*: aminoglycosides, chloramphenicol

Clinical Pearl(s)

- Bacteremia is uncommon in cellulitis (positive blood cultures in only 4% of patients). Culture of aspirates of bullae may be useful to identify causative organisms. Surface swabs are generally unhelpful.

28. CHANCROID

General Comments

Definition

- Chancroid is a sexually transmitted disease characterized by painful genital ulceration and inflammatory inguinal adenopathy.

Etiology

- Chancroid is caused by *Haemophilus ducreyi*, a gram-negative facultative anaerobic bacillus.

Keys to Diagnosis

Clinical Manifestation(s)

- Chancroid occurs more commonly in men (male:female ratio of 10:1).
- There is a higher incidence in uncircumcised men and in tropical and subtropical regions.
- The incubation period is 4 to 7 days but may take up to 3 weeks.

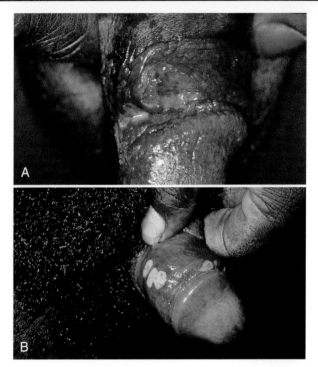

FIGURE 03-065. Chancroid. (A) A painful, solitary, foul-smelling ulcer. (B) Multiple ulcers of chancroid. *(Courtesy Michael O. Murphy, MD. From White GA, Cox NH: Diseases of the Skin: A Color Atlas and Text, ed 2, St. Louis, 2006, Mosby, Fig. 20.44.)*

Physical Examination

- One to three extremely painful ulcers are seen, accompanied by tender inguinal lymphadenopathy (especially if fluctuant).
- May present with inguinal bubo and several ulcers.

- In women the initial lesion is seen in the fourchette, labia minora, urethra, cervix, or anus, followed by an inflammatory pustule or papule that ruptures, leaving a shallow, nonindurated ulceration, usually 1 to 2 cm in diameter with ragged, undermined edges.
- Unilateral lymphadenopathy develops 1 week later in 50% of patients (**Fig. 03-065**).

Diagnostic Tests

- Darkfield microscopy of smears or aspirate
- Rapid plasma reagin (RPR)
- Herpes simplex virus (HSV) cultures
- *H. ducreyi* culture
- HIV testing

 Differential Diagnosis

- Syphilis
- HSV
- Lymphogranuloma venereum (LGV)
- Granuloma inguinale
- Traumatic ulceration
- Behçet's syndrome
- Crohn's disease

R **Treatment**

First Line

- A single dose of ceftriaxone 250 mg IM can be given.
- A single dose of azithromycin 1 g PO can be given.
- HIV-infected patients may need more prolonged therapy.
- Fluctuant nodes should be aspirated through healthy adjacent skin to prevent formation of draining sinus. Incision and drainage (I&D) is not recommended because it delays healing. Use warm compresses to remove necrotic material.

Second Line

- Ciprofloxacin 500 mg PO BID for 3 days
- Erythromycin 500 mg PO QID for 7 days
   NOTE: Ciprofloxacin is contraindicated in patients who are pregnant, lactating, or younger than 18 years old.

Third Line

- Triamphenicol
- Spectinomycin

🗨 **Clinical Pearl(s)**

- All sexual partners should be treated.
- A high incidence of HIV infection is associated with chancroid.

29. CICATRICIAL PEMPHIGOID

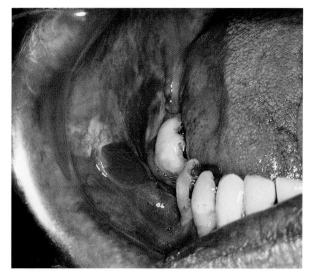

FIGURE 03-066. Cicatricial pemphigoid. Erosion of the buccal mucosa can be seen. *(Courtesy P. Morgan, FRCPath, London, UK. From McKee PH, Calonje JE, Granter SR: Pathology of the Skin, ed 3, St. Louis, 2005, Mosby, Fig. 3.102.)*

📗 **General Comments**

Definition

- Cicatricial pemphigoid is a rare blistering disorder (incidence 1:15,000) often presenting in females in the seventh decade.

Etiology
- This is an autoimmune disorder.
- Oral lesions occur in 85% to 95% of patients and commonly follow mild trauma.

 Keys to Diagnosis

Clinical Manifestation(s)
- Insidious onset of painful blisters in mucous membranes, usually in elderly patients.
- The oral cavity is affected in 90% of cases and the conjunctiva in 70%. Other sites of involvement include the upper airway (45%), skin (30%), and genitalia (15%).
- Desquamative gingivitis is the most common manifestation. Lesions present as painful areas of erosion, erythema, and ulceration.
- Patients with this condition present with painful, swollen, erythematous lesions of the gums, which may be associated with bleeding, blistering, erosions, and ulcerations.

Physical Examination
- Bullae, erosions, and erythema most commonly affect the gingival or buccal mucosa, but the hard and soft palate, tongue, and lips are also often involved (**Fig. 03-066**).

Diagnostic Tests
- Biopsy and direct immunofluorescence studies

 Differential Diagnosis

- Bullous pemphigoid
- Erythema multiforme
- Dermatitis herpetiformis
- Linear IgA dermatosis
- Pemphigus
- Stevens-Johnson syndrome
- HSV, herpes zoster

 Treatment

First Line
- Topical corticosteroids (fluocinonide 0.05% gel applied QID to mucous membranes)

Second Line
- Systemic corticosteroids

Third Line
- Dapsone
- Cyclophosphamide
- Azathioprine

 Clinical Pearl(s)

- Cicatricial pemphigoid is often associated with severe morbidity, largely due to the effects of the scarring associated with it.

30. CONDYLOMA ACUMINATUM (GENITAL WARTS)

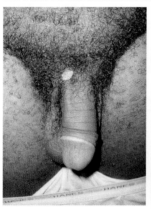
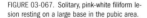

FIGURE 03-067. Solitary, pink-white filiform lesion resting on a large base in the pubic area.

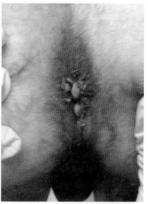

FIGURE 03-068. Multiple, large, painful perianal warts that should be monitored for HPV dysplastic changes with periodic Papanicolau (pap) tests. Two hemorrhoids at 6 and 12 o'clock are also seen.

 General Comments

Definition
- Condyloma acuminatum is a sexually transmitted viral disease of the vulva, vagina, and cervix that is caused by HPV.

Etiology
- HPV DNA types 6 and 11 are usually found in exophytic warts and have no malignant potential.

- HPV types 16 and 18 are usually found in flat warts and are associated with increased risk of malignancy.
- Virus is shed from both macroscopic and microscopic lesions.
- Predisposing conditions include diabetes, pregnancy, local trauma, and immunosuppression (e.g., transplant patients, those with HIV infection).

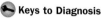 Keys to Diagnosis

Clinical Manifestation(s)

- Condyloma acuminatum is seen mostly in young adults, with a mean age of onset of 16 to 25 years.
- The average incubation time is 2 months (range: 1-8 months).
- Lesions are usually found in the genital area (**Fig. 03-067**) but can be present elsewhere **Fig. 03-068**).
- Lesions are usually in similar positions on both sides of perineum.
- The condition is usually asymptomatic, but if infected, the lesions can cause pain, odor, or bleeding.
- Vulvar condyloma is more common than vaginal and cervical.

Physical Examination

- Initial lesions are pedunculated, soft papules about 2 to 3 mm in diameter, 10 to 20 mm long; they may occur as single papule or in clusters.
- Size of the lesions varies from pinhead to large cauliflower-like masses.
- There are four morphologic types: condylomatous, keratotic, papular, and flat warts.

Diagnostic Tests

- Colposcopic examination of the lower genital tract from cervix to perianal skin with 3% to 5% acetic acid
- Biopsy of vulvar lesions that lack the classic appearance of warts and that become ulcerated or fail to respond to treatment
- Biopsy of flat white or ulcerated cervical lesions

DDx Differential Diagnosis

- Abnormal anatomic variants or skin tags around labia minora and introitus
- Pearly penile papules
- Dysplastic warts
- Seborrheic keratosis
- Erythroplasia of Queyrat
- Lichen planus
- Verrucous carcinoma
- Bowenoid papulosis
- Syphilis

Treatment

- Colposcopic examination of lower genital tract from cervix to perianal skin with 3% to 5% acetic acid
- Biopsy of vulvar lesions that lack the classic appearance of warts and that become ulcerated or fail to respond to treatment
- Biopsy of flat white or ulcerated cervical lesions

First Line
- Cryotherapy
- Electrodesiccation and curettage

Second Line
- Podofilox
- Imiquimod

Third Line
- CO$_2$ laser ablation

 Clinical Pearl(s)

- This condition is highly contagious, with 25% to 65% of sexual partners developing it.

31. CONTACT DERMATITIS (CONTACT ECZEMA)

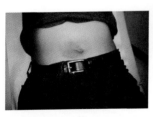

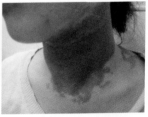

FIGURE 03-069. Classic erythematous, pruritic confluent papules of contact dermatitis caused by a metal belt buckle.

FIGURE 03-070. Intense erythema, itching, and irritation after repeated applications of the offending allergen, tea tree oil.

  General Comments

Definition
- Contact dermatitis is an acute or chronic skin inflammation, usually eczematous dermatitis resulting from exposure to substances in the environment. It can be

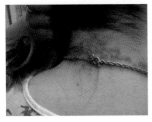

FIGURE 03-071. Papular, erythematous confluent neck rash secondary to the nickel alloy in this patient's metal necklace.

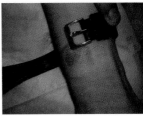

FIGURE 03-072. Scaly, erythematous, pruritic patch just under this patient's leather watchband and metal clasp.

subdivided into "irritant" contact dermatitis (nonimmunologic physical and chemical alteration of the epidermis) and "allergic" contact dermatitis (delayed hypersensitivity reaction).

Etiology

■ Irritant contact dermatitis: cement (construction workers), rubber, ragweed, malathion (farmers), orange and lemon peels (chefs, bartenders), hair tints, shampoos (beauticians), rubber gloves (medical, surgical personnel), belt buckles (**Fig. 03-069**)
■ Allergic contact dermatitis: poison ivy, poison oak, poison sumac, oils (**Fig. 03-070**), rubber (shoe dermatitis), nickel (jewelry) (**Fig. 03-071**), balsam of Peru (hand and face dermatitis), neomycin, formaldehyde (cosmetics), acrylic in adhesive tape

Keys to Diagnosis

Clinical Manifestation(s)

■ Mild exposure may result in dryness, erythema, and fissuring of the affected area (e.g., hand involvement in irritant dermatitis caused by exposure to soap, genital area involvement in irritant dermatitis caused by prolonged exposure to wet diapers).
■ Poison ivy dermatitis can present with vesicles and blisters; linear lesions (as a result of dragging of the resins over the surface of the skin by scratching) are a classic presentation.

Physical Examination

■ The pattern of lesions is asymmetric; itching, burning, and stinging may be present.
■ The involved areas are erythematous, warm to touch, and swollen and may be confused with cellulitis.

Diagnostic Tests

- A diagnosis of contact dermatitis is made from the history and distribution of lesions (**Fig. 03-072**) and is confirmed by patch testing to the suspected allergen.
- Patch testing is useful to confirm the diagnosis of contact dermatitis; it is indicated particularly when inflammation persists despite appropriate topical therapy and avoidance of suspected causative agent. Patch testing should not be used for irritant contact dermatitis because this is a nonimmunologic-mediated inflammatory reaction.

DDx Differential Diagnosis

- Impetigo
- Lichen simplex chronicus
- Atopic dermatitis
- Nummular eczema
- Seborrheic dermatitis
- Psoriasis
- Scabies
- Insect bites
- Sunburn
- Candidiasis

R Treatment

First Line

- Removal of the irritant substance by washing the skin with plain water or mild soap within 15 minutes of exposure is helpful in patients with poison ivy, poison oak, or poison sumac dermatitis.
- Patients with shoe allergy should change their socks at least once a day; use of aluminum chloride hexahydrate in a 20% solution QHS will also help control perspiration.
- Use hypoallergenic surgical gloves in patients with rubber and surgical glove allergy.
- Cold or cool water compresses for 20 to 30 minutes five to six times a day for the initial 72 hours are effective during the acute blistering stage.
- Colloidal oatmeal (Aveeno) baths can also provide symptomatic relief.
- Patients with mild to moderate erythema may respond to topical steroid gels or creams.
- Oral antihistamines will control pruritus, especially at night. Calamine lotion is also useful for pruritus; however, it can lead to excessive drying.
- Topical corticosteroids can provide temporary relief for pruritus.

Second Line

- Oral corticosteroids are generally reserved for severe, widespread dermatitis.
- Intramuscular steroids are used for severe reactions and in patients requiring oral corticosteroids but unable to tolerate them by mouth.

Third Line
- Phototherapy
- Azathioprine
- Cyclosporine

 Clinical Pearl(s)

32. CRYOGLOBULINEMIA

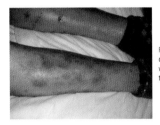

FIGURE 03-073. Resolving hyperpigmented patches of palpable purpura caused by hypersensitivity vasculitis associated with type 3 cryoglobinemia in this patient with underlying hepatitis C.

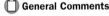 **General Comments**

Definition
- Cryoglobulins are immunoglobulins that precipitate at low temperatures (4° C) and that resolve with rewarming.

Etiology
- Cryoglobulins may be divided into three classes:
  - Type I, composed solely of monoclonal immunoglobulin (either kappa or lambda) and usually associated with lymphoproliferative disorders (multiple myeloma, Waldenstrom's macoglobulinemia)
  - Type II (mixed) cryoglobulin, composed of monoclonal (usually IgM) immunoglobulin
  - Type III (polyclonal) cryoglobulin, composed of immunoglobulins IgG and IgM.
- The last two subtypes (mixed cryoglobulins) function as immune complexes and clinical manifestations are due, at least in part, to allergic vasculitis.

 Keys to Diagnosis

Clinical Manifestation(s)
- The eponym *Meltzer's triad* has been applied to the combined features of purpura, arthralgias, and weakness, which are often present.

- Cutaneous manifestations are common to all classes of cryoglobulinemia and are often the presenting complaint.
- Type I cryoglobulinemia is usually characterized by purpuric lesions, including inflammatory macules and papules on the extremities, accompanied by foci of ulceration.
- Mixed cryoglobulinemia is characterized by joint involvement (arthralgia and arthritis), Raynaud's phenomenon, fever, purpura, weakness, renal involvement, hepatosplenomegaly, necrosis of extremities and general vasculitis. Cutaneous manifestations include palpable purpura, inflammatory macules and papules, necrotizing vasculitis, and, occasionally, cold urticaria. Renal involvement may be identified by proteinuria, hematuria, and red cell casts. Patients may also have polyneuropathies.

Physical Examination
- Purpura (**Fig. 03-073**) is the most common initial sign.
- Additional features may include livedo reticularis, Raynaud's phenomenon, scarring, and infarction, which particularly affects the digits, ears, and nose.

Diagnostic Tests
- Serum cryoglobulin level
- Skin biopsy

DDx Differential Diagnosis

- Serum sickness
- Antiphospholipid antibody syndrome
- Sarcoidosis
- Waldenstrom's hyperglobulinemia
- Septic vasculitis
- Polyarteritis nodosa

Rx Treatment

First Line
- Elimination of triggers by minimizing cold exposure
- Systemic corticosteroids (prednisone 1 mg/kg PO QD)
- NSAIDs

Second Line
- Azathioprine
- Mycophenolate mofetil
- Dapsone

Third Line
- Methotrexate
- Cyclophosphamide

Clinical Pearl(s)

- Cryoglobulins may be associated with hepatitis C, hepatitis B, SLE, lymphoreticular neoplasms, and infective processes (e.g., infective endocarditis).
- Prognosis is variable. Renal involvement, which occurs in 50% of cases, is associated with high morbidity and mortality.

33. CUTIS LAXA

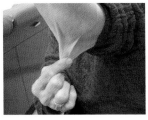 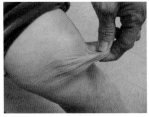

FIGURE 03-074. Cutis laxa is characterized by skin that is loose, hanging, and lacking in elasticity.

FIGURE 03-075. Severe decrease in elastic recoil of the skin in this patient with cutis laxa.

 General Comments

Definition
- Cutis laxa is a disorder manifested by wrinkling and sagging of the skin resulting in a prematurely aged appearance.

Etiology
- The condition is caused by a defect in the elastic tissue.
- It may be idiopathic, hereditary, occurring with paraneoplastic disorders, or following long-term penicillamine therapy.

 Keys to Diagnosis

Clinical Manifestation(s)
- The affected individual appears much older than chronologic age.
- Associated involvement of internal organs may result in GI diverticula, hernias, emphysema, aortic aneurysms, and ligamentous laxity.

Physical Examination
- Skin is inelastic (**Fig. 03-074**), loose, wrinkling, and sagging (**Fig. 03-075**).

Diagnostic Tests
- None

DDx Differential Diagnosis

- Anetoderma (localized area of lax skin, often with herniation of underlying tissues)
- Morphea
- Atrophotoderma (disorders characterized by a depression in the skin's surface)
- Pseudoxanthoma elasticum
- Ehlers-Danlos syndrome
- Marfan syndrome

R Treatment

- There is no effective treatment.
- Reconstructive surgery may be attempted.

Clinical Pearl(s)

- Surgical approaches are generally disappointing and not permanent.

34. CYLINDROMA

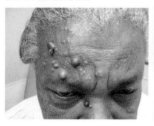

FIGURE 03-076. Cylindromas are benign, firm, rubbery nodules generally found on the head and neck.

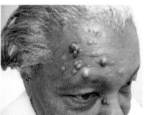

FIGURE 03-077. This patient developed multiple facial cylindromas beginning in adolescence, which is consistent with an autosomal dominant pattern of inheritance.

General Comments

Definition
- Cylindroma is a skin lesion often found on the scalp and also known as a "Turban tumor" or "Tomato tumor" due to its appearance.

Etiology
- Unknown

 Keys to Diagnosis

Clinical Manifestation(s)
- Lesions may be solitary (most common) or multiple (**Fig. 03-076** and **Fig. 03-077**).
- Lesions are most often found on the scalp, face, and neck.

Physical Examination
- Purplish to red nodule(s) with a smooth surface are present.
- Prominent surface vessels may be present.
- A rounded mass is seen, and skin may appear stretched.

Diagnostic Tests
- Biopsy of lesion

 Differential Diagnosis

- Basal cell carcinoma
- Pilar cyst
- Pilomatricoma
- Follicular neoplasm
- Eccrine spiradenoma

 Treatment

First Line
- Excision of lesion

Second Line
- CO_2 laser ablation

 Clinical Pearl(s)

- There is a familial association with multiple facial trichoepitheliomas (Spiegler-Brooke syndrome).

35. CYSTICERCOSIS

 General Comments

Definition
- Cysticercosis is an infection caused by the tissue deposition of larval forms of the pork tapeworm *Taenia solium*.

Etiology
- Humans acquire cysticercosis via fecal-oral transmission of *T. solium* eggs from human tapeworm carriers, often by ingesting tapeworm eggs or cysts in contaminated food or water. The eggs hatch in the gastrointestinal tract, and larvae migrate hematogenously to tissues and then encyst, forming cysticerci. *T. solium* cysts, or cysticerci, may accumulate in any tissue, including the eyes, spinal cord, skin, muscle, heart, and brain. Central nervous system involvement is common and is known as neurocysticercosis.

Keys to Diagnosis

Clinical Manifestation(s)
- Following ingestion of *T. solium* eggs or cysts, humans may remain asymptomatic for several years.
- The symptoms are varied and depend on the location of cysticerci. Cysticerci in muscles and skin may form "cold" nodules, which are usually asymptomatic but may calcify.

Physical Examination
- The cutaneous manifestations consist primarily of subcutaneous nodules.

Diagnostic Tests
- Definitive diagnosis is based on the histopathologic demonstration of cysticerci in the tissue involved.
- Peripheral eosinophilia is absent.

DDx Differential Diagnosis

- Epidermoid cysts
- Sarcoidosis
- Toxoplasmosis
- CNS neoplasm
- Tuberculosis

℞ Treatment

First Line
- Asymptomatic cysticercosis: There is no evidence that administering antiparasitic therapy is beneficial.
- Symptomatic cysticercosis: Patients with active lesions, with evidence of surrounding edema and/or inflammation, generally warrant treatment with antiparasitics (albendazole, praziquantel), corticosteroids, and anticonvulsants.

Second Line
- Surgical excision can remove solitary lesions.

Clinical Pearl(s)

■ Undercooked pork is the most commonly identified food source.

36. DARIER'S DISEASE

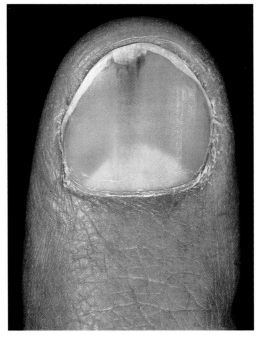

FIGURE 03-078. Darier's disease. Parallel white and red longitudinal streaks are pathognomonic features. *(Courtesy the Institute of Dermatology, London, UK. From McKee PH, Calonje JE, Granter SR: Pathology of the Skin, ed 3, St. Louis, 2005, Mosby, Fig. 4.47.)*

General Comments

Definition
- Darier's disease is a rare skin disorder characterized by abnormal keratinocyte adhesion.

Etiology
- The condition is transmitted in an autosomal dominant pattern.

Keys to Diagnosis

Clinical Manifestation(s)
- Lesions may be induced or exacerbated by stress, heat, sweating, and maceration.

Physical Examination
- The nail changes in Darier's disease include longitudinal red and/or white streaks (**Fig. 03-078**) that terminate in a notch on the free margin of the nail plate, splitting, and subungal hyperkeratosis with associated wedge-shaped onycholysis.
- The lesions are often itchy and characterized by greasy, crusted, keratotic yellow-brown papules and plaques found particularly on the scalp, forehead, ears, nasolabial folds, upper chest, back, and supraclavicular fossae.

Diagnostic Tests
- Skin biopsy reveals focal acantholytic dyskeratosis.

DDx Differential Diagnosis

- Pemphigus foliaceus
- Transient acantholytic dermatosis
- Seborrheic dermatitis
- Follicular eczema
- Folliculitis

Treatment

First Line
- Emollients, cool cotton clothing
- Topical retinoids (tretinoin 0.025% cream HS)

Second Line
- Oral retinoids (isotretinoin 0.3 mg/kg QD)
- Tazarotene

Third Line
- Topical 5-fluorouracil
- Cyclosporine

- Oral contraceptives
- Laser
- Dermabrasion

Clinical Pearl(s)

- Patients with Darier's disease are susceptible to bacterial (particularly *S. aureus*), dermatophyte, and viral infections.

37. DECUBITUS ULCER

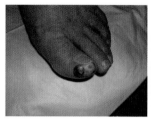

FIGURE 03-079. Stage II decubitus or pressure sore of the great toe with incipient shallow ulcer and necrosis of the dermis as evidenced by black discoloration.

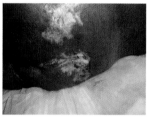

FIGURE 03-080. The uppermost decubitus ulcer has caused necrosis to the level of subcutaneous tissue (but not into the underlying fascia) and is assessed as stage III.

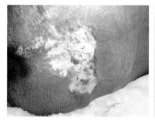

FIGURE 03-081. Stage IV decubitus ulcer with necrosis extending from skin through subcutaneous tissue, muscle, and finally to bone. Treatment included debridement of necrotic tissue and removal of infected area of sacral bone.

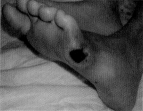

FIGURE 03-082. Stage IV ulcer, lateral foot, with dark eschar extending to the level of bone in a bedridden stroke patient.

General Comments

Definition

■ Decubitus ulcers (pressure ulcers or bed sores) are any damage to the skin and the underlying tissue or both that results from pressure, friction, or shearing forces.

Etiology

■ Decubitus ulcers are caused by pressure, friction, or shearing forces that usually occur over bony prominences such as the sacrum or heels.

Keys to Diagnosis

Clinical Manifestation(s)

■ All pressure ulcers should be staged according to depth and type of tissue damage (see physical examination).

Physical Examination

Stage I	Nonblanchable erythema of intact skin or boggy, mushy feeling of skin
Stage II	Partial-thickness skin loss involving the epidermis, dermis, or both (Fig. 03-079)
Stage III	Full-thickness skin loss involving damage or necrosis of subcutaneous tissue that may extend down to, but not through, underlying fascia or muscle (Fig. 03-080)
Stage IV	Full-thickness skin loss with extensive destruction and tissue damage to muscle, bone, or supporting structures (e.g., tendons, joint capsule) (Fig. 03-81, Fig. 03-082)

Diagnostic Tests

■ Tests are directed at identifying the cause of risk factors or any complications arising from the pressure ulcer (e.g., abscess or osteomyelitis); cultures of the wound bed are not helpful and should not be performed.
■ Nutritional laboratory tests may reveal malnutrition such as prealbumin.
■ CBC should be obtained if infection is suspected.
■ MRI or bone scans may help identify osteomyelitis when clinically suspected.

Differential Diagnosis

■ Stasis ulcer
■ Burns
■ Contact dermatitis
■ Pyoderma gangrenosum
■ Squamous cell carcinoma
■ Bullous pemphigoid

℞ Treatment

First Line

■ The area should be cleaned at each dressing change; necrotic tissue should be removed.
■ Debridement should be performed quickly because it delays wound healing. Whirlpool debridement may be useful.

- The wound should be irrigated.
- No one dressing or product is clearly superior; dressing should be used to keep the ulcer bed moist and protect it from urine/stool. Hydrocolloid dressings are useful for stage II ulcers. Wet dressings, xerogels, or hydrogels can be used for stage III and IV ulcers. Avoid agents that are cytotoxic to epithelial cells (e.g., iodine, iodophor, sodium hypochlorite, hydrogen peroxide, acetic acid, and alcohol).
- Reduce pressure by using a foam mattress, alternating pressure mattress, or dynamic support surface (e.g., low-air-loss bed) and by frequent repositioning (e.g., Q2H).
- Correct malnutrition.
- Minimize urinary/fecal incontinence.
- Use a standardized assessment tool (e.g., Pressure Ulcer Scale for Healing [PUSH] tool) to monitor wound healing on weekly basis.

Second Line
- Negative pressure devices (vacuum-assisted closure [VAC] devices) may help for wounds that have significant drainage.

Third Line
- Hyperbaric oxygen, ultrasound, and ultraviolet and low-energy radiation either are ineffective or have not been extensively evaluated for efficacy.

 Clinical Pearl(s)
- The initial manifestation of a decubitus ulcer is erythema (blanchable and nonblanchable).

38. DERMATITIS HERPETIFORMIS

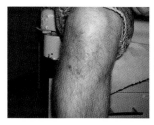

FIGURE 03-083. Intensely pruritic, grouped vesicles and papules on a red, inflamed base, found on the lower extremity in this patient with celiac sprue.

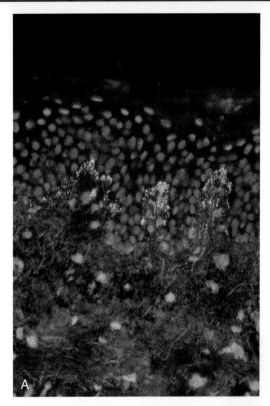

FIGURE 03-084. Dermatitis herpetiformis. Direct immunofluorescence showing (A) deposits of granular IgA in the dermal papillae; (B) fibrin deposition in the dermal papillae. *(Courtesy the Department of Immunofluorescence, Institute of Dermatology, London, UK. From McKee PH, Calonje JE, Granter SR: Pathology of the Skin, ed 3, St. Louis, 2005, Mosby, Fig. 3.144.)*

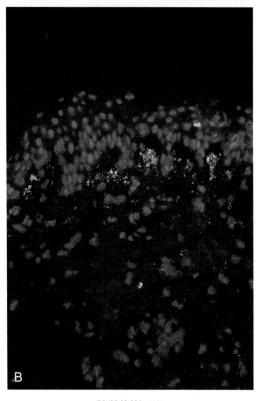

FIGURE 03-084, cont'd.

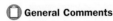 General Comments

Definition
- Dermatitis herpetiformis (DH) is a chronic skin disorder characterized by an intensely burning, pruritic, vesicular rash

Etiology
- Unknown. Increased incidence in association with HLA DRw3, B8, and DQw2.

Keys to Diagnosis

Clinical Manifestation(s)
- Pruritic, burning vesicles are seen initially; the vesicles are frequently grouped (hence the name *herpetiform*).
- May evolve in time to intensely burning urticarial papules (**Fig. 03-083**), vesicles, and, rarely, bullae.
- Celiac-type permanent-tooth enamel defects found in 53% of patients.

Physical Examination
- Symmetrically distributed vesicles and papules are seen on extensor surfaces, such as elbows, knees, scalp, nuchal area, shoulder, and buttocks, but are rarely found in the mouth.

Diagnostic Tests
- Skin biopsy should be performed for immunofluorescence studies. Diagnosis is confirmed by IgA deposits along the subepidermal basement membrane (**Fig. 03-084**). Biopsies should be taken from adjacent normal skin because the diagnostic Ig deposits are usually destroyed by the blistering process.
- Circulating antibodies include IgA antiendomysial antibody, IgA antigliadin antibodies, IgA reticulin antibody, and IgA antitissue transglutaminase.

Differential Diagnosis

- Linear IgA bullous dermatosis (not associated with gluten-sensitive enteropathy)
- Herpes simplex infection
- Herpes zoster infection
- Erythema multiforme
- Bullous pemphigoid

Ⓡ Treatment

First Line
- Adherence to a gluten-free diet has been associated with sustained remission of DH. Spontaneous remission of DH in patients on a normal diet can occur in up to 15% of cases.
- Dapsone

Second Line
- Sulfapyridine
- Systemic corticosteroids

Third Line
- Tetracycline and nicotinamide
- Cyclosporine
- Colchicine

 Clinical Pearl(s)

- DH is strongly associated with gluten-sensitive enteropathy. Up to 70% of patients with DH will have gastrointestinal symptoms, whereas approximately 10% of patients with celiac sprue will have DH.

39. DERMATOFIBROMA

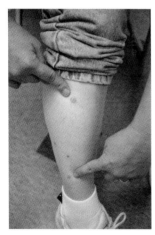

FIGURE 03-085. Asymptomatic, dome-configured 5-mm nodules on the lower extremity that recessed or dimpled when lateral pressure with thumb and index finger was applied ("dimple sign").

 General Comments

Definition
- Dermatofibroma is an extremely common benign, slow-growing asymptomatic dermal papule, also known as histiocytoma.

Etiology
- Unknown. The condition may occur spontaneously.
- Dermatofibroma may be associated with history of trauma (ruptured cyst, insect bite).

 Keys to Diagnosis

Clinical Manifestation(s)
- Papules are most often found on extremities (lower more commonly than upper) and scapulas.
- Papules are generally not tender but may be mildly tender on palpation.
- The condition is usually asymptomatic, but localized pruritus may be present when the lesion is initially detected.

Physical Examination
- Discrete firm dermal papules are 3 to 10 mm in diameter.
- Papules are flesh colored to brown.
- On palpation it feels like a button and dimples into the surrounding skin with lateral pinching (**Fig. 03-085**).

Diagnostic Tests
- Biopsy of pigmented lesions can rule out melanoma.

DDx Differential Diagnosis
- Insect bite
- Foreign body reaction
- Angioma
- Melanoma
- Wart
- Prurigo nodularis
- Basal cell carcinoma
- Scar
- Keloid
- Nevus

 Treatment

First Line
- Most lesions are innocuous and can safely be left alone.

Second Line
- Surgical excision with primary closure can be performed for symptomatic lesions.
- Surgery for cosmetic reasons is best avoided because the scar from surgery may be more prominent than original lesion.

Third Line
- Intralesional corticosteroids

Clinical Pearl(s)
- Eruption of large numbers of dermatofibromas can be seen with HIV infection.

40. DERMATOGRAPHISM

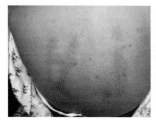

FIGURE 03-086. Dermatographism, writing on skin, is caused by the release of excessive amount of histamine in certain predisposed individuals following gentle "writing" on the skin.

General Comments
Definition
- Dermatographism is a physical urticaria manifesting with brief-lasting linear wheals at the site of stroking of the skin (**Fig. 03-086**).

Etiology
- Unknown. The condition may be associated with emotional upset, viral infections, drug reactions (antibiotics, postscabies treatment), or extreme temperature changes.

Keys to Diagnosis
Clinical Manifestation(s)
- Pruritus and scratching of the involved skin are present.
- Attacks may last from a few minutes to several hours.

Physical Examination
- Linear wheals and redness are seen at the site of stroking of the skin.

Diagnostic Tests
- Stroking of the skin with a tongue blade will elicit whealing within a few minutes.

DDx Differential Diagnosis

- Cholinergic urticaria
- Solar urticaria
- Heat urticaria
- Exercise-induced urticaria
- Cold urticaria
- Lupus
- Aquagenic urticaria
- Polymorphous light eruption

R Treatment

First Line
- Elimination of potential offending agent

Second Line
- Antihistamines

Third Line
- H2 blockers

Clinical Pearl(s)

- Although H2 blockers are sometimes added to antihistamines to treat dermatographism, some H2 blockers, such as famotidine, have been reported to cause dermatographism.

41. DERMATOMYOSITIS

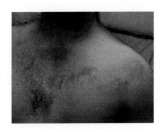

FIGURE 03-087. Photodistributed, violaceous, erythematous lesions occurring around the neck and upper shoulders ("shawl" sign).

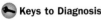 **General Comments**

Definition
- Dermatomyositis is an inflammatory eruption of the skin associated with myositis.

Etiology
- The cause is unknown, but an autoimmune etiology is suspected.

Keys to Diagnosis

Clinical Manifestation(s)
- Proximal muscle weakness, generalized pruritus, fatigue
- Itching or scaling of scalp
- Dysphagia

Physical Examination
- Purplish or faint lilac "heliotrope" discoloration around eyes, elbows, knees, and dorsum of phalanges (Grotton's sign [streaks along fingers] or Grotton's papules [presence of red flat-topped papules over bony prominences])
- Lesions possibly present around neck and upper shoulders ("shawl" sign) (**Fig. 03-087**)
- Malar and eyelid edema
- Telengiectasia of nail folds
- Calcinosis of skin (especially in juvenile disease)
- Proximal muscle weakness

Diagnostic Tests
- Skin biopsy
- Muscle biopsy
- CPK, serum aldolase
- Electromyography (EMG)
- CT of chest, abdomen, and pelvis to screen for underlying neoplasm (e.g., ovarian cancer)
- Presence of Jo-1 antibodies correlates with high risk for myositis, pulmonary disease, and arthritis

DDx Differential Diagnosis

- Lupus
- Scleroderma
- Sarcoidosis
- Lichen planus
- Trichinosis
- Drug eruption

- Psoriasis
- Mycosis fungoides
- Toxoplasmosis

Treatment

First Line

- Cutaneous disease: sunscreens, topical corticosteroids, topical pimecrolimus or tacrolimus, antimalarials (hydroxychloroquine or chloroquine)
- Muscle disease: systemic corticosteroids (prednisone 1 mg/kg PO QD), immuno-suppressants (methotrexate, azathioprine)

Second Line

- Cutaneous disease: methotrexate, mycophenolate, IVIG
- Muscle disease: mycophenolate, cyclosporine, IVIG

Third Line

- Dapsone for cutaneous disease; diltiazem for calcinosis; infliximab, etarnecept

Clinical Pearl(s)

- Approximately 25% to 40% of patients with dermatomyositis have an underlying malignancy.
- Removal of underlying malignancy (when present) may improve dermatomyositis manifestations.

42. DERMOID CYST

General Comments

Definition

- Dermoid cysts are lesions resulting from sequestration of cutaneous tissues along embryonal lines of closure.

Etiology

- Unknown

🔧 Keys to Diagnosis

Clinical Manifestation(s)

- Generally asymptomatic

Physical Examination

- The most common clinical appearance is that of a single nontender, small subcu-taneous nodule at birth on the lateral aspect of the upper eyelid (**Fig. 03-088**).

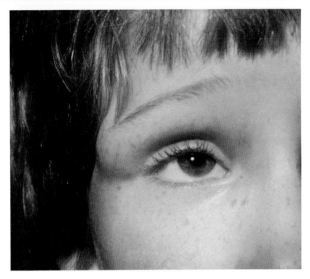

FIGURE 03-088. Dermoid cyst. Note the swelling adjacent to the upper eyelid—the external angular dermoid cyst. *(Courtesy R.A. Marsden, MD, St George's Hospital, London, UK. From McKee PH, Calonje JE, Granter SR: Pathology of the Skin, ed 3, St. Louis, 2005, Mosby, Fig. 30.26.)*

- Other potential sites of dermoid cysts include the midline of the neck, nasal root, forehead, mastoid area, and scalp. The last is a particularly important site because the lesion may occasionally show intracranial extension (dumbbell dermoid).

Diagnostic Tests
- Preoperative imaging of lesions on the nose, midline scalp, or posterior axis can exclude CNS extension.

DDx Differential Diagnosis
- Epidermoid cyst
- Nevus sebaceus
- Enlarged lymph node
- Pilomatricoma

℞ Treatment

■ Surgical excision

🧫 Clinical Pearl(s)

■ Dermoid cysts on the nose or midline scalp have a much higher likelihood of intracranial extension than those in periocular locations.

43. DISCOID LUPUS ERYTHEMATOSUS

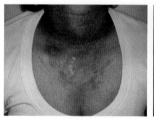

FIGURE 03-089. Fixed, indurated, erythematous plaques and papules photodistributed over V of upper chest.

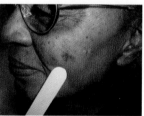

FIGURE 03-090. Facial lesions of discoid lupus causing a hyperpigmented disfiguring scar on the left cheek.

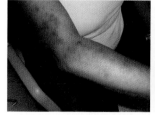

FIGURE 03-091. Hyperpigmented plaques with irregular borders widely distributed over the forearm.

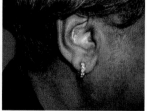

FIGURE 03-092. Longstanding, hypopigmented discoid lupus lesion in the ear with evidence of atrophy and scarring.

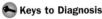 General Comments

Definition
- Discoid lupus erythematosus (DLE) is a chronic inflammatory autoimmune skin disorder. It is sometimes associated with systemic lupus erythematosus (SLE).

Etiology
- DLE is an immune complex–mediated disorder.

Keys to Diagnosis

Clinical Manifestation(s)
- DLE manifests with the appearance of single or multiple asymptomatic plaque lesions (**Fig. 03-089**).
- Alopecia can occur and is permanent.
- Urticaria is present in 5% of cases.
- DLE may be associated with other criteria for SLE (e.g., oral ulcers, arthritis, pleuritis, pericarditis).

Physical Examination
- Anatomic distribution: commonly involves the scalp, face, and ears but is not limited to these areas
- Lesion configuration: irregularly grouped
- Lesion morphology:
  - Plaque lesions with scales
  - Follicular plugging
  - Atrophy
  - Scarring (**Fig. 03-090**)
  - Telangiectasia
- Color:
  - Erythematous
  - Red to violaceous
- Hyperpigmentation (**Fig. 03-091**) or hypopigmentation (**Fig. 03-092**)

Diagnostic Tests
- Skin biopsy

DDx Differential Diagnosis

- Psoriasis
- Lichen planus
- Secondary syphilis
- Superficial fungal infections
- Photosensitivity eruption
- Sarcoidosis

- Subacute cutaneous lupus erythematosus
- Rosacea
- Keratoacanthoma
- Actinic keratosis
- Dermatomyositis

Treatment

First Line
- Sunscreens
- Topical steroids: intermediate rather than high potency; should be used on areas such as the face
- Intralesional steroids: triamcinolone acetonide 3 mg/mL with 1% Xylocaine

Second Line
- Hydroxychloroquine 400 mg PO QD for 1 month, then decrease dose to 200 mg
- Dapsone 100 mg/day can be used in patients who fail to respond to topical steroid or hydroxychloroquine
- Oral retinoids

Third Line
- Chloroquine
- Auranofin
- Thalidomide
- Azathioprine
- Mycophenolate or interferon

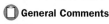 Clinical Pearl(s)

- DLE is more common in females, with a peak incidence in the fourth decade of life.
- Approximately 10% to 20% of patients with SLE will also have discoid lupus.

44. DRUG ERUPTION

General Comments

Definition
- Generally, drug eruptions are morbilliform- or urticarial-type reactions to drug therapy. Drug eruptions are the most commonly encountered adverse drug reactions. Patients who have infectious mononucleosis are particularly at risk of developing an exenthematous reaction after therapy with ampicillin or amoxicillin.

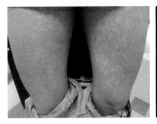

FIGURE 03-093. Erythematous, morbilliform skin reaction occurring 1 week after a course of a sulfonamide medication.

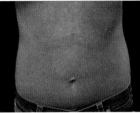

FIGURE 03-094. Pink to red morbilliform drug eruption involving the legs following administration of a sulfa drug. Sometimes referred to as a "drug red" color.

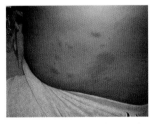

FIGURE 03-095. Generalized pruritic urticarial reaction following the ingestion of shellfish.

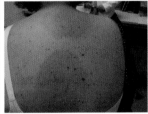

FIGURE 03-096. Several round, well-demarcated, red plaques occurring in the same areas as in the past each time the patient takes naproxen.

Etiology

- The mechanism may be immunologic or nonimmunologic. Drug eruptions most commonly develop within 1 to 2 weeks of starting the drug.
- Penicillins, sulfonamides, trimethoprim, and phenytoin are especially incriminated.

Keys to Diagnosis

Clinical Manifestation(s)

- In addition to the rash, pruritus, low-grade fever, and eosinophilia are sometimes present.
- The eruption is often morbilliform (**Fig. 03-093**) and symmetrical and usually presents on the trunk and extremities or sites of pressure and trauma.

Physical Examination

- Erythematous macules and papules (**Fig. 03-094**) are seen that, with progression, may become confluent or even acquire gyrate/polycyclic features.
- Generalized pruritic urticarial reactions (**Fig. 03-095**) are common after ingestion of shellfish.
- Red plaques may also occur (**Fig. 03-096**).
- More severe manifestations may include erythema multiforme, toxic epidermal necrolysis reactions, and exfoliative erythroderma and vessel-necrotizing vasculitis.

Diagnostic Tests

- No tests are generally necessary for morbilliform or urticarial reactions.

DDx Differential Diagnosis

- Scarlet fever
- Measles
- Rubella
- Viral exanthem such as enterovirus, echovirus, cytomegalovirus
- Kawasaki syndrome
- Juvenile rheumatoid arthritis
- Secondary syphilis
- Primary HIV disease

R Treatment

First Line

- Removal of offending agent
- Oral antihistamines
- Cooling lotions

Second Line

- Systemic corticosteroids

Third Line

- Epinephrine may be needed for severe reactions.

Clinical Pearl(s)

- Cutaneous drug reactions are seen in 3% to 5% of hospitalized patients, most of whom are on multiple medications.

45. DYSHIDROTIC ECZEMA (POMPHOLYX)

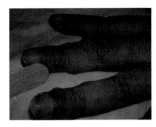

FIGURE 03-097. Clear, deep-seated, tapioca-like vesicles on the sides of fingers.

 General Comments

Definition
■ Dyshidrotic eczema is a dermatitis characterized by a recurrent pruritic vesicular eruption of the palms, soles, or digits.

Etiology
■ Unknown. Atopy, heat, and emotional stress may be contributing factors.

Keys to Diagnosis

Clinical Manifestation(s)
■ Sudden eruptions of symmetric vesicles appear on the palms of hands and plantar feet.
■ Intense pruritus often precedes and accompanies the eruptions.
■ Because of the increased thickness of the keratin layer at these sites, the vesicles appear as small pale papules before rupturing.
■ With the passage of time, the affected parts may show scaling and cracking.
■ Slow resolution of vesicles occurs over 2- to 3-week period.

Physical Examination
■ Fluid-filled vesicles 2 to 5 mm in diameter can be seen on the palms, soles, and digits (**Fig. 03-097**).
■ Rings of scale, peeling, and brown spots may all be present from previous vesiculation.

Diagnostic Tests
■ Specific investigations include patch testing for contact allergens, potassium hydroxide preparation, and bacterial culture.

Differential Diagnosis

- Contact dermatitis
- Pustular psoriasis
- Inflammatory tinea
- Bullous pemphigoid
- Id reaction

Ⓡ Treatment

First Line
- Cold wet dressings
- Topical corticosteroids
- Oral antihistamines to alleviate pruritus

Second Line
- Oral corticosteroids

Third Line
- PUVA, UVA
- Azathioprine
- Methotrexate

Clinical Pearl(s)

- Increased sweating often accompanies and may worsen this disorder.

46. ECHTYMA GANGRENOSUM

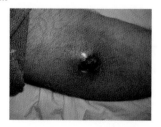

FIGURE 03-098. Painful, tender ulceration that progressed from a hemorrhagic vesicle to a necrotic ulcer with black eschar.

General Comments

Definition
- Deep necrotic ulcers that are usually seen in malnourished, immunocompromised, and debilitated hosts.

Etiology
- The cause is unknown, but this condition is often associated with widespread *Pseudomonas* sepsis.

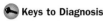 Keys to Diagnosis

Clinical Manifestation(s)
- Gradual development of edematous plaques, which evolve into hemorrhagic bullae and necrotic ulcers (**Fig. 03-098**).

Physical Examination
- Deep necrotic ulcers are often seen on lower extremities.

Diagnostic Tests
- Wound cultures usually yield mixed bacterial flora
- Blood cultures

DDx Differential Diagnosis

- Necrotizing fasciitis
- Pyoderma gangrenosum
- Trauma
- Nocardiosis, sporotrichiosis

R Treatment

- Systemic antipseudomonal antibiotics
- Nutritional support

Clinical Pearl(s)

- The mortality rate is nearly 100% if left untreated.

47. ECZEMA HERPETICUM

General Comments

Definition
- Eczema herpeticum is a herpes simplex infection of eczematous skin, also known as Kaposi's varicelliform eruption and eczema vaccinatum.

Etiology
- Herpes simplex virus

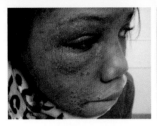

FIGURE 03-099. Acute onset of a burning, vesicular, rapidly spreading facial eruption causing facial edema and inflammation in this patient with chronic atopic dermatitis.

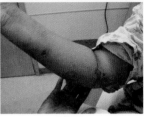

FIGURE 03-100. This patient with underlying severe eczema of the trunk and extremities developed painful shallow erosions superimposed on eczematoid lesions secondary to an acute HSV-1 infection.

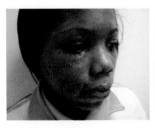

FIGURE 03-101. Marked improvement in patient from Figure 03-099 with resolution of the vesicular eruption and facial edema after a course of acyclovir.

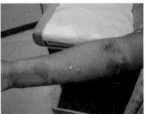

FIGURE 03-102. Same patient as Figure 03-100 showing healing of superficial ulcerations following a 7-day course of acyclovir.

Keys to Diagnosis

Clinical Manifestation(s)

- This condition is most common in areas of atopic dermatitis, often the face (**Fig. 03-099**).
- Secondary bacterial infections may occur.

Physical Examination

- Umbilicated vesicles and pustules are present in various stages.
- Crusts may coalesce and form eroded plaques (**Fig. 03-100**).
- Secondary bacterial infections may occur.

Diagnostic Tests

- Herpesvirus cultures of fluid from intact vesicles

DDx Differential Diagnosis

- Impetigo
- Contact dermatitis
- Pemphigus
- Dermatitis herpetiformis
- Bullous pemphigoid

℞ Treatment

- Systemic antiviral agents (acyclovir, valcyclovir, famcyclovir) (**Fig. 03-101**, **Fig. 03-102**).

👄 Clinical Pearl(s)

- Eczema herpeticum occurs more commonly in corticosteroid-treated skin and in immunocompromised hosts.

48. EHLERS-DANLOS SYNDROME

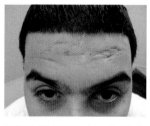

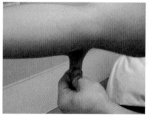

FIGURE 03-103. These scars from prior minimal forehead trauma are markedly widened secondary to impaired wound healing commonly seen with Ehlers-Danlos syndrome.

FIGURE 03-104. Velvety, soft, thin skin at the elbow with "rubber band"-like hyperextensibility.

📋 General Comments

Definition

- Ehlers-Danlos syndrome (EDS) is a group of inherited, clinically variable, and genetically heterogeneous connective tissue disorders. EDS is characterized by skin hyperextensibility, skin fragility, joint laxity, and joint hyperextensibility.

Etiology

- Defects of collagen in extracellular matrices of multiple tissues (skin, tendons, blood vessels, and viscera) underlie all forms of EDS.
- Classic EDS is associated with defects in type V collagen, corresponding to mutations of the COL5A genes.
- Vascular EDS involves a deficiency in type III collagen, and several studies suggest that mutations of gene COL3A1 lead to this deficiency.
- Arthrochalasia EDS results from a defect in type I collagen, caused by mutations in the COL1A1 and COL1A2 genes.

Keys to Diagnosis

Clinical Manifestation(s)

- Diagnosis is based solely on clinical criteria. It is important to identify patients with vascular EDS because of the grave potential complications of the disease.
- Clinical criteria for vascular EDS: two of four major diagnostic criteria establishes the diagnosis. One or more minor criteria support but are not sufficient to establish the diagnosis.
- Major criteria:
  1. Easy bruising
  2. Arterial, intestinal, or uterine fragility
  3. Thin, translucent skin
  4. Characteristic facial features (thin, delicate, and pinched nose; hollow cheeks; prominent staring eyes in 30% of patients with vascular EDS)
- Minor criteria:
  1. Small joint hypermobility
  2. Skin hyperextensibility
  3. Spontaneous pneumothorax/hemothorax
  4. Tendon or muscle rupture
  5. Early-onset varicose veins
  6. Carotid-cavernous fistula
  7. Talipes equinovarus (clubfoot)

Physical Examination

- Classic (previously types I and II): hyperextensibility (Gorlin's sign: ability to touch tip of tongue to nose); easy scarring (**Fig. 03-103**) and bruising ("cigarette-paper scars"); smooth, velvety skin; subcutaneous spheroids (small, firm, cystlike nodules) along shins or forearms
- Hypermobility (type III): joint hypermobility and some skin hypermobility (**Fig. 03-104**) with or without very smooth skin
- Vascular (type IV): thin, translucent skin with visible veins; marked bruising; pinched nose; acrogeria; generalized tissue friability; spontaneous dissection and rupture of medium and large arteries; spontaneous rupture of organs, especially sigmoid colon, spleen, liver, and uterus

- Kyphoscoliotic (type VI): joint hypermobility, progressive scoliosis, ocular fragility and possible globe rupture, mitral valve prolapse, aortic dilation
- Arthrochalasia (types VIIA and VIIB): prominent joint hypermobility with subluxations, congenital hip dislocation, skin hyperextensibility, tissue fragility
- Dermatosparaxis (type VIIC): severe skin fragility with decreased elasticity, bruising, hernias
- Unclassified types: types V and IX: classic characteristics; type VIII: classic characteristics and periodontal disease; type X: mild classic characteristics, mitral valve prolapse; type XI: joint instability.

Diagnostic Tests

- Biochemical and gene testing for known molecular defects is recommended to confirm the diagnosis of vascular EDS.
- Plain radiographs may reveal calcified nodules along the shin or forearms, corresponding to the subcutaneous spheroids.
- Echocardiogram can identify mitral valve prolapse (MVP) and aortic dilation.

DDx Differential Diagnosis

- Marfan syndrome
- Osteogenesis imperfecta
- Autosomal dominant cutis laxa
- Familial joint hypermobility
- Pseudoxanthoma elasticum

℞ Treatment

- Management of most skin and joint problems should be conservative and preventive. Joint hypermobility and pain in EDS usually does not require surgical intervention. Physical therapy to strengthen muscles is helpful. Surgical repair and tightening of joint ligaments can be performed but ligaments often will not hold sutures. Surgical intervention should be considered on an individual basis.
- For patients with vascular EDS:
  - Special surgical care is required because of increased tissue friability.
  - Patients should be advised to avoid contact sports.
  - Elevated blood pressure should be aggressively treated with beta-blockers given the risk of arterial dissection.

Clinical Pearl(s)

- Women with vascular EDS should be counseled about the risk of uterine, intestinal, and arterial rupture. Pregnancy is associated with an 11% mortality rate, and there is a 50% chance that the child will be affected.

49. EPHELIDES (FRECKLES)

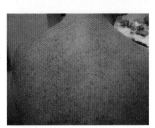

FIGURE 03-105. Multiple 1- to 2-mm tan macules on the back of this adult, which were more prominent in the summer and are beginning to fade slightly in the early winter.

 General Comments

Definition
- Ephelides are extremely common lesions that present as clusters of small (approximately 2-mm diameter), uniformly pigmented macules.

Etiology
- They are directly related to exposure to sunlight and are much more conspicuous in summer than in winter.
- They are more common in and numerous in individuals with red hair and blue eyes, where there is probably an autosomal mode of inheritance.

 Keys to Diagnosis

Clinical Manifestation(s)
- Sites of predilection include the nose, cheeks, shoulders, and dorsal aspects of the hands and arms.
- Ephelides present in childhood, increasing in frequency in adults, and typically regressing in the elderly. There is a predilection for females.

Physical Examination
- Clusters of small (approximately 2-mm diameter), uniformly pigmented macules (**Fig. 03-105**).

Diagnostic Tests
- None necessary

 Differential Diagnosis

- Melanocytic nevus
- Lentigo

- Tinea versicolor
- Seborrheic keratosis
- Café au-lait spots

℞ Treatment

First Line
- Although a cosmetic nuisance, they are of no clinical importance and no treatment is necessary.

Second Line
- Hydroquinone solutions
- Tretinoin
- Glycolic acid peels
- Azelaic acid

Third Line
- Cryosurgery

😄 Clinical Pearl(s)

- High levels of freckling may indicate a raised susceptibility to the later development of melanoma. Similarly, increasing numbers of freckles correlate with a higher frequency of acquired melanocytic nevi.

50. EPIDERMOID CYST (SEBACEOUS CYST, EPIDERMAL INCLUSION CYST)

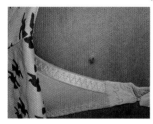

FIGURE 03-106. Firm, subcutaneous, dome-shaped nodule that often has a comedonal opening to the surface. Keratinaceous, odorous (like "rancid cheese") material can be expressed from the cyst by application of firm lateral pressure.

📋 General Comments

Definition
- An epidermoid cyst is a smooth, dome-shaped swelling occurring predominantly on the face, neck, and upper trunk resulting from damage to the pilosebaceous units. A punctum is usually present.

- Histologically the cysts are lined by an epidermis-like epithelium including a granular cell layer. The cysts contain laminated keratin.

Etiology
- Damage to the pilosebaceous units can cause epidermoid cysts.
- Epidermoid inclusion cysts may also complicate penetrating trauma to the skin, such as by a sewing needle, with resultant implantation of squamous epithelium into the dermis.

Keys to Diagnosis

Clinical Manifestation(s)
- This condition is usually asymptomatic.
- Acute inflammation, usually due to bacteria, may result in the subsequent disruption of the cyst wall, with the development of an intense foreign body giant cell reaction.
- Young and middle-aged adults are most often affected.

Physical Examination
- White or pale yellow, smooth, dome-shaped swellings occur predominantly on the face, neck, and upper trunk. A punctum is usually present (**Fig. 03-106**).
- Cheeselike, foul-smelling material will exude from it with lateral pressure.

Diagnostic Tests
- None necessary

Differential Diagnosis

- Insect bite
- Cylindroma
- Trichilemmoma
- Pylar cyst
- Granuloma annulare
- Dermoid cyst
- Lipoma
- Milia

Treatment

First Line
- Excision with narrow margins

Second Line
- Intralesional corticosteroid (for inflamed lesion)

Third Line
- Simple drainage (may lead to recurrence)

🔵 Clinical Pearl(s)

- The presence of multiple lesions may suggest the possibility of Gardner's syndrome, which includes polyposis coli, jaw osteomas, and intestinal fibromatoses in addition to cutaneous cysts.

51. EPIDERMOLYSIS BULLOSA

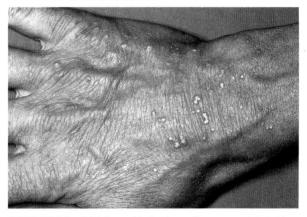

FIGURE 03-107. Epidermolysis bullosa acquisita. Conspicuous milia are present on the back of the hand. *(Courtesy the Institute of Dermatology, London, UK. From McKee PH, Calonje JE, Granter SR: Pathology of the Skin, ed 3, St. Louis, 2005, Mosby, Fig. 3.121.)*

🔵 General Comments

Definition
- Epidermolysis bullosa is a rare disorder presenting in adults with the development of blisters on the hands, feet, elbows, and knees following mild trauma. There are three major types based on the blister formation: dystrophic (dermolytic), junctional, and simplex (epidermolytic).

Etiology
- This is an inherited disorder.

Keys to Diagnosis

Clinical Manifestation(s)

- The condition is marked by development of painful blisters on the hands, feet, elbows, and knees following mild trauma.
- It may be complicated by atrophic scarring, milia formation (**Fig. 03-107**), and nail dystrophy.

Physical Examination

- Blisters on the hands, feet, elbows, and knees are seen.

Diagnostic Tests

- Skin biopsy and serum for direct and indirect immunofluorescence can detect skin basement membrane–specific autoantibodies.

DDx Differential Diagnosis

- Bullous pemphigoid
- Pemphigus vulgaris
- Linear IgA bullous dermatosis
- Porphiria cutanea tarda
- Chemical burn
- Thermal burn
- Blisters due to trauma (friction blisters)
- Cicatricial pemphigoid

R Treatment

First Line

- Nutritional support, avoidance of trauma
- Topical antibiotics, sterile dressing

Second Line

- Systemic corticosteroids
- Dapsone

Third Line

- Azathioprine
- Colchicine
- Cyclosporine

Clinical Pearl(s)

- Workup for inflammatory bowel disease and ELISA for type VII collagen-specific autoantibodies should also be considered.

52. ERYSIPELAS

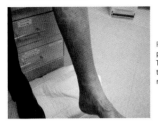

FIGURE 03-108. Superficial, rapidly spreading plaque of erysipelas involving the upper dermis. This soft tissue infection is characterized by tenderness, induration, edema, and intense redness with a raised, advancing border.

 General Comments

Definition
- Erysipelas is an infection of the dermis and superficial subcutis.

Etiology
- Usually group A beta-hemolytic streptococci
- Less often group B, C, or G streptococci
- Rarely *S. aureus*
- Risk factors: impaired lymphatic or venous drainage (mastectomy, saphenous vein harvesting), immunocompromised state; athlete's foot is a common portal of entry

 Keys to Diagnosis

Clinical Manifestation(s)
- The most common sites are the lower extremities and face.
- Systemic signs of infection (fever) are often present.

Physical Examination
- Distinctive red, warm, tender skin lesion with induration and a sharply defined, advancing, raised border is present (**Fig. 03-108**).
- Vesicles or bullae may develop.
- After several days, lesions may appear ecchymotic.
- After 7 to 10 days, desquamation of the affected area may occur.

Diagnostic Tests
- Diagnosis is usually made by characteristic clinical setting and appearance.
- CBC and white blood cell count (WBC) often elevated.
- Blood cultures are positive in 5% of patients.
- Gram's stain and culture of any drainage from skin lesions should be performed.
- Culture of aspirated fluid from the leading edge of skin lesion has a low yield.

DDx Differential Diagnosis

- Other types of cellulitis
- Necrotizing fasciitis
- DVT
- Contact dermatitis
- Erythema migrans (Lyme disease)
- Insect bite
- Herpes zoster
- Erysipeloid
- Acute gout
- Pseudogout

℞ Treatment

For typical erysipelas of the extremity in a nondiabetic patient, treat as follows:
- PO: penicillin V 250 mg to 500 mg QID
- IV: penicillin G (aqueous) 1 to 2 million units Q6H
  NOTE: Use erythromycin or cephalosporin in patients allergic to penicillin.
  For facial erysipelas (include coverage for *S. aureus*), treat as follows:
- Dicloxacillin 500 mg PO Q6H
- Nafcillin or oxacillin 2 g IV Q4H

Clinical Pearl(s)

- Consider early surgical referral when necrotizing fasciitis is suspected.
- Consider skin biopsy when the patient does not respond to appropriate antibiotics.

53. ERYTHEMA MULTIFORME

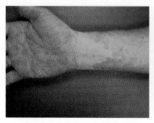

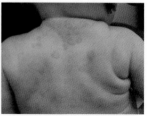

FIGURE 03-109. Polycyclic, raised, targetlike lesions involving the palms and forearm and occurring after the ingestion of shellfish.

FIGURE 03-110. Multiple urticarial-like, dull-red, round, iris-shaped macular and papular lesions over the upper back of this infant. These "target lesions" occurred several days after the administration of TDaP.

General Comments

Definition

- Erythema multiforme (EM) is an inflammatory disease believed to be secondary to immune complex formation and subsequent deposition in the skin and mucous membranes. It is considered to be a hypersensitivity reaction to infection or drugs. It is often associated with herpes simplex and other infectious agents, drugs, and connective tissue diseases.

Etiology

- Immune complex formation and subsequent deposition in the cutaneous microvasculature may play a role in the pathogenesis of erythema multiforme.
- The majority of EM cases follow outbreaks of herpes simplex virus 1 and 2.
- *Mycoplasma pneumoniae,* fungal infections, medications, (bupropion, sulfonamides, penicillins, NSAIDs, barbiturates, phenothiazines, hydantoins) are also possible causes.
- In more than 50% of patients, no specific cause is identified.

Keys to Diagnosis

Clinical Manifestation(s)

- Prodromal symptoms are mild or absent. Itching or burning at the site of eruption may occur.
- Lesions are most common in the back of the hands and feet and extensor aspect of the forearms (**Fig. 03-109**) and legs. Trunk involvement can occur in severe cases.
- Individual lesions heal in 1 or 2 weeks without scarring.

Physical Examination

- Symmetric skin lesions with a classic "target" appearance (caused by the centrifugal spread of red maculopapules to circumference of 1 to 3 cm with a purpuric, cyanotic, or vesicular center) are present (**Fig. 03-110**). The papules may enlarge into plaques measuring a few centimeters in diameter with a dark or red central portion. Target lesions may not be apparent for several days.
- Urticarial papules, vesicles, and bullae may also be present and generally indicate a more severe form of the disease.
- Bullae and erosions may also be present in the oral cavity.

Diagnostic Tests

- Medical history with emphasis on drug ingestion
- Laboratory evaluation in patients with suspected collagen-vascular diseases
- Skin biopsy when diagnosis is unclear
- CBC with differential
- ANA
- Serology for *M. pneumoniae,* HSV-1, HSV-2
- Urinalysis

Differential Diagnosis

- Chronic urticaria
- Secondary syphilis
- Pityriasis rosea
- Contact dermatitis
- Pemphigus vulgaris
- Lichen planus
- Serum sickness
- Drug eruption
- Granuloma annulare
- Polymorphic light eruption
- Viral exanthem

℞ Treatment

First Line

- Mild cases generally do not require treatment; lesions resolve spontaneously within 1 month.
- Potential drug precipitants should be removed.
- Recurrent EM may be treated with valacyclovir 500 to 1000 mg/day, famcyclovir 125 to 250 mg/day, or acyclovir 400 mg BID.

Second Line

- Dapsone, antimalarials, azathioprine, or cyclosporine use is reserved for cases resistant to antivirals.

Third Line

- Prednisone 40 to 80 mg/day for 1 to 3 weeks may be tried in patients with many target lesions; however, the role of systemic steroids remains controversial.
- Levamisole, an immunomodulator, may be effective in treatment of patients with chronic or recurrent oral lesions (dose is 150 mg/day for 3 consecutive days used alone or in combination with prednisone).

😮 Clinical Pearl(s)

- The rash of EM generally evolves over a 2-week period and resolves within 3 to 4 weeks without scarring. A severe bullous form can occur (see "Stevens-Johnson Syndrome").
- The risk of recurrence of erythema multiforme exceeds 30%.

54. ERYTHEMA NODOSUM

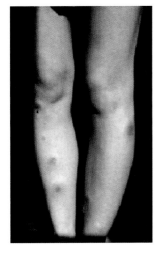

FIGURE 03-111. Tender, pink-to-red nodules, without ulceration, arising on the pretibial surface of the legs. In this 22-year-old patient, oral contraceptives were the putative cause.

 General Comments

Definition

- Erythema nodosum is characterized by panniculitis manifesting with tender erythematous nodules on the lower extremities.

Etiology

- This cell-mediated hypersensitivity reaction is seen more frequently in persons with human leukocyte antigen (HLA) B8. The lesion results from an exaggerated interaction between an antigen and cell-mediated immune mechanisms leading to granuloma formation. Up to 55% of cases of erythema nodosum are idiopathic. Other causes include sarcoidosis; infections (bacteria, fungi, viruses); drugs (sulfonamides, penicillin, oral contraceptives); cancer, usually lymphoma; ankylosing spondylosis; and reactive arthropathies (e.g., associated with inflammatory bowel disease).

Keys to Diagnosis

Clinical Manifestation(s)

- Erythema nodosum manifests with an acute onset of tender nodules that are typically located on shins (**Fig. 03-111**) and occasionally seen on thighs and forearms.

- Associated findings include the following:
  Fever
  Lymphadenopathy
  Arthralgia
  Signs of the underlying illness

Physical Examination

- The nodules are usually ⅛ to 1 inch in diameter but can be as large as 4 inches. They begin as light red lesions, then become darker and often ecchymotic. The nodules heal within 8 weeks without ulceration.

Diagnostic Tests

- ESR
- Throat culture and antistreptolysin O titer
- Purified protein derivative (PPD)
- Others depending on index of suspicion (e.g., stool culture and evaluation for ova and parasites in patients with diarrhea and GI symptoms)
- Skin biopsy in doubtful cases:
  Early lesion: inflammation and hemorrhage in subcutaneous tissue
  Late lesion: giant cells and granulomata

DDx Differential Diagnosis

- Insect bites
- Posttraumatic ecchymoses
- Vasculitis
- Weber-Christian disease
- Fat necrosis associated with pancreatitis
- Necrobiosis lipoidica
- Scleroderma
- Lupus panniculitis
- Subcutaneous granuloma
- Alpha-1 antitrypsin deficiency

Rx Treatment

First Line

- Treatment of underlying disorders
- Avoidance of contact irritation of affected areas
- NSAIDs for pain

Second Line

- Systemic steroids (prednisone 1 mg/kg of body weight/day, tapered over several days) may be useful in severe cases if the underlying risk of sepsis and malignancy has been excluded.

Third Line
- Dapsone

 Clinical Pearl(s)

- The disease is self-limited and treatment is symptomatic. Erythema nodosum nodules develop in pretibial locations and resolve spontaneously over several weeks without scarring or ulceration.

55. ERYTHRODERMA

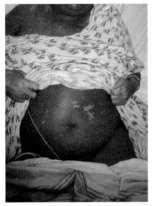

FIGURE 03-112. A rare generalized, papulosquamous eruption, with reddish-orange skin discoloration proceeding from the head downward. Areas of unaffected skin have sharp borders (a classic sign known as "nappes claires"), as noted on the abdomen of this patient. Multiple therapeutic attempts (keratolytics, retinoids, methotrexate) failed in this patient.

 General Comments

Definition
- Erythroderma is a persistent severe generalized inflammation of the skin. When it is associated with increased scale, it is called exfoliative dermatitis or exfoliative erythroderma.

Etiology
- Eczema
- Psoriasis
- Drug eruptions
- Sezary syndrome, cutaneous lymphomas
- Pemphigus foliaceus

Keys to Diagnosis

Clinical Manifestation(s)
- The skin becomes reddened, thickened, inflamed, and exfoliated continuously.
- Onset can be slowly progressive or rapid.
- Systemic symptoms may be present, such as generalized malaise, shivering, fever, impaired sweating, fatigue, and tachycardia.
- Rapid onset with high rate of skin loss can lead to protein malnutrition, dehydration, and high-output cardiac failure.

Physical Examination
- Skin appears red, thickened, and inflamed (**Fig. 03-112**).
- Persistent exfoliation of skin may be present.

Diagnostic Tests
- Skin biopsy is helpful for suspected T-cell lymphoma

Differential Diagnosis
- Atopic eczema
- Seborrheic dermatitis
- Drug eruption (sulfonamides, allopurinol, anticonvulsants, penicillins)
- Cutaneous T-cell lymphoma
- Pityriasis rubra pilaris
- Norwegian (crusted) scabies
- Fungal infection
- Lichen planus

℞ Treatment

First Line
- Treatment of underlying etiology (e.g., immediate removal of any suspected drugs)
- Application of bland emollients (e.g., petroleum) to soothe skin and partially restore skin barrier
- Nutritional support, intravenous hydration

Second Line
- Topical corticosteroids
- PUVA

Third Line
- Cyclosporine, cytotoxic drugs, antimetabolites

Clinical Pearl(s)

- Fulminant erythroderma is a life-threatening condition.
- Systemic steroids are best avoided in erythrodermic psoriasis due to risk of pustular psoriasis on withdrawal.

56. ERYTHRASMA

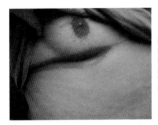

FIGURE 03-113. A hyperpigmented, clearly marginated, brownish red patch of skin commonly found in overlapping skinfolds such as under the pendulous breasts in this obese individual. It fluoresced bright coral-red under the Wood's lamp examination.

 General Comments

Definition
- Erythrasma is a bacterial skin infection.

Etiology
- The condition is caused by *Corynebacterium minutissimum,* a gram-positive bacillus.

 Keys to Diagnosis

Clinical Manifestation(s)
- It characteristically manifests as symptomatic, well-defined, scaly brownish-red patches under the breasts (**Fig. 03-113**) and on the inguinal and intergluteal skin.

Physical Examination
- Well-defined reddish-brown flexural plaques are seen on examination.

Diagnostic Tests
- Coral-red fluorescence can be demonstrated under Wood's light. It is due to production of coproporphyrin II by the organism.

Differential Diagnosis

- Intertrigo
- Tinea
- Contact dermatitis
- Eczema
- Pityriasis rosea

℞ Treatment

First Line
- Topical creams (miconazole, clotrimazole, econazole)

Second Line
- Clindamycin lotion or solution

Third Line
- Systemic antibiotics (clarithromycin, erythromycin)

🛈 Clinical Pearl(s)

- Erythrasma has a predilection for obese and diabetic patients and is more common in areas with a humid and hot climate.

57. FIFTH DISEASE (ERYTHEMA INFECTIOSUM)

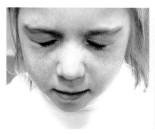

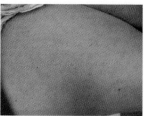

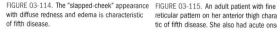

FIGURE 03-114. The "slapped-cheek" appearance with diffuse redness and edema is characteristic of fifth disease.

FIGURE 03-115. An adult patient with fine reticular pattern on her anterior thigh characteristic of fifth disease. She also had acute onset of symmetrical synovitis in her hands (metacarpophalangeal [MCP] and proximal interphalangeal [PIP]) and feet mimicking rheumatoid arthritis.

🔵 General Comments

Definition
- Fifth disease is a viral exanthem of childhood, caused by parvovirus B-19, affecting primarily school-age children. Erythema infectiosum was the "fifth" in a series of described viral exanthems of childhood and is the most common clinical syndrome associated with parvovirus B-19.

Etiology
- A typical bright red, nontender maxillary rash with circumoral pallor over cheeks is seen, producing the classic "slapped cheek" appearance.
- A reticular, nonpruritic, lacy, erythematous maculopapular rash over trunk and extremities can last for up to several weeks after the acute episode; it may be worsened by heat or sunlight.
- Polyarthritis and arthralgias are commonly seen in older patients but are less common in children. Arthritis involves small joints of extremities in symmetric fashion.
- Mild fever seen in up to one third of patients.

🔑 Keys to Diagnosis

Clinical Manifestation(s)
- This is a self-limited disease lasting 1 to 2 weeks.
- Polyarthritis and arthralgias are commonly seen in older patients but are less common in children. Arthritis involves small joints of extremities in symmetric fashion.
- Mild fever is seen in up to one third of patients.

Physical Examination
- In children, a typical bright red, nontender maxillary rash with circumoral pallor over cheeks produces the classic "slapped cheek" appearance (**Fig. 03-114**).
- In adults, a reticular, nonpruritic, lacy, erythematous maculopapular rash over trunk (**Fig. 03-115**) and extremities may last for up to several weeks after the acute episode. It may be worsened by heat or sunlight.

Diagnostic Tests
- None necessary

DDx Differential Diagnosis

- Juvenile rheumatoid arthritis (Still's disease)
- Rubella, measles (rubeola), and other childhood viral exanthems
- Mononucleosis
- Lyme disease
- Acute HIV infection
- Drug eruption

Treatment

First Line

- Treatment is supportive only.
- NSAIDs may be given for arthralgias/arthritis.

Second Line

- Intravenous immunoglobulin and transfusion support may be used in patients with an immunocompromised state with red cell aplasia.
- Consider immunoglobulin treatment or prophylaxis in pregnancy.

Clinical Pearl(s)

- Symmetric arthritis involving the small joints is common in adults, whereas facial rash is common in children.
- Can cause transient aplastic crisis in patients with underlying hematologic disorders such as sickle cell disease, in immunocompromised patients, and after transplantation.

58. FOLLICULITIS

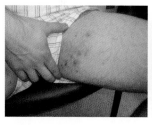
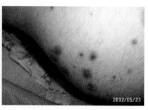

FIGURE 03-116. Chronic mechanical folliculitis in the groin secondary to chafing from undergarments with recent pustular eruptions and more remote hyperpigmented, scarred lesions.

FIGURE 03-117. *Candida albicans* folliculitis with intense erythema surrounding infected follicles in a diabetic patient.

General Comments

Definition

- Folliculitis is inflammation of the hair follicle as a result of infection, physical injury, or chemical irritation.

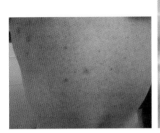

FIGURE 03-118. "Hot tub" folliculitis consisting of numerous erythematous, purulent follicles appearing 1–4 days after hot tub exposure.

FIGURE 03-119. Staphylococcal follicular infection on the anterior thigh consisting of distinct pustules with surrounding erythema.

Etiology

- *Staphylococcus* infection (e.g., sycosis barbae), *Pseudomonas aeruginosa* ("hot tub" folliculitis)
- Gram-negative folliculitis (*Klebsiella, Enterobacter, Proteus*) associated with antibiotic treatment of acne
- Chronic irritation of the hair follicle (use of cocoa butter or coconut oil, chronic chafing from clothing (**Fig. 03-116**), irritation from workplace)
- Initial use of systemic corticosteroid therapy (steroid acne), eosinophilic folliculitis (AIDS patients), *C. albicans* (immunocompromised patients) (**Fig. 03-117**)
- *Pityrosporum orbiculare*

Keys to Diagnosis

Clinical Manifestation(s)

- Patients with sycosis barbae may initially present with small follicular papules or pustules that increase in size with continued shaving; deep follicular pustules may occur surrounded by erythema and swelling; the upper lip is frequently involved
- "Hot tub" folliculitis occurs within 1 to 4 days following use of hot tub with poor chlorination, and it is characterized by pustules with surrounding erythema (**Fig. 03-118**) generally affecting torso, buttocks, and limbs.

Physical Examination
- The lesions generally consist of painful yellow pustules (**Fig. 03-119**) surrounded by erythema; a central hair is present in the pustules.

Diagnostic Tests
- Gram stain is useful to identify the infective organisms in infectious folliculitis and to differentiate infectious folliculitis from noninfectious.

Differential Diagnosis
- Pseudofolliculitis barbae (ingrown hairs)
- Acne vulgaris
- Dermatophyte fungal infections
- Keratosis biliaris
- Cutaneous candidiasis
- Superficial fungal infections
- Miliaris

R Treatment
First Line
- Prevention of chemical or mechanical skin irritation
- Glycemic control in diabetics
- Proper chlorination of hot tubs and spas
- Shaving with a clean razor
- Cleansing of the area with chlorhexidine and application of saline compresses to the involved area
- Application of 2% mupirocin ointment for bacterial folliculitis affecting a limited area (e.g., sycosis barbae)

Second Line
- Treatment of *Pseudomonas* folliculitis with ciprofloxacin
- Treatment of *S. aureus* folliculitis with dicloxacillin 250 mg QID for 10 days

Third Line
- Chronic nasal or perineal *S. aureus* carriers with frequent folliculitis can be treated with rifampin 300 mg BID for 5 days.
- Mupirocin applied to nares BID is also effective for nasal carriers.

Clinical Pearl(s)
- Staphylococcal folliculitis is the most common form of infectious folliculitis; it occurs most commonly in persons with diabetes.

59. FROSTBITE

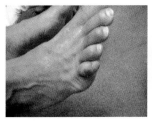
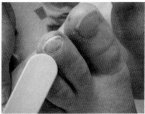

FIGURE 03-120. Bulla formation of the right fifth toe with edema and early necrotic changes characteristic of frostbite.

FIGURE 03-121. Minimal frostbite or frostnip presenting as erythema and minimal edema of the distal second toe after cold exposure.

 General Comments

Definition
- Frostbite represents tissue injury (or death) from freezing and vasoconstriction induced by severe environmental cold exposure.

Etiology
- Two distinct mechanisms are responsible for tissue injury in frostbite:
  1. Cellular death occurring at time of exposure from ice crystal damage to cells
  2. Deterioration and necrosis attributable to progressive dermal ischemia after rewarming via inflammatory mediators
- Environmental factors include wind chill factor, temperature, duration of exposure, altitude, and degree of wetness. Hands and feet account for 90% of injuries; earlobes, nose, and male genitalia are also more susceptible. Host factors include extremes of age, immobility, history of cold injuries, skin damage, psychiatric illness, neuroleptic and sedative drugs (especially alcohol), atherosclerosis, malnutrition, tobacco use, peripheral neuropathy, hypothyroidism, fatigue, and wearing constricting clothing/footwear.

 Keys to Diagnosis

Clinical Manifestation(s)
- Patients initially experience numbness, prickling, and itching. More severe injury can produce paresthesias and stiffness, with burning or throbbing pain upon thawing.

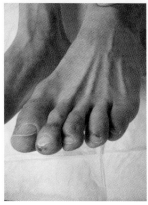

FIGURE 03-122. Distal erythema with punctate areas of early necrosis involving all toes of the left foot after a long walk in subzero temperatures.

Physical Examination

- Frostbite may be classified into degrees of injury or, more practically, into *superficial* and *deep* groups.

  Superficial frostbite involves the skin and subcutaneous tissue. The frozen part is waxy, white, and firm but soft and resilient below the surface when gently depressed. After rewarming, the frostbitten area may appear mottled and swollen, and superficial blisters (**Fig. 03-120**) with clear or milky fluid may form within 6 to 24 hours. There is no ultimate tissue loss.

  Deep frostbite extends into subcutaneous tissues and may involve muscles, nerves, tendons, or bones. The skin may be hard or wooden, without tissue resilience. Edema, cyanosis, hemorrhagic blisters (after 3-7 days), tissue necrosis (**Fig. 03-121**), and gangrene may develop. Affected tissue has a poor prognosis and debridement or amputation is generally required.

Diagnostic Tests

- Wound and blood cultures may be needed in more severe cases.
- Technetium scintigraphy, MRI, and magnetic resonance angiography (MRA) are the most promising modalities for assessment of tissue viability, but delay of 5 days is required to distinguish a level of debridement or amputation. (Some centers perform angiography within 24 hours and give thrombolytics to those with impaired blood flow.)

DDx Differential Diagnosis

Other induced cold injuries include the following:

- Frostnip (**Fig. 03-122**): transient tingling and numbness without associated permanent tissue damage
- Pernio (chilblains): a self-limited, cold-induced vasculitis of dermal vessels associated with purple plaques or nodules, often affecting dorsum of hands and feet and seen with prolonged cold exposure to above-freezing temperatures
- Cold immersion (trench) foot: caused by ischemic injury resulting from sustained severe vasoconstriction in appendages exposed to wet cold at temperatures above freezing

R Treatment

First Line

- Remove constricting or wet clothing and gently insulate, immobilize, and elevate the affected area.
- Avoid thawing if there is any risk of refreezing.
- Never rub or massage the affected area. Avoid dry heat (e.g., fires/heaters).
- If there is associated hypothermia, core temperature must first be stabilized with warmed, humidified oxygen, heated intravenous saline (45-65° C), and warming blankets before thawing of frostbitten extremities.
- Immerse affected area in circulating warm water bath with a mild antibacterial agent (e.g., hexachlorophene or povidone-iodine) maintained at 40 to 42° C for 15 to 30 minutes. Repeat until capillary refill returns and tissue is supple. Active motion during rewarming is advisable; massage is not.
- Administer intravenous narcotics for pain during thawing.

Second Line

- Tetanus prophylaxis and topical antibiotics should be given if there is a potentially contaminated skin wound.
- Streptococcal prophylaxis with intravenous penicillin for 48 to 72 hours may be advisable for severe cases.

Third Line

- Thrombolytic therapy looks promising.
- Dextran, vasodilators, hyperbaric oxygen, reserpine, and sympathectomy are of unproven benefit.

Clinical Pearl(s)

- Continuous ECG monitoring is indicated. J (Osborn) waves may be noted on ECG.

60. FURUNCLE

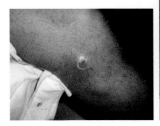

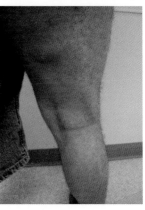

FIGURE 03-123. A firm, very tender hot nodule, warm to the touch, with a draining central necrotic plug.

FIGURE 03-124. Exquisitely painful, firm abscess on the posterior thigh with considerable edema and redness. Note the centrally located pustular plug.

General Comments

Definition
- A furuncle (boil) is a deep infection of the hair follicle.

Etiology
- Most infections are caused by *S. aureus*.

Keys to Diagnosis

Clinical Manifestation(s)
- It is more common in young adults and usually affects the skin of the face, neck, buttocks, and axillae.
- After discharge of the pustular necrotic core, the lesion heals rapidly but with scarring.

Physical Examination
- A firm, very tender hot nodule, warm to the touch, with a draining central necrotic plug (**Fig. 03-123**).
- Lesions are tender (**Fig. 03-124**) and can be up to 2 cm across. The inflammation is not confined within the follicle but is associated with much surrounding erythema and, often, systemic symptoms.

Diagnostic Tests
- Culture and sensitivity of pus
- Nasal swab
- CBC

DDx Differential Diagnosis

- Folliculitis
- Pseudofolliculitis
- Foreign body reaction
- Acne
- Hydradenitis supurativa
- Epidermoid cyst

R Treatment

First Line
- Incision and drainage

Second Line
- Topical antibiotics (2% mupirocin ointment)
- Systemic antibiotics (dicloxacillin, cephalexin, azithromycin)

Clinical Pearl(s)

- Pseudofolliculitis (pili incarnate, shaving bumps) refers to the presence of firm skin-colored or erythematous inflammatory papules or nodules in the shaving area of the face, often associated with postinflammatory hyperpigmentation. It may be caused by curly or kinky hair that tends to curve back directly into adjacent skin (extrafollicular penetration) or shaving techniques that stretch the skin and result in the cut hair end retracting under the epidermis when the skin is released (transfollicular penetration).

61. GLOMUS TUMOR

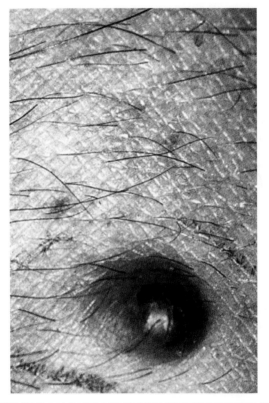

FIGURE 03-125. Glomus tumor: close-up view. *(Courtesy the Institute of Dermatology, London, UK. From McKee PH, Calonje JE, Granter SR: Pathology of the Skin, ed 3, St. Louis, 2005, Mosby, Fig. 31-478.)*

General Comments

Definition
- A glomus tumor is a relatively common benign lesions arising from glomus bodies, which are specialized arteriovenous anastomoses found most often in the fingers and palm and thought to serve as thermoregulatory receptors.

Etiology
- Unknown. The lesions arise from the neuromyoarterial apparatus.

Keys to Diagnosis

Clinical Manifestation(s)
- They classically present with paroxysmal severe pain, which is often precipitated by cold, pressure, or dependency.

Physical Examination
- Typically the tumors are small (<1 cm in diameter), reddish-blue nodules.
- The nodules may be flesh-colored but may become purple with hemorrhage (**Fig. 03-125**).

Diagnostic Tests
- Excisional biopsy

DDx Differential Diagnosis

- Schwannoma (neurilemmona)
- Eccrine spiradenoma
- Hemangioma
- Arteriovenous malformation (AVM)
- Blue nevus
- Melanoma
- Angiolipoma

R Treatment

- Surgical excision. Subungal lesions will usually require removal of the nail.

Clinical Pearl(s)

- Sometimes the nodules erode the bone of the phalanx and cause pressure dystrophy of the overlying nail.

62. GONOCOCCEMIA

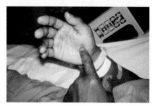

FIGURE 03-126. Tender, hemorrhagic pustules on a red-to-purple base present on the palms and soles of this patient with gonococcemia.

General Comments

Definition
- Gonorrhea is a sexually transmitted bacterial infection. It commonly manifests as urethritis, cervicitis, or salpingitis. Infection may be asymptomatic.

Etiology
- Gonococcemia is caused by *Neisseria gonorrhoeae*. The infection differs in males and females in course, severity, and ease of recognition.

Keys to Diagnosis

Clinical Manifestation(s)
- Males: Purulent discharge from anterior urethra with dysuria will appear 2 to 7 days after infecting exposure. Homosexual patients may have rectal infection causing pruritus, tenesmus, and discharge or may be asymptomatic.
- Females: Initial, often mild urethritis or cervicitis may occur a few days after exposure. In about 20% of cases, uterine invasion occurs after menstrual period with signs and symptoms of endometritis, salpingitis, or pelvic peritonitis. The patient may have purulent discharge and inflamed Skene's or Bartholin's glands.
- Classic presentation of acute gonococcal pelvic inflammatory disease (PID) is fever and abdominal and adnexal tenderness, often absent purulent discharge. Physical examination may be normal if the patient is asymptomatic.

Physical Examination
- Purulent discharge from the anterior urethra is seen in males. Females may have purulent discharge and inflamed Skene's or Bartholin's glands.
- The infection may not be limited to the genitalia. Tender, hemorrhagic pustules on a red-to-purple base may present on the palms and soles (**Fig. 03-126**).

Diagnostic Tests
- Gonorrhea culture on Thayer-Martin medium (organism is fastidious, requires aerobic conditions with increased carbon dioxide atmosphere; incubate as soon as possible)

- Serologic testing for syphilis on all patients
- Chlamydia testing on all patients
- Offer of HIV counseling and testing

DDx Differential Diagnosis

- Nongonococcal urethritis (NGU)
- Nongonococcal mucopurulent cervicitis
- *Chlamydia trachomatis*

R Treatment

For uncomplicated infections of the cervix, urethra, and rectum:
- Cefixime 400 mg PO × 1 dose *or*
- Ceftriaxone 125 mg IM × 1 dose *or*
  For uncomplicated pharyngeal infection:
- Ceftriaxone 125 mg IM × 1 dose
  Alternatives:
- Cefpodoxime 400 mg single dose *or*
- Cefuroxime 1 g PO single dose

Clinical Pearl(s)

- A rising number of cases of quinolone-resistant *N. gonorrhoeae* have been reported. Fluoroquinolones are no longer recommended to treat gonorrhea.
- Sexual partners should be identified, examined, cultured, and receive presumptive treatment.

63. GRANULOMA ANNULARE

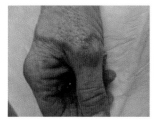

FIGURE 03-127. Annular confluent brownish-red plaques and papules, resembling ringworm, on the dorsum of the hand. These were recurrent and asymptomatic in this elderly patient.

General Comments

Definition
- Granuloma annulare (GA) is a chronic, usually self-limited inflammatory disorder of the dermis that classically presents as arciform to annular plaques located on the extremities.

Etiology
- The cause is unknown, but it may be related to vasculitis, trauma, monocyte activation, or delayed hypersensitivity.

 Keys to Diagnosis

Clinical Manifestation(s)
- The four main clinical variants of granuloma annulare are localized (75%), disseminated (>10 lesions), subcutaneous (occurring primarily in children 2-5 years of age), and perforating (rare form manifesting with 1- to 4-mm papules with a central crust).
- Most lesions resolve spontaneously after several months.

Physical Examination
- Localized granuloma annulare starts as a small ring of colored skin or pale erythematous papules.
- Lesions coalesce and evolve into annular plaques over several weeks.
- Plaques undergo central involution and increase in diameter over several months (0.5-5 cm).
- Most commonly found on the lateral and dorsal surfaces of the hands (**Fig. 03-127**) and feet.
- The generalized form of GA is characterized by hundreds to thousands of small, flesh-colored papules in a symmetric distribution on the trunk and extremities.
- Deep dermal (subcutaneous GA) presents as large, painless, skin-colored nodules that are often mistaken for rheumatoid nodules.

Diagnostic Tests
- No laboratory tests will help confirm the diagnosis.
- Biopsy shows focal degeneration of collagen and elastic fibers, mucin deposition, and perivascular and interstitial lymphohistiocytic infiltrate in the upper and mid-dermis.

DDx Differential Diagnosis

- Tinea corporis
- Lichen planus
- Necrobiosis lipoidica diabeticorum

- Sarcoidosis
- Rheumatoid nodules
- Late secondary or tertiary syphilis
- Arcuate and annular plaques of mycosis fungoides
- Annular elastolytic giant cell granuloma
  Papular GA can simulate insect bites, secondary syphilis, and xanthoma.

Treatment

First Line
- High-potency topical corticosteroids with or without occlusion
- Intralesional steroid injection into elevated border with triamcinolone 2.5 to 10 mg/mL
- Cryosurgery

Second Line
- PUVA or UVA-1 therapy and CO_2 laser treatment

Third Line
- Systemic agents (e.g., niacinamide, hydroxychloroquine, chloroquine, cyclosporine, dapsone) are generally reserved for severe cases.
- Recent case reports indicate positive outcomes with tacrolimus and pimecrolimus and with the use of the tumor necrosis factor infliximab.

Clinical Pearl(s)

- GA has been described as a paraneoplastic granulomatous reaction to Hodgkin's disease, non-Hodgkin's lymphoma (NHL), solid organ tumors, and mycosis fungoides.
- The disseminated form of GA is associated with diabetes mellitus.

64. GRANULOMA INGUINALE

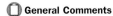 General Comments

Definition
- Granuloma inguinale is an infection manifesting with granulomatous ulcerations.

Etiology
- It is caused by a gram-negative bacterium, *Klebsiella granulomatis,* formerly called *Calymmatobacterium granulomatis,* that may be sexually transmitted, possibly by unprotected anal intercourse. It can also be spread through close, chronic nonsexual contact.

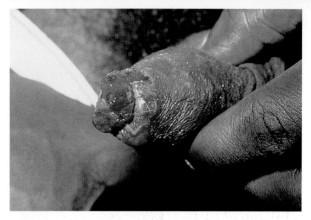

FIGURE 03-128. Granuloma inguinale. *(Courtesy Michael O. Murphy, MD. From White GA, Cox NH: Diseases of the Skin: A Color Atlas and Text, ed 2, St. Louis, 2006, Mosby, Fig. 20-45.)*

 Keys to Diagnosis

Clinical Manifestation(s)
- Lesions bleed easily. They are sharply defined and painless.
- Secondary infection may ensue.
- Inguinal involvement may cause pseudobuboes.
- Elephantiasis can result from obstruction of lymphatics.

Physical Examination
- An indurated nodule is the primary lesion and is usually painless.
- The lesion erodes to granulomatous heaped ulcer and progresses slowly (**Fig 03-128**).

Diagnostic Tests
- Microscopic examination of either biopsy specimen or tissue smears
- Wright stain: observation of Donovan bodies (intracellular bacteria); organisms in vacuoles within macrophages

DDx Differential Diagnosis

- Carcinoma
- Secondary syphilis: condylomata lata

- Amebiasis: necrotic ulceration
- Concurrent infections
- Lymphogranuloma venereum
- Chancroid
- Genital herpes

℞ Treatment

Recommended regimen:
- Doxycycline 100 mg PO BID for 3 weeks minimum

Alternative regimens:
- Ciprofloxacin 750 mg PO BID × 3 weeks
- Erythromycin base 500 mg PO OD × 3 weeks
- Azithromycin 1 g PO/wk × 3 weeks
- Add gentamicin 1 mg/kg IV q8h if no improvement within the first few days of therapy

🗨 Clinical Pearl(s)

- Sexual partners should be examined and offered therapy.
- Pregnant women should be treated with an erythromycin regimen.

65. HAIRY TONGUE

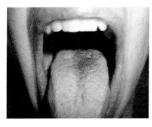

FIGURE 03-129. Yellow-brownish, painless thickening on the dorsum of the tongue following a recent course of antibiotics.

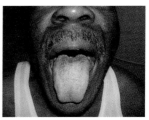

FIGURE 03-130. Marked hyperkeratosis of the filiform papillae resulting in brown hairy tongue in this chronic smoker.

🗂 General Comments

Definition

- Asymptomatic discoloration of tongue

Etiology
- Tobacco abuse, poor oral hygiene

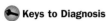 **Keys to Diagnosis**

Clinical Manifestation(s)
- Chronic, asymptomatic discoloration of dorsal surface of tongue (**Fig. 03-129**)

Physical Examination
- Brown-blackish discoloration and elongation of papillae on tongue (**Fig. 03-130**)

Diagnostic Tests
- None

DDx Differential Diagnosis
- Oral hairy leukoplakia
- Candidiasis
- Lichen planus
- Stomatitis

℞ Treatment

First Line
- Mechanical debridement of elongated papillae with toothbrush or tongue blade
- Removal of etiology (e.g., avoidance of tobacco products)

Second Line
- Mouthwashes

Third Line
- Electrodesiccation and curettage

Clinical Pearl(s)
- Improvement in mouth hygiene is essential to prevent recurrence.

66. HAND-FOOT-MOUTH DISEASE

General Comments

Definition
- Hand-foot-mouth (HFM) disease is a viral illness that is characterized by superficial lesions of the oral mucosa and of the skin of the extremities.

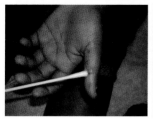

FIGURE 03-131. Painless vesicular lesion on palmar surface of the thumb. Two early pink papules are also noted.

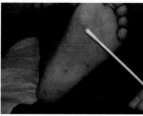

FIGURE 03-132. Linear vesicular lesion of HFM disease containing clear yellow fluid. These usually will not rupture when located on the dorsum of the foot.

Etiology

- Coxsackievirus group A, type 16, was the first and is the most common viral agent isolated.
- Coxsackieviruses A5, A7, A9, A10, B1, B2, B3, B5, and enterovirus 71 have also been implicated.

Keys to Diagnosis

Clinical Manifestation(s)

- After a 4- to 6-day incubation period, patients may complain of odynophagia, sore throat, malaise, and fever (38.3°-40° C).
- One to two days later the characteristic oral lesions appear.
- In 75% of cases, skin lesions on the extremities accompany these oral manifestations.
- Cutaneous symptoms are found in 11% of adults.
- Lesions appear over the course of 1 or 2 days.
- Involvement of the buttocks and perineum is present in 31% of cases.
- In rare cases, encephalitis, meningitis, myocarditis, poliomyelitis-like paralysis, and pulmonary edema may develop. Sporadic acute paralysis has been reported with enterovirus 71.
- Although information is limited, there is no clear evidence that pregnancy outcomes are affected.

Physical Examination

- Oral lesions, usually between five and ten, are commonly found on the tongue, buccal mucosa, gingivae, and hard palate.
- Oral lesions initially start as 1- to 3-mm erythematous macules and evolve into gray vesicles on an erythematous base.

- Vesicles are often broken by the time of presentation and appear as superficial gray ulcers with surrounding erythema.
- Skin lesions of the hands (**Fig. 03-131**) and feet (**Fig. 03-132**) start as linear erythematous papules (3-10 mm in diameter) that evolve into gray vesicles that may be mildly painful. These vesicles are usually intact at presentation and remain so until they desquamate within 2 weeks.

Diagnostic Tests

- No tests are indicated unless the diagnosis is in doubt.
- Throat culture or stool specimen may be obtained for viral testing, but results may take 2 to 4 weeks.

DDx Differential Diagnosis

- Aphthous stomatitis
- Herpes simplex infection
- Herpangina
- Behçet's syndrome
- Erythema multiforme
- Pemphigus
- Gonorrhea
- Acute leukemia
- Lymphoma
- Allergic contact dermatitis

R Treatment

First Line

- Palliative therapy is given for this usually self-limited disease.

Second Line

- Limited data suggest acyclovir may have a role in treatment of certain cases.

Clinical Pearl(s)

- HFM is transmitted primarily by the fecal-oral route and is highly contagious. Although children are predominantly affected, adults are also at risk. This disease is usually self-limited and benign.
- Frequent hand washing, disinfection of contaminated surfaces, and washing of soiled articles of clothing can help reduce transmission.
- HFM has no relationship to hoof-and-mouth disease in cattle.

67. HENOCH-SCHÖNLEIN PURPURA

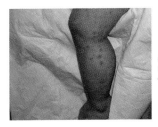

FIGURE 03-133. Classic palpable purpura on the lower extremities and buttocks of this 2-year-old child with Henoch-Schönlein purpura.

 General Comments

Definition

- Henoch-Schönlein purpura (HSP) is a systemic, small-vessel, immune complex–mediated leukocytoclastic vasculitis characterized by a triad of palpable purpura, abdominal pain, and arthritis. It may also present with gastrointestinal bleeding, arthralgias, and renal involvement.

Etiology

- Presumptive etiology is exposure to a trigger antigen that causes antibody formation.
- Antigen-antibody (immune) complex deposition then occurs in the arteriole and capillary walls of skin, renal mesangium, and GI tract. IgA deposition is most common.
- Antigen triggers postulated include drugs, foods, immunization, and upper respiratory and other viral illnesses. Group A streptococcal infection is the most common precipitant in children, seen in up to one third of cases.
- Serologic and pathologic evidence suggests an association between parvovirus B19 and HSP, which may explain observed cases of HSP that do not respond to corticosteroids or other immunosuppressive therapy.
- Case reports describing development of HSP following treatment with immunosuppressive agents such as etanercept have been published.

 Keys to Diagnosis

Clinical Manifestation(s)

- Skin manifestations are most common.
- Palpable purpura (**Fig. 03-133**) is seen in 70% of adult patients, whereas GI complaints are more common in children.
- Arthralgias and arthritis are seen in 80% of patients.

- GI symptoms are seen in approximately one third of patients. Common findings are nausea, vomiting, diarrhea, cramping, abdominal pain, hematochezia, and melena.
- Renal involvement is seen in up to 80% of older children, usually within the first month of illness. Less than 5% progress to end-stage renal failure, which is a major cause of morbidity.

Physical Examination

- Palpable purpura is seen in dependent areas, especially the lower extremities, and areas subjected to pressure such as the beltline.
- Subcutaneous edema is common.

Diagnostic Tests

- Diagnosis is clinical.
- Skin biopsy will show leukocytoclastic vasculitis.

DDx Differential Diagnosis

- Polyarteritis nodosa
- Meningococcemia
- Thrombocytopenic purpura

R Treatment

- Prednisone 1 mg/kg PO is given if there is renal or severe GI disease, although the benefits are not clear.
- A recent double-blind randomized controlled trial found that early treatment with prednisone reduced abdominal pain and joint symptoms but did not prevent development of renal disease. It was effective in treatment of renal disease once established.
- Corticosteroids and azathioprine may be beneficial if rapidly progressive glomerulonephritis is present. Pulse methylprednisolone therapy has also been proposed in patients with glomerulonephritis, mesenteric vasculitis, or pulmonary involvement.
- NSAIDs for arthritis and arthralgias.

Clinical Pearl(s)

- Prognosis is excellent, with most patients experiencing spontaneous recovery within 4 weeks.
- End-stage renal disease occurs in 5% of patients. Chronic renal insufficiency is the most common long-term morbidity.
- GI complications include mesenteric infarction, perforation, and intussusception.
- Recurrence is seen in up to one third of patients, especially within first 4 to 6 months after the initial episode, and most commonly in patients with renal involvement.

68. HERPES SIMPLEX

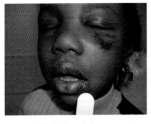

FIGURE 03-134. Autoinnoculation can occur in HSV-1 infections, as seen in this child. The crusting, vesicular lesion under the left eye occurred after self-spread from the primary perioral lesion.

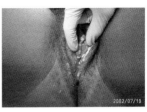

FIGURE 03-135. Recurrent painful vesicular eruption on the labia minor.

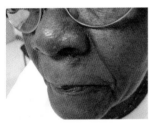

FIGURE 03-136. Recurrent, painful, grouped vesicles on an erythematous base in a patient with a recent upper respiratory infection.

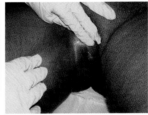

FIGURE 03-137. A cluster of painful, grouped vesicles on an erythematous base occurring on the labia majora.

General Comments

Definition
■ Herpes simplex is a viral infection caused by the herpes simplex virus (HSV). HSV-1 is associated primarily with oral infections, whereas HSV-2 causes mainly genital infections; however, each type can infect any site.

Etiology
■ HSV-1 and HSV-2 are both DNA viruses. Following the primary infection, the virus enters the nerve endings in the skin directly below the lesions and ascends to the dorsal root ganglia, where it remains in a latent stage until it is reactivated.

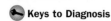

Keys to Diagnosis

Clinical Manifestation(s)

Primary infection:

- Symptoms occur from 3 to 7 days after contact (respiratory droplets, direct contact).
- Constitutional symptoms include low-grade fever, headache and myalgias, regional lymphadenopathy, and localized pain.
- Pain, burning, itching, and tingling last several hours.
- Grouped vesicles, usually with surrounding erythema, appear and generally ulcerate or crust within 48 hours (**Fig. 03-134**).
- During the acute eruption the patient is uncomfortable; involvement of lips and inside of mouth may make it unpleasant for the patient to eat; urinary retention may complicate involvement of the genital area (**Fig. 03-135**).
- Lesions generally last from 2 to 6 weeks and heal without scarring.

Recurrent infection:

- Recurrent infection is generally caused by alteration in the immune system; fatigue, stress, menses, local skin trauma, and exposure to sunlight are contributing factors.
- The prodromal symptoms (fatigue, burning and tingling of the affected area) last 12 to 24 hours.
- A cluster of lesions generally evolve within 24 hours from a macule to a papule and then vesicles surrounded by erythema (**Fig. 03-136**); the vesicles coalesce and subsequently rupture within 4 days, revealing erosions covered by crusts.
- The crusts are generally shed within 7 to 10 days, revealing a pink surface.
- Rapid onset of diffuse cutaneous herpes simplex (eczema herpeticum) may occur in certain atopic infants and adults. It is a medical emergency, especially in young infants, and should be promptly treated with acyclovir.
- Herpes encephalitis, meningitis, and ocular herpes can occur in patients with immunocompromised status and occasionally in normal hosts.

Physical Examination

- The most common location of the lesions is on the vermilion border of the lips (HSV-1), the penile shaft or glans penis and the labia (HSV-2) (**Fig. 03-137**), buttocks (seen more often in women), fingertips (herpetic whitlow), and trunk (may be confused with herpes zoster).
- The vesicles are uniform in size (differentiating it from herpes zoster vesicles, which vary in size).

Diagnostic Tests

- Direct immunofluorescent antibody slide tests will provide a rapid diagnosis.
- Viral culture is the most definitive method for diagnosis; results are generally available in 1 or 2 days; the lesions should be sampled during the vesicular or early ulcerative stage; cervical samples should be taken from the endocervix with a swab.

- Tzanck smear is a readily available test; it will demonstrate multinucleated giant cells. However, it is not a very sensitive test.
- Pap smear will detect HSV-infected cells in cervical tissue from women without symptoms.
- Serologic tests for HSV include IgG and IgM serum antibodies. Antibodies to HSV occur in 50% to 90% of adults. Routine tests do not discriminate between antibodies that are HSV-1 and HSV-2; the presence of IgM or a fourfold or greater rise in IgG titers indicates a recent infection (convalescent sample should be drawn 2 to 3 weeks after the acute specimen is drawn).

DDx Differential Diagnosis

- Impetigo
- Behçet's syndrome
- Coxsackievirus infection
- Syphilis
- Stevens-Johnson syndrome
- Herpangina
- Aphthous stomatitis
- Varicella
- Herpes zoster

℞ Treatment

First Line

- Penciclovir 1% cream can be used for recurrent herpes labialis on the lips and face. It should be applied Q2H while awake for 4 days. Treatment should be started at the earliest sign or symptom. Its use decreases healing time of orolabial herpes by about 1 day. Topical acyclovir 5% cream can also be used for herpes labialis; when started at the prodrome or papule stage, it decreases the duration of an episode by about one-half day.
- Docosanol 10% cream, a long-chain saturated alcohol, inhibits fusion between the plasma membrane and the viral envelope, blocking viral entry and subsequent replication. It is available over the counter and, when applied at the first sign of recurrence of herpes labialis, may shorten the durations of the episode by about 12 hours.
- Valacyclovir 2 g PO Q12H for 1 day or famciclovir 500 mg, 3 tablets given at once, begun within the first symptoms of herpes labialis can modestly shorten its duration.
- Acyclovir ointment or cream applied using a finger cot or rubber glove Q3H to Q6H (6 times daily) for 7 days may be useful for the first clinical episode of genital herpes.
- Primary genital infections may be treated with oral acyclovir 200 mg 5 times daily for 10 days. Valacyclovir caplets can also be used for the initial episode of genital herpes (1 g BID for 10 days). Intravenous acyclovir (5 mg/kg infused at a

constant rate over 1 hr Q8H for 7 days in patients with normal renal function) may be used for severe cases.

- Application of topical cool compresses with Burow's solution for 15 minutes 4 to 6 times daily may be soothing in patients with extensive erosions on the vulva and penis (decrease edema and inflammation, debridement of crusts and purulent material).

Second Line

- Recurrent episodes of genital herpes can be treated with acyclovir. A short course (800 mg TID for 2 days) is effective. Other treatment options include 800 mg PO BID for 3 to 5 days, generally started during the prodrome or within 2 days of onset of lesions; famciclovir is also useful for treatment of recurrent genital herpes (125 mg Q12H for 5 days in patients with normal renal function started at the first sign of symptoms), as is valacyclovir (500 mg Q12H for 3 days in patients with normal renal function).
- Patients with six recurrences of genital herpes a year can be treated with valacyclovir 1 g QD, acyclovir 400 mg BID, or famciclovir 250 mg BID.

Third Line

- Acyclovir-resistant mucocutaneous lesions in patients with HIV can be treated with foscarnet (40-60 mg/kg IV Q8H in patients with normal renal function); HPMPC has also been reported to be effective in HSV infections resistant to acyclovir or foscarnet.

Clinical Pearl(s)

- Condom use offers significant protection against HSV-1 infection.
- Patients should also avoid contact with immunocompromised hosts or neonates while lesions are present.
- Patients with herpes gladiatorum (cutaneous herpes in athletes involved in contact sports) should be excluded from participation in active sports until lesions have resolved.

69. HERPES ZOSTER (SHINGLES)

General Comments

Definition

- Herpes zoster is a disease caused by reactivation of the varicella zoster virus.

Etiology

- Reactivation of varicella-zoster virus (VZV, a human herpes virus 3) may occur several years after the primary infection (chickenpox); the virus becomes latent in the dorsal root ganglia and reemerges when there is a weakening of the immune system (secondary to disease or advanced age).

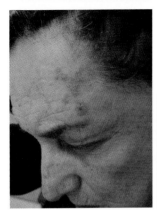

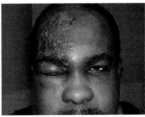

FIGURE 03-138. Following a prodrome of burning over the eye this patient experienced an outbreak of herpes zoster. These painful vesicles were limited to the V1 dermatome and spared the eye.

FIGURE 03-139. Crusted, diffuse, weeping vesicles and bullae over the ophthalmic division of the trigeminal nerve. Despite edema and closure of the eye, this patient did not suffer visual complications.

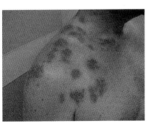

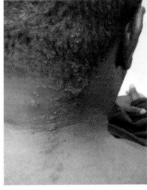

FIGURE 03-140. Clusters of painful vesicles on an erythematous base typical for herpes zoster over the C3-C4 dermatome.

FIGURE 03-141. Shingles involving the right C3 dermatome extending into the scalp with multiple clusters of yellow fluid-filled vesicles.

- Herpes zoster occurs during lifetime in 10% to 20% of the population.
- There is an increased incidence in immunocompromised patients (AIDS, malignancy), the elderly, and children who acquired chickenpox when younger than 2 months.

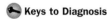 Keys to Diagnosis

Clinical Manifestation(s)

- Pain generally precedes skin manifestation by 3 to 5 days and is generally localized to the dermatome that will be affected by the skin lesions (**Fig. 03-138**).
- Constitutional symptoms are often present (malaise, fever, headache).
- Pain during and after the rash is often significant.
- Secondary bacterial infection with *S. aureus* or *Streptococcus pyogenes* may occur.
- Regional lymphadenopathy may occur.
- Herpes zoster may involve the trigeminal nerve (the most common cranial nerve involved; **Fig. 03-139**). Involvement of the geniculate ganglion can cause facial palsy and a painful ear, with the presence of vesicles on the pinna and external auditory canal (*Ramsay Hunt syndrome*).

Physical Examination

- The initial rash consists of erythematous maculopapules (**Fig. 03-140**) generally affecting one dermatome (thoracic region in majority of cases); some patients may have scattered vesicles outside the affected dermatome.
- The initial maculopapules evolve into vesicles (**Fig. 03-141**) and pustules by the third or the fourth day.
- The vesicles have an erythematous base, are cloudy, and have various sizes (a distinguishing characteristic from herpes simplex, in which the vesicles are of uniform size).
- The vesicles subsequently become umbilicated and then form crusts that generally fall off within 3 weeks; scarring may occur.

Diagnostic Tests

- Tzanck smear
- Viral culture
- Serology

Differential Diagnosis

- Herpes simplex
- Contact dermatitis
- Varicella
- Cellulitis
- Impetigo
- Pemphigus

Treatment

First Line

- Oral antiviral agents can decrease acute pain, inflammation, and vesicle formation when treatment is begun within 48 hours of onset of rash. Treatment options are as follows:
  1. Acyclovir 800 mg 5 times daily for 7 to 10 days
  2. Valacyclovir 1000 mg TID for 7 days
  3. Famciclovir 500 mg TID for 7 days
- Wet compresses (using Burow's solution or cool tap water) applied for 15 to 30 minutes 5 to 10 times a day are useful to break vesicles and remove serum and crust.
- Care must be taken to prevent any secondary bacterial infection.

Second Line

- If there are no contraindications, corticosteroids should be considered in older patients within 72 hours of clinical presentation or if new lesions are still appearing. Initial dose is prednisone 40 mg/day, decreased by 5 mg/day until finished. When used there is a decrease in the use of analgesics and time to resumption of usual activities, but there is no effect on the incidence and duration of postherpetic neuralgia.
- Immunocompromised patients should be treated with intravenous acyclovir 500 mg/m^2 or 10 mg/kg Q8H in 1-hour infusions for 7 days, with close monitoring of renal function and adequate hydration; vidarabine (continuous 12-hour infusion of 10 mg/kg/day for 7 days) is also effective for treatment of disseminated herpes zoster in immunocompromised hosts.
- Gabapentin 300 to 1800 mg QD or pregabalin 75 mg BID is effective in the treatment of pain and sleep interference associated with postherpetic neuralgia.
- Lidocaine patch 5% is also effective in relieving postherpetic neuralgia. Patches are applied to intact skin to cover the most painful area for up to 12 hours within a 24-hour period.
- Capsaicin cream can be useful for treatment of postherpetic neuralgia. It is generally applied three to five times daily for several weeks after the crusts have fallen off.

Third Line

- Patients with AIDS and transplant patients may develop acyclovir-resistant varicella zoster; these patients can be treated with foscarnet (40 mg/kg IV Q8H) continued for at least 10 days or until lesions are completely healed.
- Sympathetic blocks (stellate ganglion or epidural) with 0.25% bupivacaine and rhizotomy are reserved for severe cases of postherpetic neuralgia unresponsive to conservative treatment.

Clinical Pearl(s)

- The incidence of postherpetic neuralgia (defined as pain that persists more than 3 months after the rash has healed) increases with age (30% by age 40 years, >70% by age 70 years); antivirals reduce the risk of postherpetic neuralgia.

- Incidence of disseminated herpes zoster is increased in immunocompromised hosts (e.g., 15%-50% of patients with active Hodgkin's disease).
- Immunocompromised hosts are also more prone to neurologic complications (encephalitis, myelitis, cranial and peripheral nerve palsies, acute retinal necrosis). The mortality rate is 10% to 20% in immunocompromised hosts with disseminated zoster.
- Motor neuropathies occur in 5% of all cases of zoster; complete recovery occurs in more than 70% of patients.
- A line, attenuated vaccine aimed at boosting immunity to VZV and reducing the risk of herpes zoster is recommended for adults older than 60 years.

70. HIDRADENITIS SUPPURATIVA

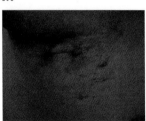

FIGURE 03-142. Painful, tender, red abscesses and nodules with numerous comedomes and hypertrophic scars from previous infections. Note the double comedomes characteristic of this disorder.

🔲 General Comments

Definition
- Hidradenitis suppurativa (HS) is a chronic, relapsing condition that occurs within the terminal follicular epithelium of the apocrine glands (axilla, inguinal folds, perineum, genitalia, and periareolar region) where keritinous materials occlude the follicles, causing secondary inflammation of the apocrine glands, resulting in chronic infection and draining abscess that lead to scarring.

Etiology
- The exact cause of hidradentis suppurativa has not been determined, though a number of theories have been proposed:
  1. Folliculitis is observed in almost all patients with HS, though whether or not this is causative has not been determined.
  2. Local friction trauma is a possible cause.
  3. Infectious agents such as *Streptococcus, Stapholoccocus,* and *Escherichia coli* have been identified in cultures, but it is uncertain whether these are cause or result.
  4. Low levels of estrogen are implicated, as are high levels of androgen.
- Predisposing factors are thought to be involved, including hyperandrogenism, obesity, and familial predilection.

- HS has been associated with other endocrine disorders, such as diabetes, Cushing's disease, and acromegaly.

Keys to Diagnosis

Clinical Manifestation(s)

- Initially there is a firm painful nodule in the groin or axilla.
- The nodule may involute slowly or discharge pus, which is often foul smelling, through the skin. In the late stages a complex interconnecting system of sinuses extends deeply into the dermis and subcutaneous fat with extensive dense fibrosis.
- There is a strong tendency toward relapse and recurrence.
- Other characteristics of the disease are poor response to conventional antibiotics and personal or family history of acne or pilonidal cysts.

Physical Examination

- Initial lesions have the appearance of "blind" boils in early adolescence.
- Skin lesions and abscesses tend to be bilateral. Multifocal involvement, bridged scarring, and sinus formation may be present. Double comedomes are characteristic of this disorder (**Fig. 03-142**).

Diagnostic Tests

- The diagnosis is primarily clinical based on the development of typical lesions.
- Any pus should be sampled for bacterial culture and sensitivity.

Differential Diagnosis

- Folliculitis and other follicular pyodermas furuncles, pilonidal cysts
- Granuloma inguinale
- Crohn's disease (perianal and vulvular manifestations)
- Bartholin's cyst infection
- Actinomycosis
- Lymphogranuloma venereum
- Furuncle
- Lymphangitis
- Cat scratch disease
- Tularemia
- Erysipelas
- Ulcerative colitis

℞ Treatment

First Line

- Topical antibiotics (2% mupirocin ointment TID or retapamulin 1% BID) applied to affected area may be effective in mild cases
- Oral antibiotics (tetracycline, doxycycline, minocycline, clindamycin)

Second Line
- Surgical intervention (incision and drainage of abscess, radical excision of at-risk tissue)
- Intralesional corticosteroids

Third Line
- Oral isotretinoin
- Dapsone

 Clinical Pearl(s)

- Treatment with oral antibiotics may be necessary for several weeks or months.

71. HISTOPLASMOSIS

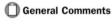 **General Comments**

Definition
- Histoplasmosis is caused by the fungus *Histoplasma capsulatum* and characterized by a primary pulmonary focus with occasional progression to chronic pulmonary histoplasmosis (CPH) or various forms of dissemination.

Etiology
- *H. capsulatum* is a dimorphic fungus present in temperate zones and river valleys worldwide.
- In the United States it is highly endemic in southeastern, mid-Atlantic, and central states.
- *H. capsulatum* exists as mold at ambient temperature and favors soils enriched with bird or bat droppings.

Keys to Diagnosis

Clinical Manifestation(s)
- Conidia are deposited in alveoli, then converted to yeast forms; they spread to regional lymph nodes and other organs, especially the liver and spleen.
- One to two weeks later, a granulomatous inflammatory response begins to contain the yeast in the form of discrete granulomas.
- Delayed-type hypersensitivity to *Histoplasma* antigens occurs 3 to 6 weeks after exposure.
- Clinical disease manifests in various forms, depending on host cellular immunity and inoculum size.

Physical Examination
- Cutaneous lesions are typically multiple small nodules, which may ulcerate.

Diagnostic Tests
- Demonstration of organism on culture from body fluid or tissues to make definitive diagnosis
  1. Especially high yield in patients with AIDS
  2. Characteristic oval yeast cells in neutrophils with Giemsa stain from peripheral smear
  3. Preparations of infected tissue with Gomori's silver methenamine for revealing yeast forms, especially in areas of caseation necrosis
- Serologic tests, including complement-fixing (CF) antibodies and immunodiffusion assays

DDx Differential Diagnosis

- Acute pulmonary histoplasmosis
  1. *Mycobacterium tuberculosis*
  2. Community-acquired pneumonias caused by *Mycoplasma* and *Chlamydia*
  3. Other fungal diseases, such as *Blastomyces dermatitidis* and *Coccidioides immitis*
- Chronic cavitary pulmonary histoplasmosis: *M. tuberculosis*
- Histoplasmomas: true neoplasms

R Treatment

First Line
- Itraconazole

Second Line
- Liposomal amphotericin B plus methylprednisolone

Third Line
- Fluconazole

Clinical Pearl(s)

- Progressive disseminated histoplasmosis (PDH) may present with a diverse clinical spectrum, including adrenal necrosis, pulmonary and mediastinal fibrosis, and ulcerations of the oropharynx and GI tract. In those patients coinfected with HIV, it is a defining disease for AIDS.

72. HORDOLEUM (STYE)

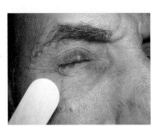

FIGURE 03-143. A tender, erythematous subcutaneous nodule on the skin side of the eyelid margin caused by an acute staphylococcal infection of the glands of Zeis or Moll.

General Comments

Definition
- A hordeolum is an acute inflammatory process affecting the eyelid and arising from the meibomian (posterior) or Zeis (anterior) glands. It is most often infectious and usually caused by *S. aureus.*

Etiology
- Approximately 75% to 95% of cases are caused by *S. aureus.*
- Occasional cases are caused by *Streptococcus pneumoniae,* other streptococci, gram-negative enteric organisms, or mixed bacterial flora.

Keys to Diagnosis

Clinical Manifestation(s)
- Abrupt onset with pain and erythema of the eyelid
- May be associated with blepharitis
- External hordeolum: points toward the skin surface of the lid and may spontaneously drain
- Internal hordeolum: can point toward conjunctival side of the lid and may cause conjunctival inflammation

Physical Examination
- Localized, tender mass on the eyelid (**Fig. 03-143**)

Diagnostic Tests
- Generally, none are necessary.
- If incision and drainage are performed, specimens should be sent for bacterial culture.

Differential Diagnosis

- Eyelid abscess
- Chalazion
- Allergy or contact dermatitis with conjunctival edema
- Acute dacryocystitis
- Herpes simplex infection
- Cellulitis of the eyelid

 Treatment

First Line
- Warm compresses
- Topical antibiotic ophthalmic ointment applied to the lid margins two to four times daily until resolution

Second Line
- Incision and drainage

Third Line
- In refractory cases, an oral antistaphylococcal agent (e.g., dicloxacillin 500 mg PO QID) possibly helpful.

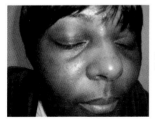 **Clinical Pearl(s)**

- Seborrheic dermatitis may coexist with hordeolum.

73. HYPERHYDROSIS

FIGURE 03-144. Excessive facial perspiration at rest in this afebrile patient with Graves' disease.

 General Comments

Definition
- Hyperhydrosis is increased sweating.

Etiology

- Idiopathic (independent of thermoregulation): symmetrical, localized to palms, soles, axillae
- Injury to the central or peripheral nervous system (e.g., syringomyelia, tabes dorsalis)
- Endocrine diseases (e.g., diabetes, hypoglycemia, hyperthyroidism, pheochromocytoma, carcinoid)
- Metabolic (e.g., alcohol intoxication)
- Febrile illness (e.g., infections, Hodgkin's lymphoma)
- Drugs (e.g., acetaminophen, cholinergic agents)
- Local heat, changes in local blood flow (e.g., arteriovenous malformations)
- Hereditary disorders (e.g., blue rubber bleb nevus syndrome)
- Exercise
- Emotional stress
- Postparotid surgery in the area of distribution of the auriculotemporal nerve (Frey's syndrome)

Keys to Diagnosis

Clinical Manifestation(s)

- Depending on the cause, hyperhydrosis may be symmetrical, generalized, or localized to palms, soles, and axillae or another specific part of the body.
- Sweating may be mainly nocturnal when due to fever from an infectious process or malignancies such as lymphoma.

Physical Examination

- Involved area reveals excessive moisture (**Fig. 03-144**) and foul odor.
- Skin maceration and bacterial or yeast overgrowth may be present.
- Superficial pits may be present with intense odor.

Diagnostic Tests

- Testing is directed by clinical suspicion of etiology (e.g., TSH, free T4 level when suspecting hyperthyroidism)

DDx Differential Diagnosis

- Infections
- Medication induced
- Metabolic/endocrine causes
- Neoplasm
- Neurologic disorders

Rx Treatment

First Line

- Topical 20% aluminum hexahydrate in an alcohol base (Drysol)
- Potassium permanganate soaks for bacterial superinfection of sweaty feet

Second Line
- Botulinum toxin injection for localized hyperhydrosis of axillae or palms
- Iontophoresis with tap water or with the anticholinergic drug glycopyronium bromide for plantar or palmar hyperhydrosis
- Oral anticholinergic agents (propantheline bromide, glycopyronium bromide)

Third Line
- Liposuction and surgical excision of axillary vault
- Sympathectomy

 Clinical Pearl(s)

- In order to be effective, the skin must be completely dry before application of topical 20% aluminum hexahydrate. Cooling of the skin and drying it with a hairdryer may be useful.

74. IMPETIGO

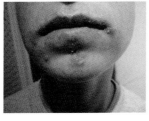 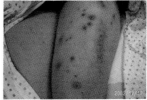

FIGURE 03-145. Honey-colored, crusted, weeping lesions of impetigo superimposed on underlying perioral atopic dermatitis.

FIGURE 03-146. Moist superficial erosions with surrounding erythema on the anterior thigh after rupture of bullous impetigo lesions.

 General Comments

Definition
- Impetigo is a superficial skin infection generally secondary to *S. aureus* and/or *Streptococcus* spp.

Etiology
- *S. aureus* coagulase positive is the dominant microorganism.
- *S. pyogenes* (group A beta-hemolytic streptococci): M-T serotypes of this organism associated with acute nephritis are 2, 49, 55, 57, and 60.

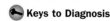 Keys to Diagnosis

Clinical Manifestation(s)

- Common presentations are bullous impetigo (generally secondary to staphylococcal disease) and nonbullous impetigo (secondary to streptococcal infection and possible staphylococcal infection); the bullous form is caused by an epidermolytic toxin produced at the site of infection.
- Constitutional symptoms are generally absent.

Physical Examination

- Nonbullous impetigo begins as a single red macule or papule that quickly becomes a vesicle. Rupture of the vesicle produces an erosion, the contents of which dry to form honey-colored crusts (**Fig. 03-145**). Multiple lesions with golden yellow crusts and weeping areas are often found on the skin around the nose, mouth, and limbs.
- Bullous impetigo is manifested by the presence of vesicles that enlarge rapidly to form bullae with contents that vary from clear to cloudy. There is subsequent collapse of the center of the bullae; the peripheral areas may retain fluid, and a honey-colored crust may appear in the center. As the lesions enlarge and become contiguous with the others, a scaling border replaces the fluid-filled rim. Erythema surrounds the lesions (**Fig. 03-146**).
- Regional lymphadenopathy is most common with nonbullous impetigo.

Diagnostic Tests

- Gram's stain and culture and sensitivity to confirm the diagnosis when the clinical presentation is unclear
- Urinalysis revealing hematuria with erythrocyte casts and proteinuria in patients with acute nephritis (most commonly occurring in children between 2 and 4 years old in the southern part of the United States)

DDx Differential Diagnosis

- Atopic dermatitis
- Herpes simplex infection
- Ecthyma
- Folliculitis
- Eczema
- Insect bites
- Scabies
- Tinea corporis
- Pemphigus vulgaris and bullous pemphigoid
- Chickenpox

Treatment

First Line

- Remove crusts by soaking with wet cloth compresses (crusts block the penetration of antibacterial creams).
- Apply to the affected area mupirocin ointment 2% TID for 10 days or retapamulin 1% BID for 5 days or until all lesions have cleared.
- Patients who are carriers of *S. aureus* in their nares should be treated with mupirocin ointment applied to their nares BID for 5 days.
- Fingernails should be kept short, and patients should be advised not to scratch any lesions to avoid spread of infection.

Second Line

- Oral antibiotics are used in severe cases: commonly used agents for *S. aureus* are dicloxacillin 250 mg QID for 7 to 10 days; cephalexin 250 mg QID for 7 to 10 days; azithromycin 500 mg on day 1, 250 mg on days 2 through 5; and amoxicillin/clavulanate 500 mg Q8H. For methicillin-resistant *S. aureus* (MRSA), use trimethoprim-sulfamethoxazole DS or minocycline. For group A streptococcal impetigo, use azithromycin or clarithromycin.

Third Line

- Rifampin

 Clinical Pearl(s)

- Bullous impetigo is most common in infants and children. The nonbullous form is most common in children ages 2 to 5 years with poor hygiene in warm climates.
- The overall incidence of acute nephritis with impetigo varies between 2% and 5%.
- Patients should be instructed on use of antibacterial soaps and avoidance of sharing of towels and washcloths because impetigo is extremely contagious.
- Children attending day care should be removed until 48 to 72 hours after initiation of antibiotic treatment.

75. KAPOSI'S SARCOMA

 General Comments

Definition

- Kaposi's sarcoma (KS) is a vascular neoplasm most commonly occurring in AIDS patients.

Etiology

- A herpesvirus (HHV-8, Kaposi's sarcoma–associated herpesvirus [KSHV]) has been isolated from patients with most forms of KS and is believe to be the causative agent. It can be transmitted sexually (homosexual or heterosexual activities) and by other forms of nonsexual contact such as maternal-infant transmission (common in African countries).

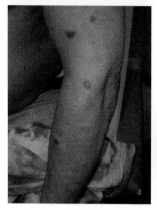

FIGURE 03-147. Subtle violaceous annular patches of Kaposi's sarcoma in this patient who has worsening resistant HIV infection.

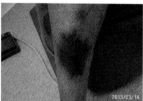

FIGURE 03-148. Asymptomatic violaceous patch on the anterior shin in a patient with HIV infection.

Keys to Diagnosis

Clinical Manifestation(s)

- KS can be divided into the following four subsets:
  1. *Classic Kaposi's sarcoma:* most commonly found in elderly Eastern European and Mediterranean males. It consists initially of violaceous macules and papules with subsequent development of plaques and red-purple nodules. Growth is slow, and most patients die of unrelated causes.
  2. *Epidemic* or *AIDS-related Kaposi's sarcoma:* most commonly occurs in homosexual men. Lesions are generally multifocal and widespread. Lymphadenopathy may be associated.
  3. *Endemic Kaposi's sarcoma:* usually affects African children and adults. An aggressive lymphadenopathic form affects African children in particular.
  4. *Immunosuppression-associated,* or *transplantation-associated, Kaposi's sarcoma:* usually associated with chemotherapy.

Physical Examination

- AIDS-related KS: Multifocal and widespread red-purple, violaceous (**Fig. 03-147**), or dark plaques (**Fig. 03-148**) and/or nodules are seen on cutaneous or mucosal surfaces.

- Generalized lymphadenopathy at the time of diagnosis is present in more than 50% of patients with AIDS-related KS. The initial lesions have a rust-colored appearance; subsequent progression to red or purple nodules or plaques occurs.
- Most commonly affected areas are the face, trunk, oral cavity, and upper and lower extremities.

Diagnostic Tests

- Diagnosis can generally be made on clinical appearance; tissue biopsy will confirm diagnosis.
- HIV serology

DDx Differential Diagnosis

- Stasis dermatitis
- Pyogenic granuloma
- Capillary hemangiomas
- Granulation tissue
- Postinflammatory hyperpigmentation
- Cutaneous lymphoma
- Melanoma
- Dermatofibroma
- Hematoma
- Prurigo nodularis

Rx Treatment

First Line

- Excisional biopsy often provides adequate treatment for single lesions and resected recurrences in classic Kaposi's sarcoma.
- Liquid nitrogen cryotherapy can result in complete response in 80% of lesions.
- Interlesional chemotherapy with vinblastine is useful for nodular lesions larger than 1 cm in diameter. Intralesional injection of interferon alfa-2b has also been reported as effective and well tolerated.
- Radiation therapy is effective in non-AIDS KS and for large tumor masses that interfere with normal function.

Second Line

- Systemic chemotherapy (vinblastine, bleomycin, doxorubicin, and dacarbazine) can be used for rapidly progressive disease and for classic and African endemic KS. Oral etoposide is also effective and has less myelosuppression than vinblastine.
- Systemic therapy with interferon is also effective in AIDS-related KS and is often used in combination with HIV antiviral medications.
- Paclitaxel is also effective in patients with advanced KS and represents an excellent second-line therapy.

Third Line

■ Sirolimus (rapamycin), an immunosuppressive drug, is effective in inhibiting the progression of dermal Kaposi's sarcoma in kidney transplant recipients.

Clinical Pearl(s)

■ Immunosuppression-associated Kaposi's sarcoma usually regresses with the cessation, reduction, or modification of immunosuppression therapy in most patients. Similarly in HIV patients, Kaposi's sarcoma responds concurrently with the decrease in serum HIV RNA and increase in the CD4 count.

76. KAWASAKI SYNDROME

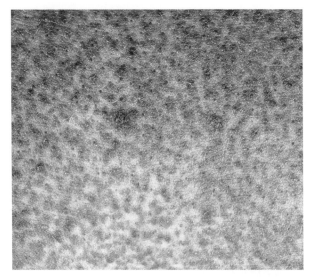

FIGURE 03-149. Kawasaki Syndrome: erythematous macular eruption. *(From McKee PH, Calonje JE, Granter SR: Pathology of the Skin, ed 3, St. Louis, 2005, Mosby, Fig. 15.61.)*

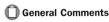 General Comments

Definition

- Kawasaki syndrome refers to a generalized vasculitis of unknown etiology and characterized by cutaneous and mucous membrane edema, rash, lymphadenopathy, and involvement of multiple organs. Kawasaki syndrome is a leading cause of acquired heart disease in children.

Etiology

- The cause of Kawasaki syndrome is not known, although evidence substantiates an infectious etiology precipitating an immune-mediated reaction. Fibrin thrombi and areas of necrosis can be found in the small vessels.

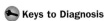 Keys to Diagnosis

Clinical Manifestation(s)

- The diagnosis of Kawasaki syndrome is based on a fever lasting more than 5 days along with four of the following five features:
  Bilateral conjunctival swelling
  Inflammatory changes of the lip, tongue, and pharynx
  Skin changes of the limbs
  Rash over the trunk
  Cervical lymphadenopathy

Physical Examination

- Bilateral conjunctivitis
- Erythema and edema of the hands and feet and desquamation
- Periungual desquamation
- Fissuring of the lips
- Erythematous pharynx
- Strawberry tongue
- Cervical adenopathy
- Truncal scarlatiniform rash, usually nonvesicular (**Fig. 03-149**)

Diagnostic Tests

- ECG, echocardiogram
- Cardiac catheterization with coronary angiography in the proper clinical setting to rule out significant obstructive coronary disease

DDx Differential Diagnosis

- Scarlet fever
- Stevens-Johnson syndrome
- Drug eruption
- Henoch-Schönlein purpura

- Toxic shock syndrome
- Measles
- Rocky Mountain spotted fever
- Infectious mononucleosis

Ⓡ Treatment

- IVIG should be given within the first 10 days of the illness.
- In patients who do not defervesce within 48 hours or have recrudescent fever after initial IVIG treatment, a second dose of IVIG 2 g/kg IV over 8 to 12 hours should be considered.
- Aspirin 30 to 100 mg/kg/day is given in four divided doses until the patient is no longer febrile.
- Oxygen may be used in selected patients.
- Patients with CHF should be placed on a salt-restricted diet.

😀 Clinical Pearl(s)

- Interventional (percutaneous transluminal coronary angioplasty) and surgical procedures (coronary bypass graft surgery) can be tried in children who have developed cardiac complications. Cardiac transplantation is an option and is indicated in patients with severe left ventricular failure, malignant arrhythmias, or multivessel distal coronary artery disease.

77. KELOID

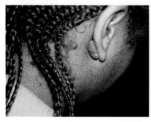

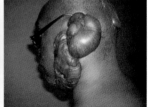

FIGURE 03-150. Skin-colored firm nodule that occurred after ear piercing.

FIGURE 03-151. Massive disfiguring tuberous keloids that followed episodes of minimal trauma in this patient with a strong family history of keloid formation.

General Comments

Definition

■ A keloid is a reactive lesion that represents exuberant (hyperproliferative growth) scar formation and typically extends beyond the site of original injury.

Etiology

■ Although keloids occasionally appear to arise spontaneously, it is believed that most develop as a direct result of local trauma, even if minor or unnoticed.
■ Keloids also develop as a result of inflammation in conditions such as acne vulgaris. The use of isotretinoin has also been linked to the development of keloids.
■ A positive family history is not uncommon and probably reflects a genetic predisposition to keloid formation.

Keys to Diagnosis

Clinical Manifestation(s)

■ Although these lesions arise at any age, they are most common in adolescents and young adults.
■ They occur four times more often in patients of African descent and are more common in females.
■ Keloids usually occur on the head and neck (especially the ear [**Fig. 03-150**]), upper chest, and arms.

Physical Examination

■ Characteristically they present as raised, well-circumscribed, rather smooth lesions, becoming progressively more indurated as time passes.
■ They are occasionally itchy or tender and may be multiple, again reflecting individual susceptibility to their development.

Diagnostic Tests

■ None necessary; skin biopsy only when diagnosis is unclear

DDx Differential Diagnosis

■ Hypertrophic scar
■ Dermatofibrosarcoma protuberans
■ Sarcoidosis
■ Squamous cell carcinoma
■ Recurrence of original tumor
■ Fibromatosis

℞ Treatment

First Line
- Intralesional corticosteroids (triamcinolone 10 mg/mL)

Second Line
- Occlusive dressing, compression
- Intralesional interferon alfa-2b

Third Line
- Radiation, laser surgery, cryosurgery

😮 Clinical Pearl(s)

- Irrespective of the treatment used, local recurrence is very common (**Fig. 03-151**).

78. KERATOACANTHOMA

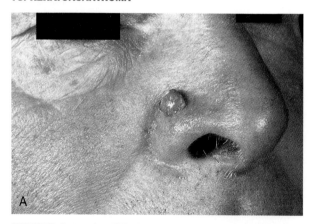

FIGURE 03-152. Keratoacanthoma. (A) A typical dome-shaped lesion on the nose, a commonly affected site. (B) In this example, the central crater is particularly well developed. *(Courtesy the Institute of Dermatology, London, UK. From McKee PH, Calonje JE, Granter SR: Pathology of the Skin, ed 3, St. Louis, 2005, Mosby, Fig. 22.178.)*

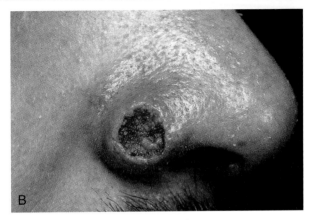

FIGURE 03-152, cont'd.

 General Comments

Definition
- Kerathoacanthoma is a rapidly growing skin tumor arising predominantly on the exposed surfaces of the body.
- A variety of subtypes have been recognized. Most common is the solitary acanthoma.

Etiology
- It usually appears to be related to excessive exposure to UVB.

Keys to Diagnosis

Clinical Manifestation(s)
- Lesions are most commonly found on sun-damaged skin, particularly of the face, forearms, wrists, and backs of the hands.

Physical Examination
- Clinically, solitary keratoacanthoma presents as a smooth, hemispherical papule that rapidly enlarges over the course of a few weeks to produce a 1- to 2-cm diameter, discrete, round or oval, often flesh-colored umbilical nodule with a central keratin-filled crater (**Fig. 03-152**).

Diagnostic Tests
- Skin biopsy

 Differential Diagnosis
- Squamous cell carcinoma
- Seborrheic keratosis
- Wart
- Molluscum contagiosum
- Basal cell carcinoma

 Treatment

First Line
- Surgical excision
- Electrodesiccation and curettage

Second Line
- Radiotherapy
- Intralesional fluorouracil or methotrexate
- Intralesional interferon alfa-2a

Third Line
- Intralesional bleomycin
- Intralesional triamcinolone

 Clinical Pearl(s)
- Although keratoacanthoma is self-limiting (rare metastatic spread), it can have an unpredictable growth and be locally destructive.

79. LENTIGO

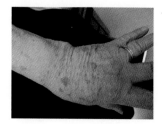

FIGURE 03-153. Benign, brown macules on the dorsum of the hand commonly found on sun-exposed skin in older patients.

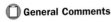 General Comments

Definition
- Lentigo simplex is a very common melanocytic lesion, generally clinically indistinguishable from ephelides (freckles). Juvenile lentigines appear in early childhood and do not increase in size or darken with sun exposure. Actinic lentigo are common brown macules occurring on sun-exposed skin of Caucasians. These lesions are not to be confused with lentigo maligna, which is a form of malignant melanoma in situ that typically develops on chronic sun-damaged skin of the elderly.

Etiology
- Actinic lentigo is associated with sun exposure.
- Juvenile lentigines may occur with some hereditary disorders.

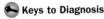 Keys to Diagnosis

Clinical Manifestation(s)
- Lentigo simplex lesions often develop at a young age and become more conspicuous during pregnancy.
- Actinic lentigo lesions are most numerous on the face and dorsal aspects of the hands and forearms (**Fig. 03-153**).

Physical Examination
- Lentigo simplex lesions are small (1-5 mm), uniformly pigmented, brown to black, sharply circumscribed macules that may be found anywhere on the integument.
- Actinic lentigo lesions measure 0.1 to 1 cm or more in diameter, have a tendency to coalesce, and vary from light to dark brown in color.

Diagnostic Tests
- Skin biopsy may be performed if there is concern about malignancy.

DDx Differential Diagnosis

- Lentigo maligna
- Ephelides
- Actinic keratosis
- Flat seborrheic keratosis
- Melanocytic nevus

R Treatment

- Sunscreens (actinic lentigo)
- Bleaching agents

- Laser ablation
- Topical retinoids
- Topical 5-fluorouracil, cryosurgery

🔵 Clinical Pearl(s)

- Hyperpigmentation and an increased number of lentigines are a feature of Addison's disease.
- Simple lentigines have no malignant potential and, in contrast to ephelides, have no connection with sunlight. They may also be associated with a variety of inherited disorders such as LEOPARD syndrome and Peutz-Jeghers syndrome.

80. LEPROSY

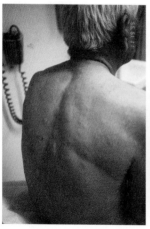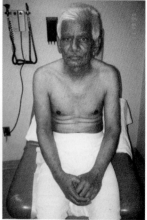

FIGURE 03-154. Multiple, hypopigmented, annular, hypesthetic plaques on the trunk and arms of this Cambodian gentleman with a longstanding history of leprosy. His sister also suffered from longstanding leprosy and had similar findings.

FIGURE 03-155. Diffuse hypopigmented plaques with loss of sensation and raised, erythematous, purplish borders in this middle-aged man with leprosy. His face has lionlike or leonine features secondary to diffuse infiltrative disease of the skin.

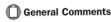 **General Comments**

Definition

■ Leprosy (Hensen's disease) is a chronic granulomatous infection of humans that primarily affects the skin and peripheral nerves.

Etiology

■ Leprosy is caused by *Mycobacterium leprae,* an obligate intracellular acid-fast rod.
■ The mode of transmission remains elusive. Spread in humans is thought to occur via the respiratory route or entry through broken skin in patients with multibacillary disease or extensive paucibacillary disease.
■ The majority of people exposed to patients with leprosy do not develop the disease because of their natural immunity.
■ Incubation period is 3 to 5 years.

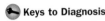 **Keys to Diagnosis**

Clinical Manifestation(s)

■ Leprosy can present along a spectrum from simple cutaneous skin lesions with minimal sensory loss to severe extensive skin involvement, painful neuritis, muscle wasting and contractures, and multiple peripheral nerve damage.

Physical Examination

■ Skin lesions may be few or multiple. Appearance may vary from hypopigmented macules and plaques (**Fig. 03-154**) to erythematous plaques and nodules.
■ Sensory loss
■ Anhidrosis
■ Neuritic pain
■ Palpable peripheral nerves
■ Nerve damage (most commonly affected nerves are ulnar, median, common peroneal, posterior tibial, radial cutaneous nerve of the wrist, facial, and posterior auricular)
■ Muscle atrophy and weakness
■ Foot drop
■ Claw hand and claw toes
■ Lagophthalmos, nasal septal perforation, collapse of bridge of nose, loss of eyebrows
■ Diffuse infiltrative disease of the skin in the face may result in "leonine" facies (**Fig. 03-155**).

Diagnostic Tests

■ The diagnosis of leprosy relies on a detailed history and physical examination and is established by the demonstration of acid-fast bacilli in skin smears or skin biopsies of the affected sites. Skin smears are taken from active sites or most commonly from the earlobe, elbows, or knees and are stained for acid-fast bacilli.

- Leprosy has been classified according to the World Health Organization (WHO) system into the following categories:
  1. Paucibacillary leprosy is defined as fewer than five skin lesions with no bacilli on skin smear.
  2. Multibacillary leprosy is defined as six or more skin lesions and may be skin-smear positive.

DDx Differential Diagnosis

- Sarcoidosis
- Rheumatoid arthritis
- Systemic lupus erythematosus
- Lymphomatoid granulomatosis
- Carpal tunnel syndrome
- Cutaneous leishmaniasis
- Fungal infections

R Treatment

- Physical therapy for patients with upper and lower extremity deformities
- Proper foot care and footwear to prevent ulcer formation

  For paucibacillary leprosy:
  - *Dapsone 100 mg PO QD for 6 months in an unsupervised setting is the treatment of choice.*
  - *Rifampin 600 mg PO QD for 6 months in a supervised setting is the recommendation by WHO.*
  - *Ofloxacin 400 mg QD or minocycline 100 mg QD are other alternatives.*

  For multibacillary leprosy:
  - *Rifampin 600 mg PO QD and clofazimine 300 mg PO qd for 24 months in a supervised setting. Rifampin can be given once monthly without loss of efficacy and at less cost.*
  - *Rifampin 100 mg PO QD and clofazimine 50 mg PO QD for 24 months in an unsupervised setting.*
  - *Dapsone 100 mg PO QD is sometimes added as triple therapy in this group of patients.*
  - *Clofazimine 50 mg daily is used with dapsone for better bacteriocidal effect.*
  - *If relapse occurs, the patient is treated with the same medical regimen; drug resistance is low.*
  - *If relapse is from paucibacillary to multibacillary, the medical regimen for multibacillary should be used for therapy.*

Clinical Pearl(s)

- The risk of transmission is low in patients with leprosy, and therefore no infection control precautions are needed for hospitalized patients.

- Family members and close contacts need to be examined frequently for the development of lesions.
- Dapsone or rifampin prophylaxis is not recommended in the prevention of leprosy.
- Bacille Calmette-Guérin (BCG) vaccination has a 50% efficacy in the prevention of leprosy and may be considered.

81. LEUKOCYTOCLASTIC VASCULITIS

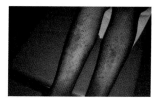

FIGURE 03-156. Palpable purpuric lesions that were mildly tender and pruritic caused by leukocytoclastic vasculitis after a course of trimethoprim-sulfamethoxazole.

General Comments

Definition
- *Leukocytoclastic vasculitis* refers to the histopathological pattern of this form of vasculitis.

Etiology
- Leukocytoclastic vasculitis is the most common form of vasculitis. It represents a vascular reaction pattern due to circulating immune complexes that may be caused by a number of disorders.

Keys to Diagnosis

Clinical Manifestation(s)
- Skin manifestations may be associated with systemic manifestations involving the joints, kidneys, and GI system in 20% to 50% of patients.

Physical Examination
- Skin manifestations are typically polymorphic, but palpable purpura (nonblanching erythematous papules; **Fig. 03-156**) is the most common manifestation.
- Urticarial, bullous or vesicular, ulceroinfarctive, nodular, pustular, livedoid, and annular lesions may be encountered.
- The lesions measure from 1 mm to several centimeters in diameter.
- The lower legs are affected most often, but lesions may be present at various other sites.

Diagnostic Tests

- Skin biopsies should be performed for routine microscopy and direct immunofluorescence.
- Immunoglobulin and complement can be identified in vitro, by immunofluorescence or immunoperoxidase techniques, and in biopsies from blood vessel wall lesions less than 24 hours old.
- Laboratory tests should include CBC, urinalysis, serum creatinine, ALT, ANA, hepatitis serology, HIV, antineutrophil cytoplasmic antibody (ANCA), and complement levels.
- Blood cultures are recommended when an infectious etiology is suspected.
- Chest radiographs should be done in all patients.
- Echocardiography is indicated in suspected infections.

DDx Differential Diagnosis

- Wegener's granulomatosis
- Infective endocarditis
- Cherry angiomas
- Insect bites
- Septic vasculitis
- Thrombocytopenia (idiopathic [ITP], thrombotic [TTP])
- Benign pigmented purpura
- Rocky Mountain spotted fever

R Treatment

First Line

- Removal/withdrawal of causative agent
- Systemic corticosteroids

Second Line

- Colchicine
- Dapsone
- Azathioprine

Third Line

- Interferon alpha
- Antihistamines
- NSAIDs

Clinical Pearl(s)

- The presence of early inflammation in the lesions is useful to distinguish them from microvascular occlusion disorders (inflammation occurs secondarily).

82. LEUKOPLAKIA, ORAL HAIRY (ORAL HAIRY CELL LEUKOPLAKIA)

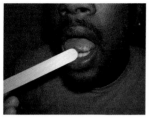

FIGURE 03-157. Painless, vertical white plaque on the lateral surface of the tongue that cannot be scraped off.

FIGURE 03-158. Verrucous white plaque suggestive of a "corduroy-like" or corrugated pattern on the side of the tongue.

General Comments

Definition

- Oral hairy leukoplakia (OHL) is a painless, white, nonremovable, plaquelike lesion typically located on the lateral aspect of the tongue.

Etiology

- Epstein-Barr virus is implicated in its etiology, and OHL is a result of replication EBV in the epithelium of keratinized cells. OHL differs from most EBV-related diseases in that infection is predominantly lytic rather than latent.

Keys to Diagnosis

Clinical Manifestation(s)

- The condition is usually asymptomatic, but some patients have mouth pain, soreness, or a burning sensation; impaired taste; or difficulty eating. Others complain of its unsightly appearance.
- Lesions may spread to cover the entire dorsal surface or spread onto the ventral surface of the tongue, where they usually appear flat.
- Rarely lesions manifest on the soft palate, buccal mucosa, and in the posterior oropharynx.
- OHL may progress to oral squamous cell carcinoma, which has a poor prognosis.

Physical Examination

- Varying morphology and appearance
- May be unilateral or bilateral

- White plaque can be small with fine vertical corrugations on the lateral margin of the tongue (**Fig. 03-157**)
- Irregular surface, verrucous white plaque suggestive of a "corduroy-like" or corrugated pattern on the side of the tongue (**Fig. 03-158**)
- May have prominent folds or projection, occasionally markedly resembling hairs

Diagnostic Tests

- Biopsy
- HIV test

DDx Differential Diagnosis

- *Candida albicans*
- Lichen planus
- Idiopathic leukoplakia
- White sponge nevus
- Focal epithelial hyperplasia
- Squamous cell carcinoma

R Treatment

First Line

- OHL is usually asymptomatic and requires no specific therapy. It may resolve spontaneously and has no known premalignant potential.
- Topical retinoids (0.1% vitamin A) may improve the appearance of OHL-affected oral surfaces through their dekeratinizing and immunomodulation effects; however, they are expensive and prolonged use may result in a burning sensation over the treated area.

Second Line

- Surgical excision and cryotherapy may help, but the lesions may recur.

Third Line

- High-dose acyclovir, ganciclovir, or foscarnet will cause lesions to resolve only temporarily.

Clinical Pearl(s)

- OHL is usually found in HIV-seropositive individuals but may also be identified in other immunocompromised patients such as transplant recipients (particularly renal) and patients taking steroids. Diagnosing OHL is an indication to institute a workup to evaluate and manage HIV disease.

83. LICHEN PLANUS

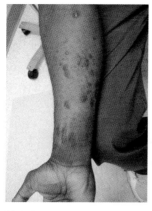

FIGURE 03-159. Multiple, flat-topped, violaceous, shiny papules and plaques developed on the arms and torso of this patient.

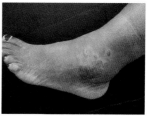

FIGURE 03-160. Grouped purple, confluent, annular, planar, pruritic papules, with crisscrossing white lines known as Wickham's striae.

General Comments

Definition

■ Lichen planus refers to a papular skin eruption characteristically found over the flexor surfaces of the extremities, genitalia, and mucous membranes.

Etiology

■ The cause of lichen planus is unknown.

Keys to Diagnosis

Clinical Manifestation(s)

■ The skin eruption usually starts on an extremity; it may remain localized, or it can spread to involve other areas over a 1- to 4-month period.
■ The affected area is highly pruritic.

Physical Examination

Physical Findings

■ Anatomic distribution:
- Flexor surface of wrists, forearms, shins, and upper thighs
- Neck and back area
- Nails
- Scalp (lichen planopilaris)
- Oral mucosa, buccal mucosa, tongue, gingiva, and lips
- Vulva, penis

Genital Mucosa

■ Lesion configuration:
- Linear
- Annular (more common)
- Reticular pattern noted on oral mucosa and genital area
■ Lesion morphology:
- Papules (flat, smooth, and shiny)—most common presentation **(Fig. 03-159)**
- Hypertrophic
- Follicular
- Vesicular
■ Color:
- Dark red, bluish red, purplish-violaceous color is noted in cutaneous lichen planus.
- Individual lesions characteristically have white lines visible (Wickham's striae) **(Fig. 03-160)**.
- Oral and genital lichen planus have a reticular network of white lines that may be raised or annular in appearance.
■ Scalp lesions may result in alopecia.

Diagnostic Tests

■ Clinical history and physical findings usually establish the diagnosis of lichen planus.
■ Skin biopsy (deep shave or punch biopsy of the most developed lesion) can be done to confirm the diagnosis.
■ Serology for hepatitis B and C

DDx Differential Diagnosis

■ Drug eruption
■ Psoriasis
■ Bowen's disease
■ Leukoplakia
■ Candidiasis
■ Lupus

- Secondary syphilis
- Seborrheic dermatitis
- Chronic graft-versus-host disease
- Scabies

 Treatment

First Line

For cutaneous lichen planus:
- Topical steroids (e.g., triamcinolone acetonide 0.1%, fluocinonide 0.05%, clobetasol propionate 0.05% cream or ointment) with occlusion can be used twice daily.
- Avoid scratching. Hydroxyzine 25 mg PO Q6H can be used for pruritus.
- Use mild soaps and emollients after bathing to prevent dryness.
  For oral lichen planus:
- Topical steroid fluocinonide in an adhesive base can be used six times a day for 9 weeks.

Second Line

- Systemic prednisone 30 to 60 mg/day as a starting dose and tapered to 15 to 20 mg/day maintenance for 6 weeks
- Intradermal steroid triamcinolone acetonide 5 mg/mL for thick hyperkeratotic lesions
- Acitretin 30 mg/day PO for 8 weeks

Third Line

- 0.1% retinoic acid in an adhesive base or gel
- Etretinate 75 mg/day for 2 months
- Topical calcineurin in steroid-unresponsive cases

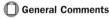 **Clinical Pearl(s)**

- Lichen planus can be remembered as purple, planar, pruritic, polygonal, papules, and plaques (*P*s).
- Lesions can develop at the site of prior skin injury *(Koebner's phenomenon)*.
- Although transformation to skin cancer has been seen in patients with lichen planus, it remains unclear if there is a true correlation.

84. LICHEN SCLEROSUS

 General Comments

Definition

- Lichen sclerosus is a chronic inflammatory condition of the skin usually affecting the vulva, perianal area, and groin.

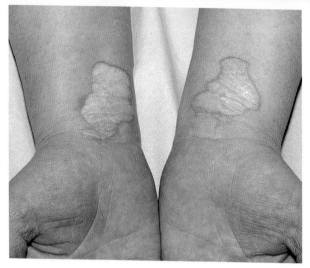

FIGURE 03-161. Lichen sclerosus is typically fairly symmetric, as shown in this case. The wrists are a relatively common site. (*From White GA, Cox NH: Diseases of the Skin: A Color Atlas and Text, ed 2, St. Louis, 2006, Mosby, Fig. 22.9.*)

Etiology

■ Unknown. There may be an autoimmune association and a genetic familial component.

 ## Keys to Diagnosis

Clinical Manifestation(s)

■ Lichen sclerosus of the vulva (kraurosis vulvae) usually occurs after menopause and is generally chronic. It can be painful and interfere with sexual activity.
■ Lichen sclerosus of the penis (balanitis xerotica obliterans) is seen more commonly in uncircumcised males. It affects the glans and prepuce and may lead to stricture if it encroaches into the urinary meatus.
■ Dyspareunia, genital bleeding, and anal bleeding are common.

Physical Examination

■ Erythema may be the only initial sign. A characteristic finding is the presence of ivory-white atrophic lesions on the involved area (**Fig. 03-161**).

- Close inspection of the affected area will reveal the presence of white-to-brown follicular plugs on the surface (dells).
- When the genitals are involved, the white parchmentlike skin assumes an hourglass configuration around the introital and perianal area ("keyhole" distribution). Inflammation, subepithelial hemorrhages, and chronic ulceration may develop.

Diagnostic Tests

- Diagnosis is based on close examination of the lesions for the presence of ivory-white atrophic lesions and typical location.
- Punch or deep shave biopsy can be used to confirm the diagnosis when in doubt.

DDx Differential Diagnosis

- Localized scleroderma (morphea)
- Cutaneous discoid lupus erythematosus
- Atrophic lichen planus
- Psoriasis
- Bowen's disease
- Vitiligo

℞ Treatment

First Line

- Application of clobetasol propionate 0.05% topically BID for up to 4 weeks is usually effective. Repeat courses of corticosteroids may be necessary because of the chronic nature of this disorder. Continual application of topical steroids may lead to atrophy of the vulva.
- Lubricants are useful to soothe dry tissues. Patients should pay attention to hygiene and eliminate irritants or excessive bathing with harsh soaps.
- Hydroxyzine 25 mg at bedtime is effective in decreasing nocturnal itching.

Second Line

- Acitretin
- Isotretinoin

Third Line

- Intralesional steroids
- Surgical management (usually reserved for refractory cases)

Clinical Pearl(s)

- Prepubertal lichen sclerosus may be confused with sexual abuse in prepubertal girls and may lead to false accusations and investigations.

85. LICHEN SIMPLEX CHRONICUS

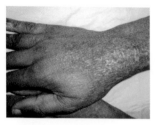

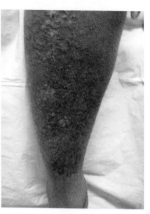

FIGURE 03-162. Longstanding pruritus and scratching resulted in this thickened, hyperpigmented skin on the wrist consisting of numerous 1- to 2-mm papules. This "follicular" pattern is more common in African Americans.

FIGURE 03-163. Lichenified skin of the lower extremity caused by habitual rubbing. The confluence of multiple scaling papules has formed a large plaque of palpably thickened skin.

 General Comments

Definition
- Lichen simplex chronicus is a neurodermatitis manifesting with localized areas of thickened scaly skin due to prolonged and severe scratching in patients with no underlying dermatologic condition.

Etiology
- Neurodermatitis

Keys to Diagnosis

Clinical Manifestation(s)
- Patients present with profound pruritus and localized scaly plaques with accentuated skin markings said to resemble tree bark (**Fig. 03-162**).

Physical Examination

- Lichenified circumscribed plaques are seen (**Fig. 03-163**).
- Commonly involved areas include hands and wrists, back and sides of neck, anterior tibias, anogenital areas, and ankles.

Diagnostic Tests

- Skin biopsy reveals hyperkeratosis, patchy parakeratosis, and elongation of the rete ridges.

 Differential Diagnosis

- Lichen planus
- Psoriasis
- Atopic dermatitis
- Insect bite
- Nummular eczema
- Contact dermatitis
- Stasis dermatitis

 Treatment

First Line

- Patient education is essential to break the itch-scratch cycle and facilitate treatment of any underlying dermatitis.
- Hydroxyzine 25 mg at bedtime is effective in decreasing nocturnal itching.
- Topical corticosteroids
- Intralesional corticosteroids

Second Line

- Flurandrenolide tape
- Doxepin cream

Third Line

- Psychotherapy
- Anxiolytics, selective serotonin reuptake inhibitors (SSRIs)

 Clinical Pearl(s)

- Significant scratching may occur during nocturnal hours.
- The involved area is always at a site that is easily reached for scratching.

86. LYME DISEASE

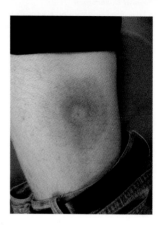

FIGURE 03-164. A slowly expanding lesion of erythema migrans consists of a circular, erythematous patch with central clearing and raised borders.

 General Comments

Definition

- Lyme disease is a multisystem inflammatory disorder caused by the transmission of a spirochete, *Borrelia burgdorferi*.

Etiology

- *B. burgdorferi* is transmitted from the bite of an *Ixodes* tick. It generally takes 36 to 48 hours for a tick to feed and transmit the infecting organism, *B. burgdorferi*, to the host.

Keys to Diagnosis

Clinical Manifestation(s)

Patients with Lyme disease may present in the following stages:

- *Early localized:* early Lyme disease, erythema migrans (EM); skin rash, often at site of tick bite; possible fever, myalgias 3 to 32 days after tick bite
- *Early disseminated:* days to weeks later; multiorgan system involvement, including CNS, joints, cardiac; related to dissemination of spirochete
- *Late persistent:* months to years after tick exposure; affects central and peripheral nervous system, heart, joints

Physical Examination
- EM starts as an erythematous papule and evolves into an annular, flat, erythematous lesion with partial central clearing (**Fig. 03-164**).
- Lymphadenopathy, pharyngeal erythema, and hepatosplenomegaly may be present.

Diagnostic Tests
- ELISA testing, Western blot IgM and IgG
- Immunofluorescent assay
- Culturing of skin lesions (EM) and PCR of skin biopsy and blood to give definitive diagnosis (available only in reference laboratories)
  Early disease is often difficult to diagnose serologically secondary to slow immune response.

DDx Differential Diagnosis
- Acute viral illnesses
- Babesiosis
- Ehrlichiosis
- Insect bite
- Granuloma annulare
- Seborrheic dermatitis
- Erythema annulare
- Erythema marginatum

Rx Treatment
First Line
- Doxycycline 100 mg BID (should be avoided in children/pregnant females) or amoxicillin 500 mg TID for 14 days

Second Line
- Alternative treatments: cefuroxime axetil 500 mg BID for 14 to 21 days, azithromycin 500 mg PO for 7 to 10 days (should not be used as a first-line agent)

Third Line
- Early disseminated and late persistent infection: 30 days of treatment necessary; doxycycline and ceftriaxone appear equally effective for acute disseminated Lyme disease.
- Arthritis: 30 days of doxycycline or amoxicillin plus probenecid.
- Neurologic involvement requires parenteral antibiotics: ceftriaxone 2 g/day for 21 to 28 days; alternative: cefotaxime 2 g Q8H; alternative: penicillin G 5 million U QID.
- Cardiac involvement: intravenous ceftriaxone or penicillin plus cardiac monitoring.

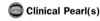 **Clinical Pearl(s)**

- A physician diagnosis of classic erythema migrans in an endemic region of Lyme disease is generally sufficient to make a definitive diagnosis.

87. LYMPHOGRANULOMA VENEREUM

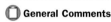 **General Comments**

Definition
- Lymphogranuloma venereum is a sexually transmitted disease caused by *Chlamydia trachomatis*.

Etiology
- *Chlamydia trachomatis*. There are three serotypes: L1, L2, and L3.

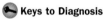 **Keys to Diagnosis**

Clinical Manifestation(s)
Primary stage:
- Primary lesion caused by multiplication of organism at site of infection
- Incubation period of 3 to 21 days
- Most common site of lesion in women: posterior wall, fourchette, or vulva
- Spontaneous healing, without scarring
Second stage:
- Inguinal syndrome: characteristic inguinal adenopathy
- Begins 1 to 4 weeks after primary lesion
- Syndrome is the most frequent clinical sign of the disease
- Unilateral inguinal adenopathy in 70% of cases
- Symptoms: painful, extensive adenitis (bubo) and suppuration may occur with numerous sinus tracts
- *"Groove sign"* signaling femoral and inguinal node involvement (20%); most often seen in men
- Involvement of deep iliac and retroperitoneal lymph nodes in women may present as a pelvic mass
Third stage (anogenital syndrome):
- Subacute: proctocolitis
- Late: tissue destruction or scarring, sinuses, abscesses, fistulas, strictures of perineum, elephantiasis

Physical Examination
- Papule, shallow ulcer
- Herpetiform lesion at site of inoculation (most common)

Diagnostic Tests
- Cell culture of *Chlamydia,* aspiration of fluctuant node yields highest rates of recovery

Differential Diagnosis

- Inguinal adenitis
- Chanchroid
- Syphilis
- Suppurative adenitis
- Retroperitoneal adenitis
- Proctitis
- Cat scratch disease
- Schistosomiasis

℞ Treatment

First Line
- Doxycycline 100 mg PO BID for 21 days
- Surgical: aspirate fluctuant nodes, incise and drain abscesses

Second Line
- Erythromycin base 500 mg PO QID for 21 days

Third Line
- Sulfisoxazole 500 mg PO QID for 21 days

Clinical Pearl(s)

- Once the scarring process begins, it cannot be reversed by antibiotic therapy.

88. MASTOCYTOSIS (URTICARIA PIGMENTOSA)

 General Comments

Definition
- Mastocytosis is a disorder of mast cell proliferation. Its most common cutaneous presentation is urticaria pigmentosa. It may be present with or without systemic manifestations.

Keys to Diagnosis

Clinical Manifestation(s)
- Lesions may be present at birth or appear during the first year of life and are pruritic. They occur predominantly on the trunk and gradually darken due to increased melanin pigmentation.
- The face, scalp, palms, and soles are usually spared.

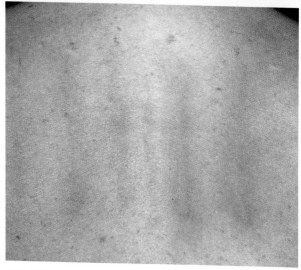

FIGURE 03-165. Urticaria pigmentosa. Gentle rubbing of the lesion typically results in erythema of the surrounding skin. *(Courtesy R. A. Marsden, MD, St. George's Hospital, London, UK. From McKee PH, Calonje JE, Granter SR: Pathology of the Skin, ed 3, St. Louis, 2005, Mosby, Fig. 25.383.)*

- Urtication at the slightest trauma (*Darier's sign*) is characteristic.
- Many patients show generalized dermatographism (whealing after stroking or gentle rubbing).
- In adults, small dark brown papules and macules are present predominantly on the trunk and extremities.

Physical Examination

- Lesions are erythematous or red-brown, round to oval macules, papules, and plaques, often measuring as much as 2 to 3 cm in diameter (**Fig. 03-165**).

Diagnostic Tests

- Skin biopsy
- Laboratory investigation: 24-hour urine histamine, histamine metabolites, prostaglandin metabolites, blood tryptase levels, bone marrow examination

Ⓓ Differential Diagnosis

- Insect bites
- Nevi and congenital pigment abnormalities
- Café-au-lait spots
- Granuloma annulare
- Lentigo
- Drug eruption
- Sarcoidosis

℞ Treatment

First Line
- H1 and H2 antihistamines

Second Line
- Topical corticosteroids with plastic film occlusion
- PUVA photochemotherapy

Third Line
- Doxepin

😊 Clinical Pearl(s)

- Avoidance of triggers (friction, temperature extremes, physical exertion, alcohol, NSAIDs) is an important component of effective treatment.

89. MELANOCYTIC NEVI (MOLES)

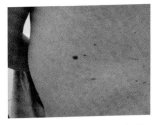

FIGURE 03-166. Slightly raised tan macule with a uniform brown color and a distinct border.

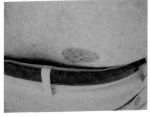

FIGURE 03-167. Light brown, flat, well-demarcated melanocytic lesion speckled internally with darker brown macules.

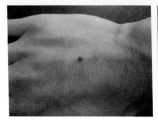

FIGURE 03-168. Blue-black, round papular blue nevus that has remained unchanged for years in this 25-year-old patient.

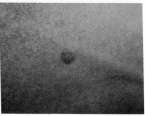

FIGURE 03-169. Brown-tan, dome-shaped papule found on the neck.

General Comments

Definition

- Melanocytic nevi are skin lesions appearing initially in childhood and increasing in number during the second and third decades.
- They generally involute during middle age and may regress completely in the elderly.

Etiology

- Congenital
- Development of acquired melanocytic nevi is related to the extent of sun exposure during the first two decades of life. Intermittent intense sunlight is of greater importance than chronic exposure.

Keys to Diagnosis

Clinical Manifestation(s)

- In males, the head, neck, and trunk (**Fig. 03-166**) are particularly affected, whereas in females the upper and lower limbs are more often involved.

Physical Examination

- Melanocytic nevi present a variety of features depending upon their stage of evolution (**Fig. 03-167**, **Fig. 03-168**, **Fig. 03-169**).
- *Junctional nevi* are usually macular or slightly raised, up to 0.5 cm in diameter, and from light to dark brown in color. They are well circumscribed with a regular border and are usually uniformly pigmented, but sometimes the central area is darker. Typically the skin lines can be clearly discerned on the surface of the lesion.
- The *compound nevus* is raised, sometimes dome shaped or warty, and often still deeply pigmented. Occasionally, coarse hairs project from its surface.

■ The *intradermal nevus* is often devoid of pigment and may present as a dome-shaped nodule or a pedunculated skin tag. Malignant transformation is rare. It has been estimated that the likelihood of one nevus evolving into melanoma is roughly 1/100,000.

Diagnostic Tests
■ Biopsy only if diagnosis is in doubt

DDx Differential Diagnosis
■ Actinic keratosis
■ Melanoma
■ Lentigines
■ Ephelides
■ Seborrheic keratosis
■ Basal cell carcinoma

R Treatment
■ Surgical excision only when diagnosis is in doubt or for cosmetic reasons

Clinical Pearl(s)
■ An average Caucasian can expect to develop 15 to 40 such lesions during life.

90. MELANOMA

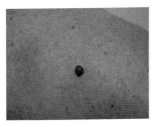

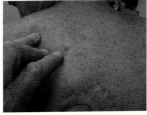

FIGURE 03-170. Round, smooth-bordered, 6-mm black nodular melanoma on the back of this 30-year-old man.

FIGURE 03-171. Remnant scar after removal of a nodular melanoma (thickness < 1 mm). According to the surgical guidelines for the removal of melanoma, the excision was performed with a 1-cm margin from the lesion edge.

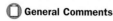 General Comments

Definition

Melanoma is a skin neoplasm arising from the malignant degeneration of melanocytes. It is classically subdivided in four types:
- Superficial spreading melanoma (70%)
- Nodular melanoma (15%-20%)
- Lentigo maligna melanoma (5%-10%)
- Acral lentiginous melanoma (7%-10%)

Etiology

- UV light is the most important cause of malignant melanoma.
- There is a modest increase in melanoma risk in patients with small nondysplastic nevi and a much greater risk in those with dysplastic lesions.
- The CDKN2A gene, residing at the 9p21 locus, is often deleted in people with familial melanoma.

Keys to Diagnosis

Clinical Manifestation(s)

- Melanoma has doubled to tripled in incidence over the past 25 years (annual incidence is 13 cases/100,000 persons). Median age at diagnosis is 53 years.
- Melanoma is the most common cancer among women 20 to 29 years.
- Melanoma is much more common in Caucasians (17.2/100,000 Caucasian men) than in African Americans (1/100,000 African-American men).
- The warning signs that a lesion may be a melanoma can be summarized with the ABCD rules:
  A: Asymmetry (e.g., lesion is bisected and halves are not identical)
  B: Border irregularity (uneven, ragged border)
  C: Color variegation (presence of various shades of pigmentation)
  D: Diameter enlargement (>6 mm)
- Recent data regarding small-diameter melanoma suggest that the ABCD criteria for gross inspection of pigmented skin lesions and early diagnosis of cutaneous melanoma should be expanded to ABCDE to include *Evolving* (i.e., lesions that have changed over time).

Physical Examination

Findings on physical examination are variable depending on the subtype of melanoma:
- *Superficial spreading melanoma* is most often found on the lower legs, arms, and upper back. It may have a combination of many colors or may be uniformly brown or black.

- *Nodular melanoma* (**Fig. 03-170**) can be found anywhere on the body, but it most commonly occurs on the trunk on sun-exposed areas. It is dark-brown or red-brown and can be dome shaped or pedunculated; lesions are frequently misdiagnosed because they may resemble a blood blister or hemangioma and may also be amelanotic.
- *Lentigo maligna melanoma* is generally found in older adults in areas continually exposed to the sun and often arising from lentigo maligna (*Hutchinson's freckle*) or melanoma in situ. Lesions might have a complex pattern and variable shape; color is more uniform than in superficial spreading melanoma.
- *Acral lentiginous melanoma* often occurs in soles, subungual mucous membranes, and palms (sole of the foot is the most prevalent site). Unlike other types of melanoma, it has a similar incidence in all ethnic groups.

Diagnostic Tests

- Perform excisional biopsy (**Fig. 03-171**) with elliptical excision that includes 1 to 2 mm of normal skin surrounding the lesion and extends to the subcutaneous tissue; incisional punch biopsy is sometimes necessary in surgically sensitive areas (e.g., digits, nose).
- Sentinel lymph node dissection (SLND) should be considered in patients with intermediate (1-4 mm) melanomas or high-risk skin tumors to obtain information regarding a patient's subclinical lymph node status with minimal morbidity. It involves the use of radiologic lymphoscintigraphy to map lymphatic drainage from the site of the primary melanoma to the first "sentinel" lymph node in the region. When properly performed, if the sentinel node is negative, the remaining lymph nodes in the region will not have metastases in more than 98% of cases. The staging of intermediate thickness (1.2-3.5 mm) primary melanomas, according to the results of sentinel node biopsy, provides important prognostic information and identifies patients with nodal metastases whose survival can be prolonged by immediate lymphadenectomy.
- The staging system for melanoma adapted by the American Joint Committee on Cancer (AJCC) follows TNM classification. The pathology report should indicate the following:
  - Tumor thickness (Breslow microstage)
  - Tumor depth (Clark level): The depth of invasion is the most important histologic prognostic parameter in evaluating the primary tumor.
  - Mitotic rate: tabulated as mitosi per mm^2 in the dermal part of the tumor in which most mitoses are identified.
  - Radial growth rates vs. vertical growth rate: Radial growth phase describes the growth of melanoma within the epidermis and along the dermal-epidermal junction.
  - Tumor infiltrating lymphocytes: They have a strong predictive value in vertical growth phase melanomas and are defined as brisk, nonbrisk, and absent.

- Histologic regression: characterized by the absence of melanoma in the epidermis and dermis flanked on one or both sides by melanoma.
■ Reverse transcriptase–polymerase chain reaction (RT-PCR) assay for tyrosine messenger RNA is a useful marker for the presence of melanoma cells. It is performed on sentinel lymph node biopsy and is useful for detection of submicroscopic metastases.

DDx Differential Diagnosis

■ Dysplastic nevi
■ Lentigo
■ Vascular lesions
■ Blue nevus
■ Basal cell carcinoma
■ Seborrheic keratosis
■ Cherry hemangioma
■ Keratoacanthoma
■ Pyogenic granuloma
■ Dermatofibroma
■ Squamous cell carcinoma
■ Subungual hematoma

R Treatment

First Line

■ Initial excision of the melanoma
■ Re-excision of the involved area after histologic diagnosis:
  1. The margins of re-excision depend on the thickness of the tumor.
  2. Low-risk or intermediate-risk tumors require excision of 1 to 3 cm.
  3. Melanomas of moderate thickness (0.9-2.0 mm) can be excised safely with 2-cm margins.
  4. A 1-cm margin of excision for melanoma with a poor prognosis (as defined by a tumor thickness of at least 2 mm) is associated with a significantly greater risk of regional recurrence than is a 3-cm margin, but with a similar overall survival rate.
■ Lymph node dissection: recommended in all patients with enlarged lymph nodes. Lymph node evaluation is important in patients with melanoma 1 mm in depth because it determines the overall prognosis and need for therapeutic lymph node dissection or adjuvant treatment.
  1. Elective lymph node dissection remains controversial.
  2. It is indicated with positive sentinel node. It may be considered in those with a primary melanoma that is between 1 and 4 mm thick (especially in patients <60 years old).

Second Line
- Adjuvant therapy with interferon alfa-2b (Intron A) in patients with metastatic melanoma is approved by the Food and Drug Administration (FDA) for AJCC stages IIb and III melanoma; however, its statistical benefit remains unclear.
- Dacarbazine (DTIC) and interleukin 2 (IL-2) can be used in metastatic melanoma. Results are generally poor, with median survival in patients with distant metastatic melanoma approximately 6 months.
- Recent attention has focused on combinations of dacarbazine and cisplatin with interleukin-2 and interferon alfa (biochemotherapy).

Third Line
- Novel therapeutics involve cancer vaccines and use of granulocyte-macrophage colony-stimulating factor (GM-CSF) and angiogenesis inhibitors.
- Treatment of advanced disease consists (in addition to surgical excision and lymph node dissection) of chemotherapy, immunotherapy, and radiation therapy.

🟢 Clinical Pearl(s)
- Superficial spreading melanoma occurs most often in young adults on sun-exposed areas, whereas acral lentiginous melanoma is most often found in Asian Americans and African Americans and is not related to sun exposure.
- Approximately 8% to 10% of melanomas arise in people with a family history of the disease.
- Prognosis varies with the stage of the melanoma. The 5-year survival related to thickness is as follows: smaller than 0.76 mm, 99% survival; 0.6 to 1.49 mm, 85%; 1.5 to 2.49 mm, 84%; 2.5 to 3.9 mm, 70%; larger than 4 mm, 44%.

91. MELASMA (CHLOASMA)

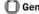 General Comments

Definition
- Common, usually symmetric, acquired hypermelanosis characterized by irregular light to dark-brown confluent or speckled macules with sharply demarcated margins involving sun-exposed skin.

Etiology
- The exact pathogenesis is unknown but there is a clear etiologic link to female hormones and to sun exposure.

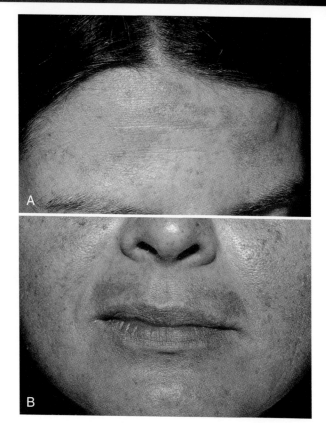

FIGURE 03-172. (A) Melasma on the forehead. Darker patches are quite common on the face of a woman. They seem to result from a combination of female hormones and the sun. (B) Melasma of the upper lip in a woman. This change often gives the appearance of a mustache. *(From White GA, Cox NH: Diseases of the Skin: A Color Atlas and Text, ed 2, St. Louis, 2006, Mosby.)*

- Histologically there is an increase in content of melanin in keratinocytes at all levels of the epidermis and an increase in the number of epidermal melanocytes.
- An association has also been documented with cosmetics, phototoxic drugs, isotretinoin, and anticonvulsants.

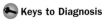 Keys to Diagnosis

Clinical Manifestation(s)
- There is a marked predilection for the face.

Physical Examination
- Irregular light to dark-brown confluent or speckled macules with sharply demarcated margins involving sun-exposed skin
- Symmetric involvement; irregular, "moth-eaten" border (**Fig. 03-172**)

Diagnostic Tests
- TSH, microsomal thyroid autoantibodies

DDx Differential Diagnosis
- Poikiloderma of Civatte
- Postinflammatory hyperpigmentation
- Photolichenoid drug reaction

R Treatment

First Line
- Avoidance of sun exposure, sunscreens to block both ultraviolet A and ultraviolet B

Second Line
- Bleaching creams that contain hydroquinone
- Tretinoin

Third Line
- Azelaic acid

Clinical Pearl(s)
- Women (particularly Hispanic or Indian) are more commonly affected than men. Melasma usually develops in association with oral contraceptives and pregnancy and is worsened by sun exposure.

92. MILIARIA

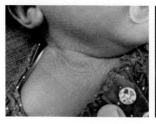

FIGURE 03-173. Multiple, clear vesicles in the intertriginous area subject to excessive perspiration, between the neck and shoulder, caused by obstruction of the eccrine sweat glands in this newborn with miliaria crystallina.

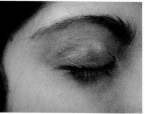

FIGURE 03-174. Multiple white papules or microcysts, 1 to 2 mm, that have persisted on the eyelids of this young woman.

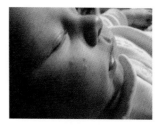

FIGURE 03-175. Several erythematous vesicles characteristic of miliaria rubra on the cheek of this neonate.

 General Comments

Definition

■ Miliaria is a papulovesicular eruptive dermatitis also known as "prickly heat."

Etiology

■ Miliaria is usually due to a combination of heat and occlusion of the skin. It involves retention of sweat in occluded eccrine glands.

Keys to Diagnosis

Clinical Manifestation(s)

■ Miliaria may represent primary lesions when no cause can be identified or secondary variants following skin trauma or other injury.
■ The presentation may be accompanied by a stinging or prickling sensation.

Physical Examination
- Superficial keratinous cysts are seen that present as white or yellow dome-shaped nodules measuring 1 to 3 mm in diameter (**Fig. 03-173**).
- These lesions are most often apparent on the face (forehead, eyelids [**Fig. 03-174**], and cheeks [**Fig. 03-175**]) and the external genitalia.

Diagnostic Tests
- Microbiology swab for bacteria and yeasts; histology when diagnosis is unclear

DDx Differential Diagnosis

- Viral exanthem
- Drug eruption
- Candidiasis
- Insect bites
- Milia
- Folliculitis

R Treatment

First Line
- Frequent showering, air-conditioned environment
- Limit activity, remove occlusive clothing
- Topical antiseptics, oatmeal baths

Second Line
- Topical corticosteroids

Third Line
- Systemic antibiotics
- Anhydrous lanolin/isotretinoin

Clinical Pearl(s)

- Miliaria are seen in up to 50% of newborns on the face, upper trunk, and extremities. They typically regress spontaneously. Children and adults can also be affected.

93. MOLLUSCUM CONTAGIOSUM

General Comments

Definition
- Molluscum contagiosum is a viral infection characterized by discrete skin lesions with central umbilication.

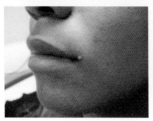

FIGURE 03-176. Solitary, pearly white papule arising at the corner of the mouth of a 35-year-old woman. Her child had multiple mollusca lesions.

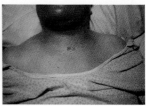

FIGURE 03-177. Cluster of molluscum contagiosum lesions in a mosaic pattern over the upper chest in an HIV-infected individual. These appeared after the patient shaved this area for cosmetic reasons.

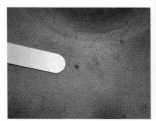

FIGURE 03-178. Several umbilicated lesions of molluscum contagiousm appearing as shiny, flesh-colored papules. Note the adjacent papules, which have healed, leaving areas of hyperpigmentation.

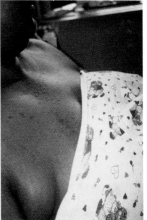

FIGURE 03-179. Rapid onset of multiple umbili-cated papules of molluscum contagiosum spread over the anterior chest of an adult patient. This clinical scenario should raise the suspicion of HIV infection.

Etiology
- This viral infection of epithelial cells is caused by a poxvirus.
- Molluscum contagiosum spreads by autoinoculation, scratching, or touching a lesion.

Keys to Diagnosis

Clinical Manifestation(s)
- This condition usually occurs in young children. It is also common in sexually active adults and patients with HIV infection.
- Incubation period varies between 4 and 8 weeks.
- Typical distribution in children involves the face, extremities, and trunk. Mucous membranes are spared.
- Distribution in adults generally involves pubic and genital areas.
- Spontaneous resolution in immunocompetent patients can occur after several months.

Physical Examination
- The individual lesion appears initially as a flesh-colored, firm, smooth-surfaced papule (**Fig. 03-176**) with subsequent central umbilication. Lesions are often grouped (**Fig. 03-177**). The size of each lesion generally varies from 2 to 6 mm in diameter. Adjacent papules that have healed will leave areas of hyperpigmentation (**Fig. 03-178**).
- Erythema and scaling at the periphery of the lesions may be present as a result of scratching or hypersensitivity reaction.
- Lesions are not present on the palms and soles.

Diagnostic Tests
- Diagnosis is usually established by the clinical appearance of the lesions (distribution and central umbilication). A magnifying lens can be used to observe the central umbilication. If necessary, the diagnosis can be confirmed by removing a typical lesion with a curette and examining the content on a slide after adding potassium hydroxide and gentle heating. Staining with toluidine blue will identify viral inclusions.

Differential Diagnosis

- Verruca plana (flat warts): no central umbilication, not dome shaped, irregular surface, can involve palms and soles
- Herpes simplex: lesions rapidly become umbilicated
- Varicella: blisters and vesicles are present
- Folliculitis: no central umbilication, presence of hair piercing the pustule or papule
- Cutaneous cryptococcosis in AIDS patients: budding yeasts will be present on cytologic examination of the lesions
- Basal cell carcinoma: multiple lesions are absent

Ⓡ Treatment

First Line

- Therapy is individualized depending on number of lesions, immune status, and patient's age and preference.
- Observation for spontaneous resolution is reasonable in patients with few, small, not irritated, and not spreading lesions. Genital lesions should be treated in all sexually active patients.
- Liquid nitrogen cryotherapy can be used to remove lesions.
- Curettage after pretreatment of the area with combination prilocaine 2.5% with lidocaine 2.5% cream (EMLA) for anesthesia is useful for treatment of few lesions. Curettage should be avoided in cosmetically sensitive areas because scarring may develop.

Second Line

- Application of cantharidin 0.7% to individual lesions covered with clear tape will result in blistering over 24 hours and possible clearing without scarring. This medication should be avoided on facial lesions.

Third Line

- Other treatment measures include use of imiquimod cream or tretinoin 0.025% gel or 0.1% cream at bedtime, daily use of salicylic acid (Occlusal) at bedtime, and use of laser therapy.
- Trichloroacetic acid peel generally repeated every 2 weeks for several weeks is useful in immunocompromised patients with extensive lesions.

🔵 Clinical Pearl(s)

- Genital molluscum contagiosum in children may be indicative of sexual abuse.
- Rapid onset of multiple, umbilicated papules of molluscum contagiosum spread over the anterior chest of an adult patient should raise the suspicion of HIV infection (**Fig. 03-179**).

94. MONGOLIAN SPOT

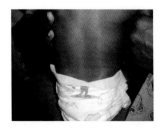

FIGURE 03-180. Characteristic lumbosacral location for this gray to blue-black Mongolian spot.

General Comments

Definition
- A Mongolian blue spot is a dermal melanocytic lesion presenting as relatively uniform slate-blue areas of discoloration most often situated over the sacral region.

Etiology
- Mongolian blue spots are believed to represent arrested transdermal migration of melanocytes from the neural crest to the epidermis.

 Keys to Diagnosis

Clinical Manifestation(s)
- Asymptomatic lesion

Physical Examination
- The lesion is benign and characterized by variably pigmented melanocytes, which tend to be orientated parallel to the skin surface (**Fig. 03-180**) and situated predominantly in the deep reticular dermis. The overlying epithelium is normal. Lesions are most often located on the buttocks, flank, and shoulders.

Diagnostic Tests
- None necessary

 Differential Diagnosis

- Nevus of Ito
- Dermal melanocytic hamarthoma (macular blue nevus)
- Late-onset dermal melanosis
- Trauma
- Acquired bilateral nevus of Otalike macules

 Treatment

- None necessary

 Clinical Pearl(s)

- These skin lesions are more common in people of Japanese and Chinese descent and other pigmented races.

95. MORPHEA

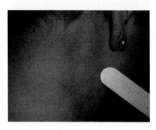

FIGURE 03-181. Smooth, shiny sclerotic plaque with ill-defined borders and underlying induration proved to be morphea on biopsy.

 General Comments

Definition
- Morphea is a connective tissue disorder affecting the skin and subcutaneous tissue. It is a localized form of scleroderma affecting the skin but causing no internal sclerosis (no association with any systemic disease).

Etiology
- Unknown

Keys to Diagnosis

Clinical Manifestation(s)
- Onset is variable, but most often is gradual and asymptomatic.
- The most common presentation is with one or more localized plaques (**Fig. 03-181**).
- Presentation with multiple tiny spots is known as guttate morphea.
- Uncommon presentations include nodular morphea (lesions resemble keloids) and generalized or diffuse morphea (involves a large portion of body surface area); frontoparietal linear variant morphea affects the forehead and scalp, is also known as *en coup de saber*, and may be a variant of facial hemiatrophy (Parry-Romberg syndrome).
- Subcutaneous or deep morphea and bullous morphea are very rare presentations.

Physical Examination
- Early lesions have a violaceous or lilac color.
- The border has an active inflammatory appearance.
- Poorly defined areas of nonpitting edema with induration are seen.
- Skin atrophy and softening may occur after several months or years.

Diagnostic Tests
- Skin biopsy
- ANA

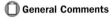 Differential Diagnosis

- Granuloma annulare
- Lichen sclerosus
- Hypertrophic scar
- Scleroderma
- Eosinophilic fasciitis
- Porphyria cutanea tarda
- Atrophoderma
- Nephrogenic fibrosing dermopathy
- Necrobiosis lipoidica

Ⓡ Treatment

First Line
- Topical corticosteroids
- Skin emollients
- Intralesional corticosteroids (e.g., triamcinolone 5-10 mg/mL)
- Calcipotriene ointment

Second Line
- PUVA-bath photochemotherapy
- Low-dose UVA phototherapy

Third Line
- Methotrexate
- Methotrexate plus pulse corticosteroids

🦷 Clinical Pearl(s)

- Linear scleroderma is more common in children. About 30% of patients with linear morphea have positive ANA.

96. MUCORMYCOSIS

📋 General Comments

Definition
- Mucormycosis is a fungal infection by *Zygomycetes* fungi, which include *Mucorales* spp. (*Mucor, Rhizopus, Absidia, Cunninghamella, Mortierella, Saksenaea, Syncephalastrum, Apophysomyces,* and *Thamnidium*) and *Entomophthorales* spp. (*Conidiobolus* and *Basidiobolus*).

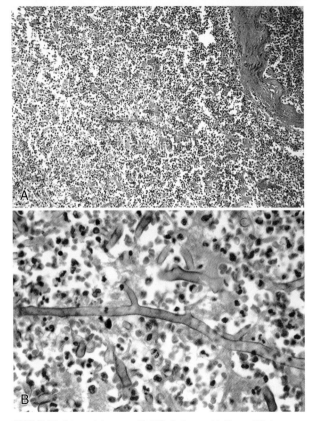

FIGURE 03-182. Zygomycosis (mucormycosis). (A) The fungi are recognizable even at this low-power magnification. (B) The hyphae are very broad (much more than *Aspergillus*), are nonseptate, and branch at 90 degrees. *(Courtesy R. Hay, MD, Institute of Dermatology, London, UK. From McKee PH, Calonje JE, Granter SR: Pathology of the Skin, ed 3, St. Louis, 2005, Mosby, Fig. 17.334.)*

Etiology
- The cause of mucormycosis is infection by a fungus of the *Zygomycetes* class (see "Definition").
- Infection by these ubiquitous organisms occurs in association with underlying conditions including diabetes mellitus, lymphoma, severe burns or trauma, prolonged postoperative course, multiple myeloma, hepatitis, cirrhosis, renal failure, steroid treatment, immunodeficiency states (e.g., AIDS), and use of contaminated Elastoplast bandages. Immunocompetent hosts may become infected in tropical climates.

Keys to Diagnosis

Clinical Manifestation(s)
- Most commonly the fungus gains entry to the body through the respiratory tract. The spores are deposited in the nasal turbinates and may be inhaled into the pulmonary alveoli. In cases of cutaneous mucormycosis, the spores are introduced directly into the skin lesion.

Physical Examination
- Cutaneous zygomycosis presents as nodular lesions (hematogenous seeding) or a wound infection. It involves primarily the epidermis and dermis following use of occlusive dressings that have not been properly sterilized (**Fig. 03-182**).

Diagnostic Tests
- Biopsy of infected tissue with direct light microscopy examination establishes the diagnosis within minutes of the biopsy in the case of nasopharyngeal infection. Typically the fungi appear as broad (10-20 μm in diameter) nonseptate hyphae with branches occurring at right angles.

DDx Differential Diagnosis

- Infection of the sites described previously by other organisms (bacterial [including tuberculosis and leprosy], viral, fungal, or protozoan)
- Noninfectious tissue necrosis (e.g., neoplasia, vasculitis, degenerative) of the sites described previously

Treatment

First Line
- Standard therapy for invasive mucormycosis is treatment with amphotericin B. Lipid preparations of amphotericin B may be less toxic (i.e., amphotericin B lipid complex, amphotericin B colloidal dispersion, and liposomal amphotericin B).

Second Line
- The role of flucytosine, rifampin, and tetracycline is controversial.

Third Line
- Surgical debridement or radical resection may be necessary.

Clinical Pearl(s)

- The hallmark of mucormycosis is vascular invasion and tissue necrosis. Black eschars and discharges should be closely evaluated. Diagnosis depends on the demonstration of the organism in the tissue of a biopsy specimen.

97. MYCOSIS FUNGOIDES

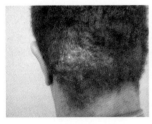

FIGURE 03-183. Weeping, nodular, spongy, violaceous lesion on the scalp of this patient with multiple oozing sites.

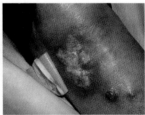

FIGURE 03-184. Advanced stage of mycosis fungiodes with ulcerated, indurated, necrotic tumor nodules on the leg of this elderly patient.

General Comments

Definition
- Mycosis fungoides is a T-cell lymphoproliferative disorder with characteristic cutaneous skin lesions and the potential to disseminate into lymph nodes and viscera.

Etiology
- The specific cause of mycosis fungoides is not known. Infection with the retrovirus HTLV-1 has been suspected, given the association of individuals infected with HTLV-1 and those with T-cell leukemia.

Keys to Diagnosis

Clinical Manifestation(s)

Mycosis fungoides characteristically progresses through three phases:

- A *premycotic phase* featuring scaly, erythematous patches that can last from months to years. During this stage the diagnosis can only be suspected because the histopathologic features are not definitive for mycosis fungoides. Lesions are pruritic and can appear anywhere but are usually found in sun-shielded areas. Parapsoriasis en plaques, poikilodermatous parapsoriasis, parapsoriasis lichenoides, and variegata are skin lesions suspicious of representing premycotic cutaneous T-cell lymphoma.

- The *infiltrative plaque phase* features raised, indurated erythematous palpable plaques that are pruritic and may be associated with alopecia (**Fig. 03-183**).

  Stage IA disease is defined as a patch or plaque skin disease involving less than 10% of the skin surface area and with absence of blood involvement or with low blood tumor burden (<5% of atypical T-cells [Sézary cells] in the peripheral blood).

  Stage IB disease is defined as a patch or plaque skin disease involving more than 10% of the skin surface area with absence of blood involvement or low blood tumor burden (<5% Sézary cells).

- The *tumor phase* is characterized by large, lumpy nodules arising from a premycotic patch, plaque, or unaffected skin and represents systemic infiltration and spreading. The tumors can be pruritic and large (>10 cm) and ulceration can occur (**Fig. 03-184**).

  Stage IIA and stage IIB diseases are defined by the presence of tumors with or without clinically abnormal peripheral lymph nodes with absence of blood involvement or low blood tumor burden.

  Stage III disease is defined by the presence of generalized erythroderma.

- Lymphadenopathy can occur during the plaque or tumor stages and may be regional or diffuse.

  Stage IVA disease is defined as a lymph node biopsy showing large clusters of atypical cells, more than six cells, or total effacement by atypical cells.

- Infiltration of the liver, spleen, lungs, bone marrow, kidney, stomach, and brain can occur.

- Stage IVB disease is defined by the presence of visceral involvement.

Physical Examination

- Findings on physical examination are variable depending on the stage (see "Clinical Manifestations").

Diagnostic Tests

- The diagnosis of mycosis fungoides is established by skin biopsy. This may be difficult to differentiate from other skin lesions in the early phases of the disease (e.g., premycotic patch or early plaque lesions) and therefore the diagnosis can only be suspected.

DDx Differential Diagnosis

- Contact dermatitis
- Atopic dermatitis
- Nummular dermatitis
- Parapsoriases
- Superficial fungal infections
- Drug eruptions
- Psoriasis
- Photodermatitis
- Alopecia mucinosa
- Lymphomatoid papulosis

R Treatment

- For dry, cracking skin, emollients (e.g., lanolin and petrolatum) are applied BID.
- Moisturizing lotion (e.g., ammonium lactate) is applied BID.
- Topical antibiotics are used on ulcerative tumors.
- Treatment of patients with stage IA limited patch or plaque phase include topical nitrogen mustard and PUVA therapy.
- Treatment of patients with stage IB and IIA disease is similar to stage IA, with topical nitrogen mustard or PUVA.
  Total skin electron beam therapy is considered in patients with thick plaques.
  Interferon alfa 5 million units SQ 3 times weekly can be considered in patients with stage IB or IIA disease.
  Retinoids in combination with PUVA are used in refractory cases. Isotretinoin 1 mg/kg/day or acitretin 25 to 50 mg/day is the standard dosing.
- Treatment of patients with stage IIB disease with generalized tumor and plaque disease includes total skin electron beam therapy in doses of 3000 to 3600 cGy given over 8 to 10 weeks, followed by adjuvant therapy with topical mustard.
- In patients developing diffuse erythroderma, stage III disease (e.g., Sézary syndrome, extracorporeal photopheresis), 8-methoxypsoralen is ingested and peripheral blood is exposed to UVA through a membrane filter.
- Interferon and other systemic chemotherapeutic agents (e.g., methotrexate, cyclophosphamide, doxorubicin, vincristine, and prednisone) are considered in disseminated mycosis fungoides, stage IV disease.

Clinical Pearl(s)

- In approximately 5% of cases of mycosis fungoides, the presentation may be a diffuse, painful, pruritive erythroderma with Sézary cells in the peripheral blood (known as *Sézary syndrome*).

98. NECROBIOSIS LIPOIDICA

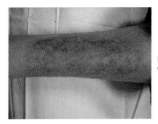

FIGURE 03-185 Atrophic, smooth, shiny lesion with telangiectasias in a diabetic patient.

 General Comments

Definition

■ Necrobiosis lipoidica is an inflammatory condition (also known as necrobiosis lipoidic diabeticorum) usually seen in diabetics. It is characterized by collagen degeneration manifesting primarily with pretebial skin lesions.

Etiology

■ The disease has a strong association with diabetes mellitus. It has been suggested that the lesions develop as a consequence of diabetic microangiopathy.

 Keys to Diagnosis

Clinical Manifestation(s)

■ The lesion usually manifests in the pretibial area (**Fig. 03-185**) in a diabetic patient.

Physical Examination

■ The characteristic lesion, sometimes referred to as a sclerodermatous plaque, is round or oval, circumscribed, and often has a slightly elevated rim. It is typically a few millimeters to several centimeters in diameter.
■ Newly acquired lesions are often red-brown, but with progression the center of the lesion becomes yellowish and the peripheral border may acquire a violaceous hue.
■ Larger plaques are usually irregular and more variably shaped. Scaling and telangiectasia may become evident.
■ Ulceration appears to be relatively common and has been reported in up to 13% of patients.

Diagnostic Tests

■ Skin biopsy
■ Fasting blood sugar, 2-hour postprandial glucose

Differential Diagnosis

- Xanthoma
- Morphea
- Granuloma annulare
- Vasculitis
- Lichen sclerosus

℞ **Treatment**

First Line
- Topical corticosteroids
- Improved glycemic control

Second Line
- Intralesional corticosteroids
- Systemic corticosteroids

Third Line
- Ticlopidine, pentoxifylline, aspirin, and dipyridamole

😀 **Clinical Pearl(s)**

- Fewer than 5% of diabetics have necrobiosis but more than 50% of patients with necrobiosis will have diabetes. Smoking and history of trauma may play a contributing role to the development of these lesions in diabetics.

99. NEVUS FLAMMEUS

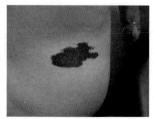

FIGURE 03-186. Red to purple port wine stain with irregular borders that has remained unchanged in this middle-aged man.

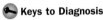 General Comments

Definition
- Nevus flammeus are congenital capillary malformations of the superficial cutaneous vasculature, also known as *port wine stains* (PWS).

Etiology
- Dilated dermal capillaries

Keys to Diagnosis

Clinical Manifestation(s)
- Initially, light pink to red macules appear, often following a dermatome distribution. Most commonly they affect the head and neck, but they can also affect other areas.
- Macules may undergo color change with time and may become studded with angiomatous nodules.

Physical Examination
- Pink/violaceous to red macules (**Fig. 03-186**). The size varies from barely noticeable to severely disfiguring.

Diagnostic Tests
- Ophthalmologic examination
- Brain MRI

Differential Diagnosis

- Capillary hemangioma
- Salmon patch
- Cherry angiomas
- Glomus tumor
- Lymphocytoma cutis

R Treatment

First Line
- Pulsed-dye laser started in infancy

Second Line
- Intense pulsed light source (IPLS)

Clinical Pearl(s)

- Nevus flammeus may be associated with ocular abnormalities or Sturge-Weber syndrome when involving the forehead, upper and lower eyelid, and side of the nose.

100. NEVI OF OTA AND ITO

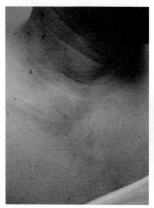

FIGURE 03-187. Hyperpigmentation of the right anterior chest and neck area due to excessive deposition of dermal melanocytes.

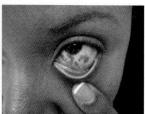

FIGURE 03-188. Blue-black pigmentation involving the sclera of the left eye in the distribution of the ophthalmic division of the trigeminal nerve, a common pattern for the nevus of Ota.

 General Comments

Definition

■ Nevi of Ota and Ito are dermal melanocytic lesions located on the face (nevus of Ota) or shoulders and neck (nevus of Ito). They are also known as nevus fuscocereleus, Hori nevus, and oculodermal melanosis.

Etiology

■ Unknown. Both lesions can be congenital or acquired.

Keys to Diagnosis

Clinical Manifestation(s)

■ Often present at birth, the lesions may enlarge and darken until the adult years.

■ These lesions are rare in those of Northern European descent and are more common in Asians and Japanese in particular.

Physical Examination
- Unilateral dark bluish pigmentation is seen affecting the cheek and eye (nevus of Ota) or the chest and shoulder region (nevus of Ito) (**Fig. 03-187**).
- Ocular involvement may reveal hyperpigmentation of the sclera (**Fig. 03-188**), iris, or conjunctiva.

Diagnostic Tests
- Generally none; biopsy if suspecting melanoma

 Differential Diagnosis

- Melanoma
- Blue nevus
- Melasma
- Late-onset dermal melanosis

 Treatment

First Line
- Laser ablation
- Topical bleaching

Clinical Pearl(s)

- These lesions are typically benign; however, rare malignant degeneration has been reported.

101. NOCARDIOSIS

General Comments

Definition
- Nocardiosis is an infection caused by aerobic actinomycetes found in soil and characterized by lung, soft tissue, or CNS involvement.

Etiology
- The most common *Nocardia* species leading to infection in humans are as follows:
  1. *N. asteroides* (causing more than 80% of the cases of pulmonary nocardiosis)
  2. *N. brasiliensis* (most common cause of mycetoma)
  3. *N. otitibiscaviarum*
- *N. asteroides* has two subgroups:
  1. *N. farcinica*
  2. *N. nova*

Keys to Diagnosis

Clinical Manifestation(s)

- Inhalation of *Nocardia* organisms is the most common mode of entry, and pneumonia is the most common presentation, with 75% manifesting with fever, chills, dyspnea, and a productive cough.

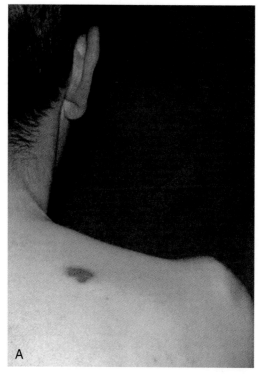

FIGURE 03-189. Nocardiosis. (A) This cutaneous nodule developed in an immunocompromised young male; (B) a different lesion is shown in close-up. *(Courtesy R. A. Marsden, St George's Hospital, London, UK. From McKee PH, Calonje JE, Granter SR: Pathology of the Skin, ed 3, St. Louis, 2005, Mosby, Fig. 17.220.)*

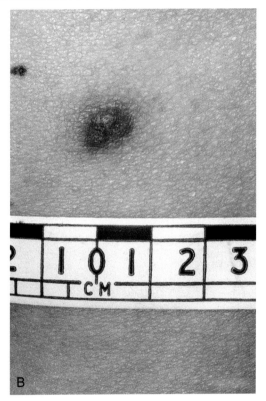

FIGURE 03-189, cont'd.

1. Presentation can be acute, subacute, or chronic.
2. Nocardiosis should be suspected if soft tissue abscesses or CNS tumors or abscesses form in conjunction with the pulmonary infection.
3. Pulmonary infection may spread into the pericardium, mediastinum, and superior vena cava.

Physical Examination

- Cutaneous disease usually occurs via direct inoculation of the organism as a result of skin puncture by a thorn or splinter, surgery, intravenous catheter use, or animal scratches or bites manifesting in the following conditions:
  1. Cellulitis
  2. Lymphocutaneous nodules appearing along lymphatic sites draining the infected puncture wound
  3. Mycetoma (*Madura foot*), a chronic, deep nodular infection usually involving the hands or feet that can cause skin breakdown, fistula formation, and spread along the fascial planes to infect surrounding skin, subcutaneous tissue, and bone (**Fig. 03-189**)

Diagnostic Tests

All patients with suspected nocardiosis need laboratory identification of the microorganism by obtaining sputum in the case of pneumonia, cultures of the infected skin lesions in mycetoma or lymphocutaneous disease, or the sampling of any purulent material (e.g., brain abscess, lung abscess, and pleural effusion).

- Gram's stain shows gram-positive beaded filaments with multiple branches.
- Gomori methenamine silver staining may detect the organism.
- *Nocardia* species are acid-fast on a modified Ziehl-Neelsen stain.
- *Nocardia* are slow-growing organisms, and colony growth in cultures may take up to 2 to 3 weeks.

DDx Differential Diagnosis

- Tuberculosis
- Lung abscess
- Lung tumor
- Other causes of pneumonia
- Actinomycosis
- Mycosis
- Cellulitis
- Coccidioidomycosis
- Histoplasmosis
- Aspergillosis
- Kaposi's sarcoma

℞ Treatment

- For any abscess formation: surgical drainage (e.g., skin, lung, or brain)
- For cutaneous infection: trimethoprim-sulfamethoxazole (TMX-SMX) (5 mg/kg/day divided in 2 doses)
- For severe infection, life-threatening pulmonary or disseminated disease, or CNS disease or in immunocompromised patients: two-drug therapy with TMP-SMX 15 mg/kg/day divided into 4 to 6 doses and amikacin 7.5 mg/kg/IV

every 12 hours; in patients with CNS disease, ceftriaxone 2 g/IV daily is substituted for amikacin

Clinical Pearl(s)

- Nocardiosis is not transmitted from person to person.
- Nocardiosis is found most commonly in patients who are immune compromised (e.g., patients receiving steroids or immunosuppressive therapy; those with lymphoma, leukemia, or lung cancer; transplant patients; and those with other pulmonary infections).

102. NUMMULAR ECZEMA

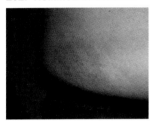

FIGURE 03-190. Pruritic, round, scaly erythematous lesion on the trunk with indistinct borders that help differentiate it from tinea corporis (potassium hydroxide preparation was also negative), which has sharper borders.

General Comments

Definition
- Nummular eczema, also known as discoid eczema, is a dermatitis manifesting with pruritic, coin-shaped lesions (**Fig. 03-190**).

Etiology
- Unknown. Chronic stress is often present.

Keys to Diagnosis

Clinical Manifestation(s)
- There are two peak ages of onset: it affects young women (15-30 years old) and middle-aged adults of both sexes.
- Early lesions are seen as papules or vesicles. Lesions may be exudative and crusted.

Physical Examination
- Patients present with single or multiple pruritic, coin-shaped, erythematous plaques with vesiculation, particularly involving the lower legs, forearms, and backs of hands.

Diagnostic Tests
- Usually no tests are necessary. Biopsy may be performed when diagnosis is in doubt. Patch testing is positive in nearly 30% of patients.

 Differential Diagnosis
- Psoriasis
- Atopic dermatitis
- Contact dermatitis
- Stasis dermatitis
- Tinea infection
- Scabies

R **Treatment**

First Line
- Topical corticosteroids

Second Line
- Topical steroid-antiseptic combination
- Topical steroid-antibiotic combination

Third Line
- Systemic corticosteroid

Clinical Pearl(s)
- The absence of a raised border distinguishes nummular eczema from ringworm.
- Secondary infection may result in disease flares. Lesions often yield staphylococci on cultures.

103. ONYCHOMYCOSIS (TINEA UNGUIUM)

 General Comments

Definition
- Onychomycosis is defined as a persistent fungal infection affecting the toenails and fingernails.

Etiology
- The most common causes of onychomycosis are dermatophyte, yeast, and nondermatophyte molds.
- The dermatophyte *Trichophyton rubrum* accounts for 80% of all nail infections caused by fungus.
- *Trichophyton interdigitale* and *Trichophyton mentagrophytes* are other fungi causing onychomycosis.

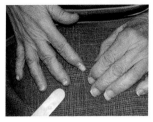

FIGURE 03-191. Tinea unguium of all nails of the right hand causing yellow-brown discoloration of the distal plate with elevation of the nail bed secondary to deposition of keratotic debris. Mycotic fingernail infection is usually unilateral and associated with bilateral involvement of the feet (referred to as "one-hand, two feet").

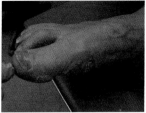

FIGURE 03-192. Onychomycosis commonly occurs in association with tinea pedis, as seen on the medial aspect of this patient's foot.

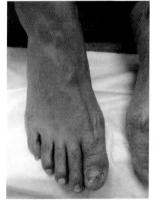

FIGURE 03-193. Tinea unguium occuring in association with tinea corporis seen more proximally on the dorsum of this patient's foot in an easily recognized ringworm configuration.

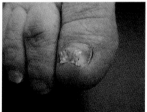

FIGURE 03-194. Distal and lateral subungual onychomycosis (DLSO) causing extensive hyperkeratosis and separation of the distal nail bed.

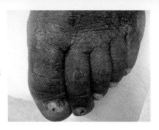

FIGURE 03-195. Proximal subungual onychomycosis (PSO), which starts at the nailfold and results in ultimate destruction of the entire nail. Note the aggressive tinea pedis infection involving the dorsum of the foot in this immunocompromised patient with HIV infection.

- The yeast *C. albicans* is responsible for 5% of the cases of onychomycosis.
- Nondermatophyte molds *Scopulariopsis brevicaulis* and *Aspergillus niger,* although rare, can also cause onychomycosis.

Keys to Diagnosis

Clinical Manifestation(s)

- Onychomycosis is most commonly found in people between the ages of 40 and 60 years.
- Onychomycosis rarely occurs before puberty.
- The incidence is 20 to 100 cases/1000 population.
- Toenail infection is four to six times more common than fingernail infection (**Fig. 03-191**).
- Onychomycosis affects men more often than women.
- Onychomycosis occurs more commonly in patients with diabetes, peripheral vascular disease, and any conditions resulting in the suppression of the immune system.
- Occlusive footwear, physical exercise followed by communal showering, and incompletely drying the feet predispose the individual to developing onychomycosis.
- Onychomycosis commonly occurs in association with tinea pedis (**Fig. 03-192**) and tinea corporis (**Fig. 03-193**)
- Onychomycosis is classified according to the clinical pattern of nail bed involvement. The main types are as follows:
  1. Distal and lateral subungual onychomycosis (DLSO) (**Fig. 03-194**)
  2. Superficial onychomycosis
  3. Proximal subungual onychomycosis (**Fig. 03-195**)
  4. Endonyx onychomycosis
  5. Total dystrophic onychomycosis

Physical Examination

- Onychomycosis causes nails to become thick, brittle, hard, distorted, and discolored (yellow to brown). Eventually, the nail may loosen, separate from the nail bed, and fall off.

Diagnostic Tests
- The diagnosis of onychomycosis is based on the clinical nail findings and confirmed by direct microscopy and culture.
- The workup of suspected onychomycosis is directed at confirming the diagnosis of onychomycosis by visualizing hyphae under the microscope or by culturing the organism.

 Differential Diagnosis
- Psoriasis
- Contact dermatitis
- Lichen planus
- Subungual keratosis
- Paronychia
- Infection (e.g., *Pseudomonas*)
- Trauma
- Peripheral vascular disease
- Yellow nail syndrome

 Treatment

First Line
- Terbinafine
  For toenails: 250 mg/day for 3 months
  For fingernails: 250 mg/day for 6 weeks
- Topical antifungal creams are used for early superficial nail infections.
  Miconazole 2% cream applied over the nail plate BID
  Clotrimazole 1% cream BID
- Ciclopirox, a topical nail lacquer antifungal agent (Penlac), is FDA approved for treatment of mild to moderate disease not involving the lunula.
- Poiatric debridement

Second Line
- Itraconazole
  For toenails: 200 mg QD for 3 months
  For fingernails: 200 mg PO BID for 7 days, followed by 3 weeks of no medicine, for two pulses
- Itraconazole is contraindicated in patients taking cisapride, astemizole, triazolam, midazolam, and terfenadine. Statins should be discontinued during itraconazole therapy. Itraconazole requires gastric acidity for absorption; patients should be advised not to take oral antacids, H2 blockers, or proton pump inhibitors while taking itraconazole.

Third Line
- Fluconazole
  For toenails: 150 to 300 mg once weekly, until infection clears
  For fingernails: 150 to 300 mg once weekly until infection clears

- Fluconazole is contraindicated in patients taking cisapride and terfenadine.
- All oral agents used for onychomycosis require periodic monitoring of liver function blood tests. Patients should be advised to watch for symptoms of drug-induced hepatitis (anorexia, fatigue, nausea, right upper quadrant pain) while taking these oral antifungal agents. They should stop their medication and contact their physician immediately if symptoms occur.
- Oral antifungal agents should not be initiated during pregnancy.
- Surgical removal of the nail plate is a treatment option; however, the relapse rate is high.

Clinical Pearl(s)

- Podiatry consultation is indicated in diabetic patients for proper instruction in foot care, footwear, and nail debridement or surgical removal of the toenail.
- Patients can attempt to prevent reinfection by wearing properly fitted shoes, avoiding public showers, and keeping feet and nails clean and dry.
- A disease-free toenail is reported to occur in approximately 25% to 50% of patients treated with the oral antifungal agents mentioned previously.

104. OSLER-RENDU-WEBER DISEASE

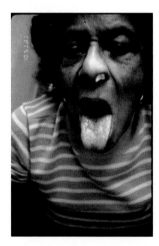

FIGURE 03-196. Multiple telangiectases are evident on the tongue and in the nose (recent epistaxis left nostril) of this patient with Osler-Rendu-Weber syndrome.

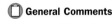 General Comments

Definition
- Osler-Rendu-Weber syndrome, also known as hereditary hemorrhic telengiectasia, is a disorder characterized by the appearance of multiple telengiectases on the face, mouth, lips, and other areas.

Etiology
- This is an autosomal dominant disorder with incomplete penetrance.

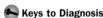 Keys to Diagnosis

Clinical Manifestation(s)
- Recurrent epistaxes and GI bleeds due to lesions on the oropharyngeal epithelium and gut are seen.

Physical Examination
- Telengiectasia lesions may be present on the lips, tongue (**Fig. 03-196**), nasal mucosa, retina, hands, chest, and lower extremities.

Diagnostic Tests
- CBC (including platelet count)
- Ferritin level, stool for occult blood
- Endoscopy (upper and lower)
- Angiography

DDx Differential Diagnosis

- Generalized essential telengiectasia
- Unilateral nevoid telengiectasia
- Scleroderma with CREST syndrome
- Rosacea
- Actinic keratosis
- Ataxia telengiectasia
- Venous hypertension
- Cushing's syndrome

R Treatment

First Line
- Laser ablation of symptomatic lesions

Second Line
- GI bleeding prophylaxis
- Angiographic embolization
- Segmental bowel resection

🦷 Clinical Pearl(s)

- Vascular abnormalities may result in portal hypertension, pulmonary AVMs with hemoptysis, cerebrovascular accidents, and hematuria in addition to GI bleeding and anemia.
- Genetic screening of first-degree relatives should be performed.

105. PAGET'S DISEASE OF THE BREAST

🗋 General Comments

Definition
- Paget's disease of the breast is a dermatologic manifestation of intraductal breast carcinoma.

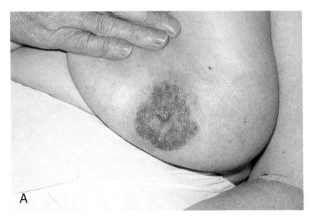

FIGURE 03-197. (A) Paget's disease affecting the areola, again strictly unilateral. (B) By contrast, this patient with eczema on the breast has sparing of the nipple and areola. *(Panel B courtesy Dr. G. Dawn. From White GA, Cox NH: Diseases of the Skin: A Color Atlas and Text, ed 2, St. Louis, 2006, Mosby, Fig. 33.50.)*

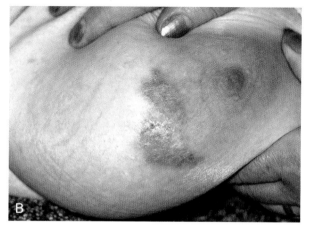

FIGURE 03-197, cont'd.

Etiology

■ The exact origin are unknown. Possibly, migration of either in situ or invasive carcinoma cells in the breast to nipple skin produces Paget's disease. Microscopically, typical large clear cells (Paget's cells) with pale and abundant cytoplasm and hyperchromatic nuclei with prominent nucleoli are found in the epidermal layer.

Keys to Diagnosis

Clinical Manifestation(s)

■ Onset is insidious, and the condition is often confused with eczema. Serosanguinous discharge may be present.

Physical Examination

■ A scaly, sore, eroding, bleeding ulcer of the nipple is seen on examination (**Fig. 03-197**).

Diagnostic Tests

■ Deep biopsy of nipple lesion
■ Mammography

DDx Differential Diagnosis

- Chronic dermatitis
- Florid papillomatosis of the nipple or nipple adenoma
- Eczema
- Lichen simplex
- Bowen's disease
- Intertrigo
- Melanoma
- Basal cell carcinoma
- Contact dermatitis
- Seborrheic dermatitis

R Treatment

- In some patients, Paget's disease of the nipple is the only finding when the breast is mammographically negative. Consideration should be given to wide excision of the nipple with or without radiation.
- In other patients, an additional invasive or in situ carcinoma is recognized. Either modified mastectomy or breast conservation treatment is warranted.
- The presence of underlying in situ or invasive carcinoma in the mastectomy specimen is seen in the majority of patients. In these cases, systemic adjuvant therapy is needed, depending on the extent of invasive carcinoma found.

Clinical Pearl(s)

- Paget's disease is more often associated with primary invasive or in situ carcinoma of the breast.

106. PARONYCHIA

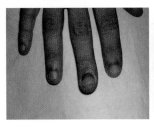

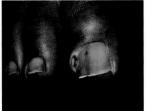

FIGURE 03-198. Chronic nail changes in a dishwasher with disappearance of the cuticle rendering this moist space vulnerable to *Pseudomonas* infection (hence the green discoloration under the nailplate of the third digit).

FIGURE 03-199. Acute onset of pain, redness, and swelling of the great toe with accumulation of pus in the lateral nail fold.

📋 General Comments

Definition

- Paronychia is a localized superficial infection or abscess of the lateral and proximal nail fold. Paronychia may be acute or chronic.

Etiology

- Any disruption of the seal between the proximal nail fold and the nail plate can cause paronychial infections.
- Acute paronychia is almost always bacterial in origin (e.g., *S. aureus* [most common], *Streptococcus pyogenes, Enterococcus faecalis, Proteus* and *Pseudomonas* species, and anaerobes).
- Chronic paronychia is commonly caused by *C. albicans* (70%), with bacterial organisms accounting for the remaining 30%.
- Trauma, nail biting, hangnails, diabetes, and chronic exposure to water (**Fig. 03-198**) are common predisposing features of paronychia.

🔑 Keys to Diagnosis

Clinical Manifestation(s)

- Acute paronychia affects males and females equally.
- Chronic paronychia more common in females than males (9:1).
- Acute paronychia most often occurs in children.
- Chronic paronychia usually presents in the fifth or sixth decade of life.
- Paronychia is the most common infection of the hand.
- Acute paronychia usually involves only one finger.
- Chronic paronychia may involve more than one finger.
- Acute paronychia usually involves the thumb.
- Chronic paronychia commonly involves the middle finger.
- Most acute paronychias with appropriate treatment resolve within 7 to 10 days.
- Untreated chronic paronychia leads to thickening and discoloration with eventual nail loss.

Physical Examination

- Acute paronychia usually presents with the sudden onset of redness, swelling, and pain with abscess or cellulitis formation in the nail fold. Fluid with purulence is often present (**Fig. 03-199**).
- Chronic paronychia is insidious, presenting with mild swelling and erythema of the nail folds.

Diagnostic Tests

- The diagnosis of paronychia is self-evident on physical examination.

Differential Diagnosis

- Herpetic whitlow
- Pyogenic granuloma
- Viral warts
- Ganglions
- Squamous cell carcinoma

℞ Treatment

First Line

- For acute paronychia without purulent drainage, warm soaks TID or QID are helpful. If pus is present, surgical drainage is required.
- For chronic paronychia, avoid chronic immersion in water or exposure to moisture.
- First-generation cephalosporin (e.g., cephalexin 250-500 mg QID) or penicillinase-resistant penicillin (e.g., dicloxacillin 250-500 mg QID) are usually the antibiotics of choice for acute paronychia.
- Surgical drainage is indicated if purulent discharge is noted.
- A no. 11 blade scalpel is used to lift the lateral perionychium and proximal eponychium off the nail, facilitating drainage.
- If the pus is located beneath the nail, the lateral edge of the nail can be lifted off the nail bed and excised.
- If no fungal organism is found, tincture of iodine (2 drops BID) helps keep the nail and skin dry.

Second Line

- Alternative antibiotic choices include clindamycin and amoxicillin-clavulanate potassium
- Chronic paronychia caused by *C. albicans* is treated with topical antifungal agents (e.g., miconazole or ketoconazole applied TID).

Third Line

- Unresponsive cases may be treated with itraconazole or fluconazole but should be done in consultation with an infectious disease specialist.

Clinical Pearl(s)

- The GI tract, including the mouth and bowel, or the genitourinary (GU) tract in women, are the usual sources of *C. albicans* in chronic paronychia.
- Osteomyelitis is a potential complication of paronychia.

107. PEDICULOSIS (LICE)

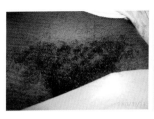

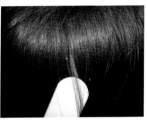

FIGURE 03-200. Heavy infestation of pubic lice, *Phthirus pubis*, with obvious presence of multiple nits on hair shafts.

FIGURE 03-201. Head lice infestation consisting of small, flaky-appearing, white, oval lice eggs on the hair shaft, commonly referred to as nits.

General Comments

Definition

- Pediculosis is lice infestation. Humans can be infested with three kinds of lice: *Pediculus capitis* (head louse), *Pediculus corporis* (body louse), and *Phthirus pubis* (pubic, or crab, louse (**Fig. 03-200**). Lice feed on human blood and deposit their eggs (nits) on the hair shafts (head lice and pubic lice) and along the seams of clothing (body lice). Nits generally hatch within 7 to 10 days. Lice are obligate human parasites and cannot survive away from their hosts for longer than 7 to 10 days.

Etiology

- Lice are transmitted by close personal contact or use of contaminated objects (e.g., combs, clothing, bed linen, hats).

Keys to Diagnosis

Clinical Manifestation(s)

- Pruritus with excoriation may be caused by hypersensitivity reaction, inflammation from saliva, and fecal material from the lice.
- Head lice is most commonly found in the back of the head and neck, behind the ears.
- Scratching can result in pustules and crusting.

Physical Examination

- Nits can be identified by examining hair shafts (**Fig. 03-201**).
- The presence of nits on clothes is indicative of body lice.

- Lymphadenopathy may be present (cervical adenopathy with head lice, inguinal lymphadenopathy with pubic lice).

Diagnostic Tests

- Diagnosis is made by seeing the lice or their nits. Combing hair with a fine-toothed comb is recommended because visual inspection of the hair and scalp may miss more than 50% of infestations.
- Wood's light examination is useful to screen a large number of children: live nits fluoresce, empty nits have a gray fluorescence, nits with unborn louse reveal white fluorescence.

DDx Differential Diagnosis

- Seborrheic dermatitis
- Scabies
- Eczema
- Other: pilar casts, trichonodosis (knotted hair), monilethrix

R Treatment

- Patients with body lice should discard infested clothes and improve their hygiene.
- Combing out nits is a widely recommended but unproven adjunctive therapy.
- Personal items such as combs and brushes should be soaked in hot water for 15 to 30 minutes.
- Close contacts and household members should also be examined for the presence of lice.

First Line

- Permethrin is available over the counter (1% permethrin) or by prescription (5% permethrin). It should be applied to the hair and scalp and rinsed out after 10 minutes. A repeat application is generally not necessary in patients with head lice. It can be applied to clean, dry hair and left on overnight (8-14 hours) under a shower cap.
- Lindane 1% are pyrethrin S are available as shampoos or lotions. They are applied to the affected area and washed off in 5 minutes; treatment should be repeated in 7 to 10 days to destroy hatching nits. Resistance to this medication is increasing. Lindane is potentially neurotoxic and should be avoided in infants and children weighing less than 50 kg.
- Malathion is effective in head lice. It is available by prescription. Use should be avoided in children younger than 2 years. It is not commonly used due to its objectionable odor, fear of flammability, and prolonged application time (8-12 hours).
- Eyelash infestation can be treated with the application of petroleum jelly rubbed into the eyelashes three times a day for 5 to 7 days. The application of baby shampoo to the eyelashes and brows three or four times a day for 5 days is also effective. The use of fluorescein drops applied to the lids and eyelashes is also toxic to lice.

Second Line

■ In patients who have previously failed treatment or in whom resistance with 1% permethrin cream rinse occurs, a 10-day course of trimethoprim-sulfamethoxazole (TMP-SMX) 8 mg/kg/day in divided doses is an effective treatment for head lice infestation, especially for eyelash infestations with *Phthirus pubis*.

Third Line

■ Ivermectin, an antiparasitic drug, given in a single oral dose of 200 mcg/kg is effective for head lice resistant to other treatments (currently not FDA approved for pediculosis).

🝰 Clinical Pearl(s)

■ Infestation of the eyelashes is most often seen in children and may indicate sexual abuse.
■ The chance of acquiring pubic lice from one sexual exposure with an infested partner is greater than 90% (most contagious STD known).
■ Body lice is most common in conditions of poor hygiene.
■ Patients with pubic lice should notify their sexual contacts. Sex partners within the last month should be treated.
■ Parents of patients should also be educated that head lice infestation (unlike body lice) does not indicate poor hygiene.

108. PEMPHIGUS VULGARIS

🛈 General Comments

Definition

■ Pemphigus refers to a group of rare, potentially fatal, chronic, autoimmune blistering diseases of the skin and mucous membranes.
■ Pemphigus has four main subtypes:
  1. Pemphigus vulgaris (PV)
     Pemphigus vegetans, a rare clinical variant of PV
  2. Pemphigus foliaceus (PF)
     Pemphigus erythematosus, a variant of PF
  3. Paraneoplastic pemphigus
  4. IgA pemphigus
■ Pemphigus vulgaris is the most common form of pemphigus and refers to an intraepidermal autoimmune mucocutaneous blistering disorder characterized by the formation of a flaccid blister.

Etiology

■ Pemphigus is an autoimmune disease caused by autoantibodies binding to antigens within the epithelial layer of the skin.

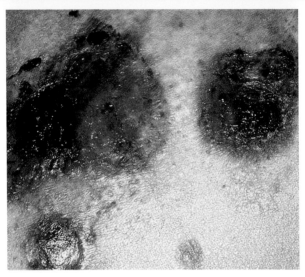

FIGURE 03-202. Pemphigus vulgaris. Because the blisters are superficial, erosions are more commonly encountered. *(Courtesy the Institute of Dermatology, London, UK. From McKee PH, Calonje JE, Granter SR: Pathology of the Skin, ed 3, St. Louis, 2005, Mosby, Fig. 4.4.)*

🦴 Keys to Diagnosis

Clinical Manifestation(s)

History

- Multiple oropharyngeal mucosal lesions typically occur first; these are followed within several weeks or months by a generalized bullous eruption involving the skin.
- Lesions are fragile and rupture easily, leaving painful, denuded, crusted erosions, which may be the only presenting symptom.
- Pain associated with oral mucosal blistering often results in dysphagia and hoarseness in voice.
- Pemphigus is usually not pruritic.

Physical Examination
- Anatomic distribution:
  - Oral mucosa
  - Can also involve the pharynx, larynx, vagina, penis, anus, and conjunctival mucosa
  - Generalized cutaneous involvement
- Lesion configuration:
  - All stratified squamous epithelium can become involved
- Lesion morphology:
  - Flaccid bullae
  - Commonly, denuded crusting and erosion
- *Nikolsky's sign:* nonspecific but clinically sensitive sign in which clinician applies sliding pressure to skin, causing separation of superficial epidermal layer of skin from basal layer (**Fig. 03-202**)

Diagnostic Tests
- The diagnosis of pemphigus vulgaris should be suspected in patients with oral lesions and flaccid bullae on the skin.
- Specific laboratory tests and histology and immunofluorescence testing of skin biopsy specimens can establish the diagnosis.
- Autoantibodies can be detected in the serum by indirect immunofluorescence assays.
- Skin biopsy reveals intraepidermal bulla formation, also called acantholysis (loss of cell adhesion between the epidermal cells).
- Direct and indirect immunofluorescence studies of the lesion show deposits of IgG and C3 in the epidermal layers of the skin.

DDx Differential Diagnosis
- Bullous pemphigoid
- Cicatricial pemphigoid
- Behçet's syndrome
- Erythema multiforme
- Systemic lupus erythematosus
- Aphthous stomatitis
- Dermatitis herpetiformis
- Drug eruptions

R Treatment
First Line
- For mild cases, topical or intralesional steroids, triamcinolone acetonide 5 to 10 mg/mL can be used for individual lesions. Topicals used for prevention of secondary infections on skin lesions include gentamicin and tetracycline.

- Systemic corticosteroids are the cornerstone of therapy and critical to eliminating the inflammatory component of PV. They are very effective and work rapidly but are associated with significant complications, such as secondary infections, hypertension, osteoporosis, aseptic necrosis, and Cushing's syndrome.
- For more severe cases of PV, systemic corticosteroids are indicated at high dosages: prednisone 1 mg/kg/day, titrating the dose to a clinical response. The drug is tapered as the condition is improved. The duration of treatment is variable; however, one should expect long-term management. Initial treatment duration and dosing changes usually occur at 6 to 8 weeks.

Second Line
- Adjuvant therapy such as immunosuppressants, antiinflammatories, chemotherapeutic agents, and biologics (e.g., Rituximab) are tried in patients as a steroid-sparing mechanism:
  Azathioprine 50 to 100 mg/day; treatment duration and dosing is determined by clinical response
  Cyclophosphamide 1 to 3 mg/kg/day
  Cyclosporine, mycophenolate

Third Line
- Dapsone 25 to 100 mg/day, low-dose methotrexate, hydroxychlorine, and rituximab (monoclonal antibody) are third-line treatments.

 Clinical Pearl(s)
- PV, unlike bullous pemphigoid, rarely occurs in the elderly population.

109. PEUTZ-JEGHERS SYNDROME

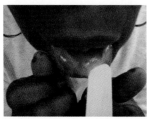

FIGURE 03-203. Hyperpigmented macules on the thumbs of both hands and lower lip in a patient with Peutz-Jeghers syndrome.

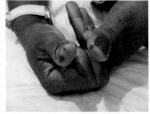

FIGURE 03-204. Dark macules on both thumbs of a patient who has had multiple hamartomas removed from the large and small bowel.

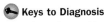 **General Comments**

Definition
- Peutz-Jeghers is a hereditary polyposis syndrome characterized by periorifacial pigmentation and GI polyps.

Etiology
- Autosomal dominant with incomplete penetrance

Keys to Diagnosis

Clinical Manifestation(s)
- The syndrome manifests with gastrointestinal symptoms, small bowel obstruction, intussusception, and GI bleeding.
- Disease expression can be characterized by the following:
- Small and large intestinal hamartomas with bands of smooth muscle in the lamina propria
- Pigmented lesions around the mouth (lips and buccal mucosa [**Fig. 03-203**]), nose, hands, feet, genital, and perineal areas
- Ovarian tumors
- Sertoli cell testicular tumors
- Airway polyps
- Pancreatic cancer
- Breast cancer
- Urinary tract polyps

Physical Examination
- Pigmented macules around the mouth, eyes, hands (**Fig. 03-204**), and anus are seen.

Diagnostic Tests
- Colonoscopies with polypectomies
- Screening for breast cancer, testicular cancer, possibly ovarian cancer

DDx Differential Diagnosis

- Familial adenomatous polyposis
- Juvenile polyposis
- Turcot syndrome
- Cowden diseae

Treatment

First Line
- For GI lesions: colonoscopies with polypectomies
- For skin lesions: Ruby laser

Second Line
- For skin lesions: Q-switched Nd:YAG laser, carbon dioxide laser

Third Line
- For skin lesions: cryosurgery, surgical excision, dermabrasion

 Clinical Pearl(s)

Cumulative lifetime cancer risk is as follows:
- Colon cancer: 39%
- Stomach cancer: 29%
- Small intestine cancer: 13%
- Pancreatic cancer: 36%
- Breast cancer: 54%
- Ovarian cancer: 10%
- Sertoli cell tumor: 9%
- Overall cancer risk: 93%

110. PILAR CYST (WEN)

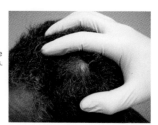

FIGURE 03-205. A dome-shaped, painless nodule on the scalp with atrophy of overlying hair follicles. Note the lack of a central punctum, which distinguishes a wen from an epidermal cyst.

 General Comments

Definition
- Pilar cysts, also known as wen or trichilemmal, are lesions found on the scalp in 90% of cases (**Fig. 03-205**).

Etiology
- Unknown

 Keys to Diagnosis

Clinical Manifestation(s)
- They present as smooth, yellowish, dome-shaped intradermal swellings and are more common in females.

Physical Examination
- Typically the cyst is encapsulated, and uncomplicated lesions readily shell out at surgery.

Diagnostic Tests
- None

DDx Differential Diagnosis

- Epidermoid cyst
- Lipoma
- Sebaceous cyst
- Dermoid cyst
- Pilomatricoma

R Treatment

- Surgical excision

Clinical Pearl(s)

- In contrast to epidermoid cysts, pilar cysts are characteristically devoid of a punctum.

111. PINWORMS

General Comments

Definition
- Pinworms are a noninvasive infestation of the intestinal tract.

Etiology
- Pinworms are caused by *Enterobius vermicularis,* a helminth of the nematode family. It is the most common intestinal nematode, with approximately 30,000 cases/year in the United States. They are distributed worldwide but are most common in temperate climates.
- The prevalence of pinworm infection is lowest in infants and reaches highest infection rate in school-age children (5-14 years old).
- Eggs are infective within 6 hours of oviposition and may remain so for 20 days.
- Clusters are found in families, institutionalized persons, and homosexual men.

Keys to Diagnosis

Clinical Manifestation(s)
- Most infested persons are asymptomatic.
- Perianal itching is the most common reported symptom, with scratching leading to excoriation and sometimes secondary infection.
- Rarely, insomnia, irritability, anorexia, and weight loss are described.

Physical Examination
- Perianal excoriation from scratching is seen on examination.

Diagnostic Tests
- Adult worms or eggs must be identified. *E. vermicularis* ova are ovoid but flattened on one side and measure approximately 56 by 27 μm.

 Differential Diagnosis
- Perianal itching related to poor hygiene
- Hemorrhoidal disease and anal fissures
- Perineal yeast/fungal infections

℞ **Treatment**

First Line
- A single dose of albendazole (400 mg) with a second dose given 2 weeks later is highly effective.
- Other infected family members, classmates, or residents of long-term care facilities should be treated at the same time as the index case.

Second Line
- A single dose of mebendazole (100 mg) can be given, with a repeat dose given after 2 weeks.

Third Line
- Pyrantel pamoate (11 mg/kg up to 1 g) can prevent against *E. vermicularis* infestation. It is available as a suspension and has minimal toxicity (mild transient GI symptoms, headache, drowsiness). A repeat dose after 2 weeks is recommended because of the frequency of reinfection and autoinfection.

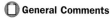 **Clinical Pearl(s)**
- The eggs can be identified on transparent tape placed on the perianal skin upon awakening. (NOTE: Five consecutive negative tests rule out the diagnosis.) A single examination detects 50% of infections, three examinations detect 90%, and five examinations detect 99%.

112. PITYRIASIS ALBA

📋 **General Comments**

Definition
- Pityriasis alba is a common form of chronic dermatitis usually affecting the face of preadolescent children and manifesting with hypopigmented lesion with indistinct borders.

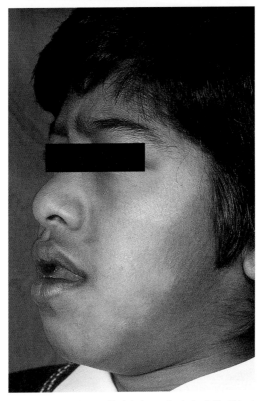

FIGURE 03-206. Pityriasis alba. There is striking leukoderma on the cheek and chin, which are commonly affected sites. *(Courtesy R. A. Marsden, MD, St George's Hospital, London, UK. From McKee PH, Calonje JE, Granter SR: Pathology of the Skin, ed 3, St. Louis, 2005, Mosby, Fig. 5.48.)*

Etiology
- Unknown. Prevalence in the U.S. population is 2%.

 Keys to Diagnosis

Clinical Manifestation(s)
- The skin lesions are seen most commonly in the face.
- The condition usually resolves spontaneously after months or years.

Physical Examination
- Early lesions present as slightly scaly, asymptomatic or mildly pruritic, round to oval pink plaques measuring from 0.5 to more than 5 cm in diameter, which later appear as scaly, hypopigmented lesions (**Fig. 03-206**).

Diagnostic Tests
- No tests are usually necessary. A potassium hydroxide preparation can be used to rule out superficial fungal infections.

 Differential Diagnosis

- Eczema
- Tinea
- Vitiligo
- Psoriasis
- Chemical leukoderma

 Treatment

First Line
- Observation (benign, self-resolving lesions)

Second Line
- Topical corticosteroids

 Clinical Pearl(s)

- Gentle sunlight exposure following use of topical steroids may accelerate resolution of hypopigmented lesions.

113. PITYRIASIS ROSEA

 General Comments

Definition
- Pityriasis rosea is a common, self-limiting skin eruption of unknown etiology.

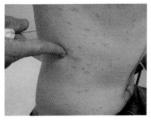

FIGURE 03-207. The earliest lesion of pityriasis rosea is referred to as the herald patch. Multiple smaller lesions subsequently follow and are distributed mainly on the trunk.

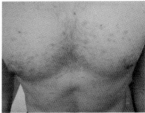

FIGURE 03-208. Multiple, oval-shaped, salmon-colored, scaling patches associated with mild pruritus and low-grade fever.

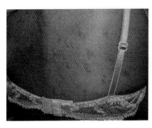

FIGURE 03-209. Violaceous to dark brown lesions in an African-American patient distributing along skin lines in a drooping pine tree fashion. Note the fine scale confined to the interior of the lesion, referred to as the collarette.

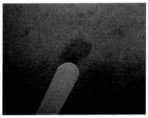

FIGURE 03-210. Raised, fine scale within the confines of the lesion is often called the collarette. This helps to distinguish pityriasis rosea from ringworm in which scale forms at the leading edge.

Etiology

■ Unknown, possibly viral (picornavirus)

Keys to Diagnosis

Clinical Manifestation(s)

■ Most cases of pityriasis rosea occur between ages 10 and 35 years; mean age is 23 years.
■ The incidence of disease is highest in the fall and spring.
■ Most patients are asymptomatic; pruritus is the most common symptom.
■ History of recent fatigue, headache, sore throat, and low-grade fever is present in approximately 25% of cases.

Physical Examination

- The initial lesion (herald patch) (**Fig. 03-207**) precedes the eruption by approximately 1 to 2 weeks; it typically measures 3 to 6 cm, is round to oval, and most commonly is located on the trunk.
- The eruptive phase follows within 2 weeks and peaks after 7 to 14 days.
- Lesions are most commonly located in the lower abdominal area. They have a salmon-pink appearance in Caucasians (**Fig. 03-208**) and a hyperpigmented appearance in African Americans (**Fig. 03-209**).
- Most lesions are 4 to 5 mm in diameter. The center has a "cigarette paper" appearance, and the border has a characteristic ring of scale (collarette) (**Fig. 03-210**).
- Lesions occur in a symmetric distribution and follow the cleavage lines of the trunk (Christmas tree pattern)
- The number of lesions varies from a few to hundreds.

Diagnostic Tests

- The presence of a herald lesion and characteristic rash are diagnostic. Skin scrapings for mycologic examination and biopsy are generally reserved for atypical cases.

DDx Differential Diagnosis

- Tinea corporis (can be ruled out by potassium hydroxide examination)
- Secondary syphilis (absence of herald patch, positive serologic test for syphilis)
- Psoriasis
- Nummular eczema
- Drug eruption: medications that may cause rashes similar to pityriasis rosea include clonidine, captopril, interferon, bismuth, barbiturates, gold, hepatitis B vaccine, and imatinib mesylate
- Viral exanthem
- Eczema
- Lichen planus
- Tinea versicolor (lesions are more brown and borders are not as ovoid)

R Treatment

First Line

- The disease is self-limited and generally does not require any therapeutic intervention. Emollients may be helpful.
- Topical corticosteroids may be used.
- Direct sun exposure or use of ultraviolet light within the first week of eruption is beneficial in decreasing the severity of disease.
- Oral antihistamines may be used in patients with significant pruritus.

Second Line

- UVB phototherapy

Third Line
- Prednisone tapered over 2 weeks in patients with severe pruritus

Clinical Pearl(s)
- The patient should experience spontaneous complete resolution of the rash within 4 to 8 weeks.
- Reassure the patient that the disease is not contagious and its course is benign.

114. POLYARTERITIS NODOSA

General Comments

Definition
- Polyarteritis nodosa (PAN) is a vasculitic syndrome involving medium to small arteries, characterized histologically by necrotizing inflammation of the arterial media and inflammatory cell infiltration.

Etiology
- Unknown. Hepatitis B virus–associated PAN appears to be an immune complex–mediated disease.

Keys to Diagnosis

Clinical Manifestation(s)
- Typical presentation is subacute, with onset of constitutional symptoms over weeks to months
- Weight loss, nausea, vomiting
- Testicular pain or tenderness
- Myalgias, weakness, or leg tenderness
- Neuropathy (mononeuritis multiplex), foot drop
- Abdominal pain after meals, hematemesis, hematochezia, hypertension

Physical Examination
- Cutaneous findings include livedo reticularis and ulceration of digits and shins (**Fig. 03-211**).
- Asymmetric polyarthritis (tending to involve large joints of lower extremities) is seen; true synovitis occurs only in a minority of patients.
- Fever may be present (polyarteritis nodosa is often a cause of fever of unknown origin) and can range from intermittent, low-grade fevers to high fevers with chills.
- Tachycardia is common and often striking.

Diagnostic Tests
- Elevated BUN or creatinine and a positive test for hepatitis B virus or hepatitis C can indicate a diagnosis of PAN.

- Laboratory evaluation, arteriography, and biopsy of small or medium arteries can confirm diagnosis. Clinical manifestations are variable and depend on the arteries involved and the organs affected (e.g., kidney involvement occurs in approximately 80% of cases).
- The presence of any 3 of the following 10 items allows the diagnosis of polyarteritis nodosa with a sensitivity of 82% and a specificity of 86%:
  1. Weight loss more than 4 kg
  2. Livedo reticularis

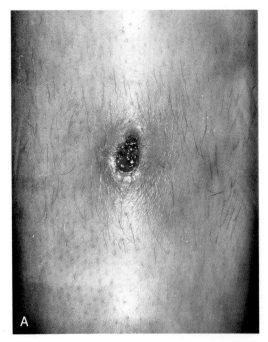

FIGURE 03-211. Polyarteritis nodosa. (A) A sharply defined ulcer with an indurated purplish border on the shin. (B) Multiple ulcers, nodules, and foci of livedo reticularis. *(Courtesy R. A. Marsden, MD, St George's Hospital, London, UK. From McKee PH, Calonje JE, Granter SR: Pathology of the Skin, ed 3, St. Louis, 2005, Mosby, Fig. 15.26.)*

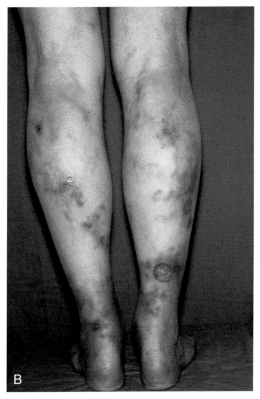

FIGURE 03-211, cont'd.

3. Testicular pain or tenderness
4. Myalgias, weakness, or leg tenderness
5. Neuropathy
6. Diastolic blood pressure greater than 90 mm Hg
7. Elevated BUN or creatinine

8. Positive test for hepatitis B virus
9. Arteriography revealing small or large aneurysms and focal constrictions between dilated segments
10. Biopsy specimen of small or medium artery containing WBC

DDx Differential Diagnosis

- Cryoglobulinemia
- SLE
- Infections (e.g., SBE, trichinosis, *Rickettsia*)
- Lymphoma

R Treatment

First Line
- Prednisone 1 to 2 mg/kg/day

Second Line
- Cyclophosphamide

Third Line
- Azathioprine, methotrexate
- Intravenous immune globulin

Clinical Pearl(s)

- The 5-year survival is less than 20% in untreated patients. Treatment with corticosteroids increases survival to approximately 50%. Usage of both corticosteroids and immunosuppressive drugs may increase 5-year survival more than 80%. Poor prognostic signs are severe renal or GI involvement.

115. POLYMORPHOUS LIGHT ERUPTION

General Comments

Definition
- Polymorhous (polymorphic) light eruption is a dermatosis following exposure to ultraviolet light.

Etiology
- Ultraviolet light exposure. The disease is more common in people residing in northern latitudes, occurring most often in spring and summer.

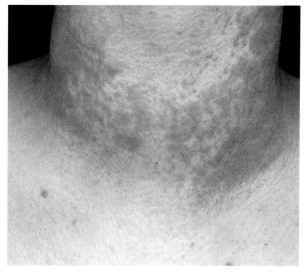

FIGURE 03-212. Polymorphous light eruption. The eruption is typically symmetric and is usually pruritic. *(Courtesy the Institute of Dermatology, London, UK. From McKee PH, Calonje JE, Granter SR: Pathology of the Skin, ed 3, St. Louis, 2005, Mosby.)*

 ## Keys to Diagnosis

Clinical Manifestation(s)

- Most patients require less than 30 minutes of associated sun exposure to elicit clinical lesions. Onset of lesions following light exposure typically takes 18 to 24 hours.

Physical Examination

- The face, chest, upper back, and extremities are the most common sites of involvement.
- Erythematous papules, vesicles, or plaques are seen following exposure to ultraviolet light (**Fig. 03-212**).

Diagnostic Tests

- If diagnosis is unclear, possible testing may include skin biopsy, phototesting, and ANA and lupus antibody tests.

- Either the UVA or UVB part of the light spectrum may cause lesions. In cases where the diagnosis is in doubt, phototesting may be necessary.

 Differential Diagnosis

- Reticular erythematous mucinosis (Clinically, polymorphous light eruption resolves once exposure to sunlight has ceased, in contrast to the persistent lesions of reticular erythematous mucinosis.)
- Lymphocytic infiltration (Histologically the presence of marked papillary edema favors polymorphic light eruption.)
- SLE (Most cases of polymorphic light eruption are negative with immunofluorescence testing.)

®️ **Treatment**

First Line
- Limit sun exposure. Use sunscreens and wear protective clothing.

Second Line
- PUVA therapy, narrowband or broadband phototherapy

Third Line
- Hydroxychloroquinine
- Beta carotene

😬 **Clinical Pearl(s)**

- The disease is more common in people residing in northern latitudes, occurring most often in spring and summer.

116. PORPHYRIA CUTANEA TARDA (PCT)

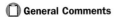 **General Comments**

Definition
- *Porphyria* is a term encompassing several related disorders caused by reduced hepatic uroporphirinogen decarboxylase enzyme activity. The resulting excess porphyrins result in cutaneous photosensitivity. PCT is the most common type of porphyria.

Etiology
- There are two main forms: familial and sporadic.
- The familial form exhibits an autosomal dominant inheritance, and its onset is earlier than the sporadic form.
- The disease is related to many different mutations in the URO-D gene. Eighty percent of patients have the sporadic form.

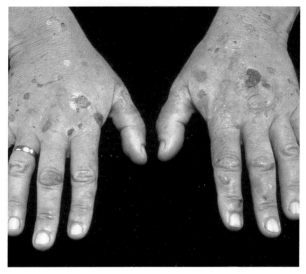

FIGURE 03-213. Porphyria cutanea tarda. There are numerous ruptured blisters. Milia are also evident. *(Courtesy the Institute of Dermatology, London, UK. From McKee PH, Calonje JE, Granter SR: Pathology of the Skin, ed 3, St. Louis, 2005, Mosby.)*

 Keys to Diagnosis

Clinical Manifestation(s)

- It usually manifests in middle age and shows a marked male predominance.
- Typically, blisters occur on light-exposed skin and are traumatically or actinically induced.
- Cutaneous fragility is usually marked. The blisters are slow to heal and leave superficial atrophic scars. Hypertrichosis and premature aging with chronic actinic damage are usual, and sclerodermatous changes may be marked.

Physical Examination

- Cutaneous bullae, hypertrichosis, scarring, sclerodermoid features, dyspigmentation, and fragility (**Fig. 03-213**) are seen on examination.

Diagnostic Tests

- Laboratory testing includes porphyrin levels in plasma, urine and feces, ALT, aspartate aminotransferase (AST), serum ferritin, hepatitis C serology, HIV, FBS, and ANA.
- Direct immunofluorescence of biopsy specimens reveals immunoglobulin (particularly IgG and to a lesser extent IgM) in the papillary dermis.
- The diagnosis is confirmed by the presence of uroporphyrin and heptacarboxylic porphyrins in urine and plasma and by the presence of isocoproporphyrin in feces.

 Differential Diagnosis

- Pseudoporphyria
- Porphyria variegata
- Polymorphos light eruption
- Bullous pemphigoid
- Bullous lupus

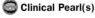 **Treatment**

First Line

- Protect skin from sunlight exposure and trauma.
- Perform ferrodepletion by serial phlebotomy.
- Administer antiviral drugs for PCT associated with hepatitis C or HIV.

Second Line

- Chelate with desferrioxamine.
- Increase porphyrin excretion with hydroxychloroquine.

Third Line

- Interferon alpha
- Plasmapherisis, plasma exchange

Clinical Pearl(s)

- PCT may be precipitated by many exogenous factors, including alcohol abuse, iron overload, childbirth, and sun exposure. Hepatitis C and HIV infection are also often associated with PCT.

117. PSEUDOFOLLICULITIS BARBAE (INGROWN HAIRS, RAZOR BUMPS)

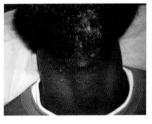 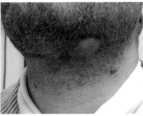

FIGURE 03-214. Painful perifollicular papules and pustules occurring commonly in the curly-haired beard area of African-American and Hispanic males.

FIGURE 03-215. Keloids and abscess formation complicating pseudofolliculitis barbae.

General Comments

Definition
■ Pseudofolliculitis is a chronic inflammatory disorder of hair-bearing areas affecting individuals who shave closely on a regular basis.

Etiology
■ Transepithelial or transfollicular penetration by the sharpened hair remnant results in a foreign body reaction.

Keys to Diagnosis

Clinical Manifestation(s)
■ Pseudofolliculitis occurs most often in individuals with curly hair. It is most common in African-American individuals.
■ The condition is seen most commonly on the neck and face and around the mouth and chin.

Physical Examination
■ The presence of papules, pustules, and postinflammatory hyperpigmentation in the shave site, most typically on the beard area (**Fig. 03-214**), is noted.
■ Hair sometimes grows sideways. Growth grooves and hypertrophic or keloidal scarring may also be present (**Fig. 03-215**). Comedones are absent.

Diagnostic Tests
■ Tests are generally not necessary. Skin biopsy may be performed in rare cases.

Differential Diagnosis

- Acne
- Folliculitis
- Tinea barbae
- Rosacea

℞ Treatment

First Line

- Stop shaving. Beard growth will lessen the number of inflammatory lesions.
- If shaving is necessary, the embedded hair should be lifted, not plucked prior to shaving. Presoaking the area with a hot, wet face cloth will allow the hairs to swell and lift.
- Proper shaving technique consists of shaving in the direction of hair growth, not against it. Shaving must be performed daily. The hairs should be shaved neither too close nor too long.
- Use of special electric razors that cut the hair above the skin surface to prevent ingrowth from below is beneficial. Use of hair clippers to cut hair not so close as to allow transfollicular penetration is also useful.

Second Line

- Laser depilation can destroy surface pigment along with the hair bulb and can result in white marks in individuals with dark skin.
- Chemical depilatories may be used to dissolve the hair.

Third Line

- Surgical depilation may be performed, but side effects may include wound edge necrosis.
- Topical antibiotic preparations (clindamycin, erythromycin, benzoyl peroxide) are sometimes used to reduce bacterial colonization, but the rationale for their use is questionable.
- Retinoic acid may be effective but can cause irritation.

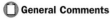 Clinical Pearl(s)

- Use of antibiotics should generally be avoided because the inflammation is due to a foreign body reaction and not a pyoderma.

118. PSEUDOXANTHOMA ELASTICUM

🗋 General Comments

Definition

- Pseudoxanthoma elasticum is a disorder of the connective tissue resulting in swelling and fragmentation of elastic fibers in the mid-dermis.

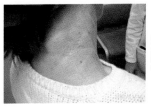

FIGURE 03-216. Thickened, yellow, pebbly plaques of skin (resembling "plucked chicken skin") in a patient with pseudoxanthoma elasticum.

Etiology
- This is a hereditary, primarily recessive disorder, but dominantly inherited cases have been reported.

Keys to Diagnosis

Clinical Manifestation(s)
- The disorder may affect the skin, blood vessels, and eyes.
- Patients are at an increased risk of hypertension and ischemic heart disease.
- GI hemorrhage, cerebral hemorrhage, retinal hemorrhage, and uterine and urogenital bleeding (increased risk of miscarriage) may occur.

Physical Examination
- A "plucked chicken" appearance of the skin (**Fig. 03-216**) is seen due to the presence of yellow plaques and papules and skin sagging. The skin may appear lax and wrinkled.
- Pseudoxanthoma is noted most commonly on the neck, axillae, and other flexural areas.
- An eye examination may reveal breaks in the retina with the presence of brown linear tears resembling vessels known as "angioid streaks".

Diagnostic Tests
- Skin punch biopsy from affected site
- Lipid panel, CBC
- Close monitoring of blood pressure
- Ophthalmology examination

DDx Differential Diagnosis

- Ehlers-Danlos syndrome
- Actinic keratosis
- Xanthomas
- Amyloidosis
- Marfan syndrome

℞ Treatment

First Line

■ Control of cardiovascular risk factors (hypertension, hyperlipidemia, tobacco abuse), dietary calcium restriction
■ Occupation and athletic activity restrictions to minimize complications

Second Line

■ Genetic counseling
■ Surgical correction of lax skin

👁 Clinical Pearl(s)

■ Diagnosis is generally delayed until the teenage years, with the initial appearance of typical skin lesions on the lateral neck.

119. PSORIASIS

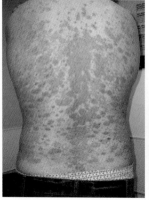

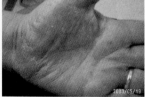

FIGURE 03-217. Advanced, severe erythrodermic psoriasis covering more than 20% of body area in a patient under consideration for systemic therapy.

FIGURE 03-218. Painful pustular psoriasis of the hand with erythema and scaling. This has a similar appearance to eczema.

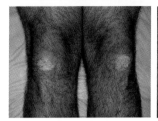

FIGURE 03-219. Well-demarcated, round, red plaques with thick silvery scale typically involving the extensor areas of the extremities.

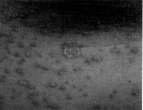

FIGURE 03-220. Silvery scale adherent to an underlying psoriatic lesion, which will bleed if forcibly removed (Auspitz sign).

 General Comments

Definition

■ Psoriasis is a chronic skin disorder characterized by excessive proliferation of keratinocytes, resulting in the formation of thickened scaly plaques, itching, and inflammatory changes of the epidermis and dermis (**Fig. 03-217**). The various forms of psoriasis include guttate, pustular (**Fig. 03-218**), and arthritis variants.

Etiology

■ Unknown, but there is a strong genetic component and high heritability. The mode of inheritance of psoriasis is complex. There is a strong association between psoriasis and HLA B13, B17, and B27 (pustular psoriasis).

■ Familial clustering is evident (genetic transmission with a dominant mode with variable penetrants).

■ One third of persons affected have a positive family history.

■ In early-onset psoriasis, carriage of HLA-Cw6 and environmental triggers such as beta-hemolytic streptococcal infections are major determinants of disease expression. Within the past decade, several putative loci for genetic susceptibility to psoriasis have been reported. One locus (psoriasis susceptibility 1 [PSORS1] locus) in the major histocompatibility complex (MHC) region on chromosome 6 is considered the most important susceptibility locus.

■ Psoriasis affects 1% to 3% of the world's population. Most patients have limited psoriasis involving less than 5% of their body surface.

■ Peak age of onset is bimodal (adolescents and at 60 years old).

 Keys to Diagnosis

Clinical Manifestation(s)

■ Chronic plaque psoriasis generally manifests with symmetric, sharply demarcated, erythromatous, silver-scaled patches affecting primarily the intergluteal folds, elbows, scalp, fingernails, toenails, and knees (**Fig. 03-219**). This form accounts for 80% of psoriasis cases.

■ Psoriasis can also develop at the site of any physical trauma (sunburn, scratching). This is known as *Koebner's phenomenon*.

■ Pruritus is variable. Soreness and bleeding may occur.

■ Joint involvement can result in sacroiliitis and spondylitis.

■ Guttate psoriasis is generally preceded by streptococcal pharyngitis and manifests with multiple droplike lesions on the extremities and the trunk.

■ Psoriasis has an adverse effect on psychologic and social functioning, with affected persons often feeling stigmatized.

Physical Examination

■ The primary psoriatic lesion is an erythematous papule topped by a loosely adherent scale. Scraping the scale results in several bleeding points (*Auspitz sign*).

■ Nail involvement is common (pitting of the nail plate), resulting in hyperkeratosis and onychodystrophy with onycholysis.

■ Silvery scale is seen adherent to an underlying psoriatic lesion, which will bleed if forcibly removed (*Auspitz sign*) (**Fig. 03-220**).

Diagnostic Tests

■ Diagnosis is clinical.

■ Skin biopsy is rarely necessary.

DDx Differential Diagnosis

■ Contact dermatitis
■ Atopic dermatitis
■ Stasis dermatitis
■ Tinea
■ Nummular dermatitis
■ Candidiasis
■ Mycosis fungoides
■ Cutaneous SLE
■ Secondary and tertiary syphilis
■ Drug eruption

R Treatment

■ Sunbathing generally leads to improvement.

■ Eliminate triggering factors (stress, certain medications [e.g., lithium, beta-blockers, antimalarials]).

■ Patients with psoriasis benefit from a daily bath in warm water followed by application of a cream or ointment moisturizer. Regular use of an emollient moisturizer limits evaporation of water from the skin and allows the stratum corneum to rehydrate itself.

- Therapeutic options vary according to the extent of disease. Approximately 70% to 80% of all patients can be treated adequately with use of topical therapy.
- Patients with limited disease (<20% of the body) can be treated with the following:
  1. Topical steroids: disadvantages are brief remissions, expense, and decreased effect with continued use. Salicylic acid can be compounded by a pharmacist in concentrations of 2% to 10% and used in combination with a corticosteroid to decrease the amount of scale.
  2. Calcipotriene: a vitamin D analogue, it is effective for moderate plaque psoriasis; adults should comb the hair, apply solution to the lesions, and rub it in, avoiding uninvolved skin; disadvantages are its cost and potential burning and skin irritation. It should not be used concurrently with salicylic acid because calcipotriene is inactivated by the acidic nature of salicylic acid. Taclonex ointment is a combination of calcipotriene and the high-potency corticosteroid betamethasone dipropionate. It is well tolerated and more effective than either agent used alone but also much more expensive.
  3. Tar products can be used overnight and are most effective when combined with UVB light (Goeckerman regimen).
  4. Anthralin is useful for chronic plaques but can result in purple/brown staining. It is best used with UVB light.
  5. Retinoids such as tazarotene 0.05% or 0.1% cream or gel are effective in thinning plaques but are expensive and can produce irritation.
  6. Other useful measures include tape or occlusive dressing, UVB and lubricating agents, and interlesional steroids.
- Therapeutic options for persons with generalized disease (affecting > 20% of the body) and for those with inadequate response to topical agents are as follows:
  1. UVB light exposure three times a week: This therapy does not require administration of a systemic drug (unlike PUVA), but to be effective, it requires removal of scale with keratolytic agents and emollients.
  2. Oral PUVA administered two to three times weekly is effective for generalized disease. It is often considered in patients for whom narrow-band UVB therapy is ineffective. However, many PUVA treatments are required, necessitating frequent office visits, and it may be associated with phototoxicity, such as erythema and blistering, and increased risk of skin cancer.
- Systemic treatments include methotrexate 25 mg every week for severe psoriasis. Etretinate (Tegison, a synthetic retinoid) is most effective for palmar-plantar pustular psoriasis; the dose is 0.5 to 1 mg/kg/day. It can cause liver enzyme and lipid abnormalities and is teratogenic.
- Cyclosporine is also effective in severe psoriasis; however, relapses are common.
- Chronic plaque psoriasis may be treated with alefacept, a recombinant protein that selectively targets T lymphocytes. Treatment with alefacept for 12 weeks (0.025, 0.075, or 0.150 mg/kg of body weight IV weekly) may result in significant improvement. Some patients also experience a sustained clinical response after the cessation of treatment. This medication is very expensive (a 12-week course may cost > $8,000). Treatment with etanercept, a tumor necrosis factor

(TNF) antagonist, for 24 weeks can also lead to a reduction in severity of plaque psoriasis. Efalizumab, a humanized monoclonal antibody that inhibits the activation of T cells, has also been reported to produce significant improvement in plaque psoriasis over a 24-week treatment period. Adalimumab—a fully human, anti-TNF-alpha monoclonal antibody—has been reported effective for joint and skin manifestations of psoriasis.

Clinical Pearl(s)

■ Hospital admission may be necessary for severe diffuse or poorly responsive psoriasis. The Goeckerman regimen combines daily application of tar with UVB exposure and can result in prolonged remissions.

120. PYODERMA GANGRENOSUM

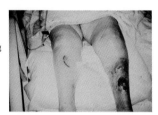

FIGURE 03-221. Large, painful, rapidly expanding ulcer of pyoderma gangrenosum in a patient with Crohn's disease. A biopsy was taken to rule out malignancy.

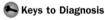 General Comments

Definition

■ Pyoderma gangrenosum is a clinical entity presenting as pustules and usually associated with other medical disorders.

Etiology

■ The condition is often associated with a variety of conditions, especially inflammatory bowel disease (**Fig. 03-221**), arthritis, and plasma cell dyscrasias and at times occurring at sites of prior surgery.

Keys to Diagnosis

Clinical Manifestation(s)

■ Typically the ulcers have undermined edges and red-purple borders.
■ They may be solitary or multiple and occur most often on the lower limbs.
■ The ulcers are painful and tender and may persist for months or years.
■ There is a risk of disfiguring scarring.

Physical Examination
- The typical lesion consists initially of a pustule that enlarges, forming an ulcer with a dark irregular margin.

Diagnostic Tests
- Investigation of other coexisting disorders (colonoscopy, protein innumoelectrophoresis, cryoglobulins, CBC, ALT, rheumatoid factor [RF])

Differential Diagnosis
- Insect (spider) bite
- Vasculitis
- Traumatic ulceration
- Vascular insufficiency
- Antiphospholipid antibody syndrome

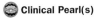 Treatment

First Line
- Treatment of associated disorders
- Topical corticosteroids, clofazimine, dapsone

Second Line
- Intralesional steroids, minocycline

Third Line
- Cyclosporine, azathioprine, cyclophosphamide, systemic corticosteroids

Clinical Pearl(s)
- Most lesions tend to resolve spontaneously; however, considerable scarring may occur.

121. PYOGENIC GRANULOMA

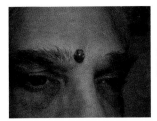

FIGURE 03-222. Red, shiny, friable, dome-shaped papule that grew rapidly on the forehead of this patient and bled profusely when traumatized.

General Comments

Definition

- Pyogenic granuloma is a benign vascular lesion of the skin and mucous membranes. It is a result of capillary proliferation generally secondary to trauma.
- It is common in children and young adults.
- It is equally prevalent in males and females and shows no racial or familial predisposition.
- It is caused by trauma or surgery.
- Gingival lesions occur more frequently during pregnancy.

Etiology

- Trauma causes focal capillary growth. These lesions are neither infectious in etiology nor granulomatous in histology.

Keys to Diagnosis

Clinical Manifestation(s)

- Most commonly found on the head, neck, and extremities
- Often found on the gingiva during pregnancy (called *epulis*)
- Extremely friable, can easily ulcerate, and may bleed profusely with minor trauma

Physical Examination

- Small (<1 cm), yellow-to-red, dome-shaped lesions (**Fig. 03-222**)
- May have surrounding scale at base

Diagnostic Tests

- Diagnosis is based on clinical history and appearance. The condition generally begins with trauma followed by the development of an erythematous papule. The lesion tends to bleed easily and develops over several days to weeks.

DDx Differential Diagnosis

- Amelanotic melanoma
- Bacillary angiomatosis
- Glomus tumor
- Hemangioma
- Irritated nevus
- Wart
- Kaposi's sarcoma

℞ Treatment

First Line

- Excision: using 1% lidocaine for anesthesia, shave or curette at base and border. Follow with electrocauterization or cryotherapy.
- Pregnancy epulis generally resolve spontaneously following childbirth.

Second Line

- Pulsed-dye laser is also a safe and effective treatment modality.

🦷 Clinical Pearl(s)

- Removal of entire lesion is essential because lesions may recur at the site of residual tissue.
- Patients and parents should be alerted to the possibility of recurrence after removal.
- Multiple satellite lesions occasionally develop near a primary pyogenic granuloma, usually after destruction of that lesion.

122. RAYNAUD'S PHENOMENON

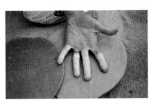
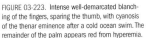
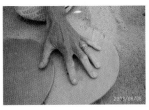

FIGURE 03-223. Intense well-demarcated blanching of the fingers, sparing the thumb, with cyanosis of the thenar eminence after a cold ocean swim. The remainder of the palm appears red from hyperemia.

FIGURE 03-224. With rewarming, the sequence of color changes persist ranging from white (vasoconstriction), to blue (cyanosis), and finally, to red (hyperemia from reperfusion)—thus its oft-quoted resemblance to the colors of the French flag.

🗔 General Comments

Definition

- Raynaud's phenomenon (RP) is a vasospastic disorder that produces an exaggerated response to cold temperatures or emotional stress, resulting in transient digital ischemia. It is manifested as a triphasic discoloration of the fingers and toes (a result of pallor, cyanosis, and rubor).

Etiology

- RP is classified clinically into primary or secondary forms and affects approximately 3% of the general population.
- Primary RP usually occurs between the ages of 15 and 25 years. It is more likely to affect women than men and appears to be more common in colder climates.
- Secondary RP tends to begin after 35 to 40 years of age.
- Secondary RP occurs in more than 90% of patients with scleroderma and in about 30% of patients with systemic lupus erythematosus and with Sjögren's syndrome.
- There is also some suggestion that secondary RP may be associated with drugs (nicotine, caffeine, ergotamine, vinyl chloride) or trauma to the hands from vibrating tools such as jack hammers.

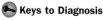 Keys to Diagnosis

Clinical Manifestation(s)

- The classic manifestation is the triphasic color response to cold exposure (**Fig. 03-223**), which may or may not be accompanied by pain:
  1. Pallor of the digit resulting from vasospasm
  2. Blue discoloration (cyanosis) secondary to desaturated venous blood
  3. Red (rubor) with or without pain and paresthesia when vasospasm resolves and blood returns to the digit. (**Fig. 03-224**)
- Initial pallor is typically necessary for the diagnosis to be made.
- The triphasic color changes can sometimes be induced in the office by placing the hand in an ice bath.
- Fingertips are most often involved, but feet, ears, and nose can be affected.
- Duration of attacks can range from seconds to hours.
- Chronic skin changes resulting from repeated attacks may include skin thickening and brittle nails. Ulcerations and, rarely, gangrene may occur.

Physical Examination

- Color changes are well delineated, symmetric, and usually bilateral involving the fingers and toes. The index, middle, and ring fingers are commonly involved.

Diagnostic Tests

- Primary RP can also be called idiopathic Raynaud's phenomenon, primary Raynaud's syndrome, or Raynaud's disease. It occurs in the absence of any associated disease.
- With primary RP, the possibility that another first-degree family member is affected is reported as approximately 25%.
- Secondary RP is associated with an underlying pathologic condition or disease and may include the following:
  - CREST syndrome (calcinosis, RP, esophageal dysmotility, sclerodactyly, and telangiectasia)
  - Scleroderma

- Mixed connective tissue disease, polymyositis, and dermatomyositis
- Systemic lupus erythematosus
- Rheumatoid arthritis
- Thromboangiitis obliterans (Buerger's disease)
- Drug induced (beta-blockers, ergotamine, methysergide, vinblastine, bleomycin, oral contraceptives, nicotine, caffeine, vinyl chloride)
- Hematologic disorders (polycythemia, cryoglobulinemia, cold agglutinins, paraproteinemia)
- Carpal tunnel syndrome
- Use of tools that vibrate
- Endocrine disorders (hypothyroidism, carcinoid syndrome)

■ The suggested criteria for primary RP are as follows:
- Symmetric attacks
- Absence of tissue necrosis, ulceration, or gangrene
- Absence of a secondary cause on the basis of a patient's history and general physical examination
- Normal nail-fold capillaries
- Negative test for antinuclear antibody (ANA)
- Normal ESR

■ Secondary RP is suggested by the following findings:
- Onset of symptoms after the age of 30 years
- Episodes that are painful, asymmetric, or associated with ischemic skin lesions
- Clinical features suggestive of a connective-tissue disease
- Elevation of specific autoantibody tests and ESR
- Evidence of microvascular disease on microscopy of nail-fold capillaries

■ CBC, serum electrolytes, BUN, creatinine, ESR, ANA, VDRL antibody test, RF, and urinalysis should be included in the initial evaluation.

■ If the history, physical examination, and initial laboratory tests suggest a possible secondary cause, specific serologic testing (e.g., anticentromere antibodies, anti-Scl 70, cryoglobulins, complement testing, and protein electrophoresis) may be indicated.

■ Noninvasive vascular testing includes finger systolic blood pressures, segmental blood pressure measurements, cold recovery time (measure vasoconstrictor and vasodilator responses of finger to cold), fingertip thermography, and laser Doppler with thermal challenge (measure relative change in skin blood flow with ambient warming).

DDx Differential Diagnosis

■ Neurogenic thoracic outlet syndrome or carpal tunnel syndrome
■ Frostbite or cold weather injury
■ Medication reaction (ergotamine, chemotherapeutic agents)
■ Atherosclerosis, thromboembolic disease
■ Buerger's disease, embolic disease

- Acrocyanosis
- Livedo reticularis
- Injury from repetitive motion

 Treatment

First Line

- Avoid drugs that may precipitate RP (see "Etiology").
- Avoid cold exposure. Use warm gloves, hats, and garments during the winter months or before going into cold environments (e.g., air-conditioned rooms). Sudden shifts in temperature are more likely to precipitate RP.
- Avoid stressful situations, and use relaxation techniques in preventing RP attacks.
- Typically, patients with RP respond well to nonpharmacologic measures.
- Medications are indicated in the treatment of RP if there are signs of critical ischemia or if the quality of life of the patient is affected to the degree that activities of normal living are no longer possible and preventative techniques do not work.
- Calcium channel blockers are the most effective treatment for RP.
- Calcium channel blockers differ in their peripheral vasodilator properties. Nifedipine, amlodipine, felodipine, nisoldipine, and isradipine appear more effective than diltiazem and verapamil in the treatment of RP.
- Nifedipine is most often prescribed at a dose of 10 to 20 mg 30 minutes before going outside. If symptoms occur with long duration, nifedipine XL 30 to 180 mg PO QD is effective.

Second Line

- Patients who do not tolerate or fail to respond to calcium channel blocker therapy can try other vasodilator drugs alone or in combination. Options include nitroglycerin, nitroprusside, hydralazine, papaverine, minoxidil, niacin, and topical nitrates.
- Agents that indirectly cause vasodilation (SSRIs, ACE inhibitors, phosphodiesterase inhibitors) may be useful, but there is no convincing evidence that they are better than calcium channel blockers alone.
- Sympatholytic agents (reserpine, guanethidine) may be helpful for acute treatment, but their effect tends to decrease with time, and they often have intolerable side effects.
- Alpha receptor blockers such as prazosin or doxazosin counteract the actions of norepinephrine, which will constrict blood vessels.

Third Line

- The prostaglandins, including inhaled iloprost, intravenous epoprostenol, and alprostadil, may be promising in severe RP. However, additional experience and controlled studies are needed to substantiate this claim.

- Phosphodiesterase inhibitors (such as cilostazol, pentoxifylline, and sildenafil and angiotensin II receptor antagonists (such as losartan) have also been used with some limited success.
- Anticoagulation with aspirin and heparin can be considered during the acute phase of an ischemic event. Aspirin (81 mg/day) therapy can be considered in all patients with secondary RP with a history of ischemic ulcers or thrombotic events; however, caution should be exercised because aspirin can theoretically worsen vasospasm via inhibition of prostacyclin. Long-term anticoagulation with heparin or warfarin is not recommended unless there is evidence of a hypercoagulable disorder.
- Bypass surgery can be performed for severe RP associated with reconstructible arterial occlusive disease.
- Sympathectomy is available for unreconstructable occlusive disease or pure vasospastic disease refractory to medical treatment.

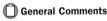 Clinical Pearl(s)

- Physical examination should also include examination for symptoms associated with autoimmune disease, such as fever, rash, arthritis, dry eyes, dry mouth, myalgias, or cardiopulmonary abnormalities.

123. REITER SYNDROME (REACTIVE ARTHRITIS)

General Comments

Definition

Reiter syndrome is one of the seronegative spondyloarthropathies, so called because serum rheumatoid factor is not present in these forms of inflammatory arthritis. There is an international consensus that the term *reactive arthritis* should replace *Reiter syndrome* to describe this constellation of signs and symptoms. Unfortunately, the original name is still associated with the syndrome. Reiter syndrome is an asymmetric polyarthritis that affects mainly the lower extremities and is associated with one or more of the following:

- Urethritis
- Cervicitis
- Dysentery
- Inflammatory eye disease
- Mucocutaneous lesions

Etiology

- Epidemic Reiter syndrome following outbreaks of dysentery has been well described.
- Genetically susceptible HLA B27 individuals are at risk for developing Reiter syndrome following infection with certain pathogens:
  - *Salmonella*
  - *Shigella*

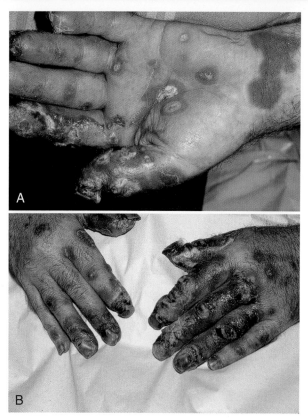

FIGURE 03-225. Reiter syndrome. (A, B) Examples of lesions on the hands. *(From White GA, Cox NH: Diseases of the Skin: A Color Atlas and Text, ed 2, St. Louis, 2006, Mosby.)*

- *Yersinia enterocolitica*
- *Chlamydia trachomatis*
- Molecular mimicry mechanism suspected
- Symptom complex indistinguishable from Reiter syndrome has been described in association with HIV infection.

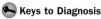 Keys to Diagnosis

Clinical Manifestation(s)
- Polyarthritis
  - Affecting the knee and ankle
  - Commonly asymmetric
- Heel pain and Achilles tendinitis, especially at the insertion of the Achilles tendon
- Plantar fasciitis
- Large effusions
- Dactylitis or "sausage toe"
- Urethritis
- Uveitis or conjunctivitis; uveitis can progress to blindness without treatment
- Aortic regurgitation similar to that seen in ankylosing spondylitis

Physical Examination
- Keratoderma blennorrhagicum, circinate balinitis
  1. Hyperkeratotic lesions on soles of the feet, toes, penis, hands (**Fig. 03-225**)
  2. Closely resembles psoriasis

Diagnostic Tests
- ESR, ANA, HLA B27, chlamidiae serology, urine and stool cultures for bacteria, HIV

DDx Differential Diagnosis

- Epidemic Reiter syndrome following outbreaks of dysentery has been well described.
- Genetically susceptible HLA B27 individuals are at risk for developing Reiter syndrome following infection with certain pathogens:
  - *Salmonella*
  - *Shigella*
  - *Yersinia enterocolitica*
  - *Chlamydia trachomatis*
  - Molecular mimicry mechanism suspected
- Symptom complex indistinguishable from Reiter syndrome has been described in association with HIV infection.

Treatment

First Line

- Cutaneous disease: Should be treated with topical corticosteroids, calcipotriene, or tazarotene.
- Systemic manifestations: Flares should be treated with NSAIDs such as indomethacin (25-50 mg PO TID).
- Enteric or urethral infection should be treated with appropriate antibiotic coverage.
- Uveitis should be treated with steroid eye drops in consultation with an ophthalmologist.
- Achilles tendinitis and plantar fasciitis should be treated with injections of methylprednisolone (40-80 mg).

Second Line

- Cutaneous disease: Can be managed with systemic retinoids or UV/PUVA.
- Systemic manifestations: Sulfasalazine (2-3 g PO TID) may be effective.

Third Line

- Cutaneous disease: Third-line treatments include methotrexate, cyclosporine.
- Systemic manifestations: Persistent and uncontrolled disease should be managed with cytotoxic drugs (methotrexate, azathioprine) in consultation with a rheumatologist.

Clinical Pearl(s)

- Reiter syndrome is strongly associated with HLA B27 (63%-96%).

124. RHUS DERMATITIS (POISON IVY, POISON OAK, POISON SUMAC)

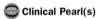 **General Comments**

Definition

- Rhus dermatitis is an acute skin inflammation resulting from exposure to poison ivy, poison oak, and poison sumac.

Etiology

- Rhus dermatitis is caused by contact with poison ivy, poison oak, or poison sumac.

Keys to Diagnosis

Clinical Manifestation(s)

- The pattern of lesions is asymmetric, often involving the extremities (**Fig. 03-226**); itching, burning, and stinging may be present. Intense erythema may be present (**Fig. 03-227**).

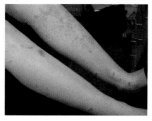

FIGURE 03-226. Rhus dermatitis is often found on exposed extremities, where contact with the plant occurs, but can be further spread via autoinoculation.

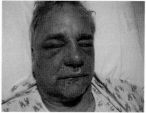

FIGURE 03-227. Intense erythema, edema of face and eyelids, and oozing blisters in this individual who burned a field containing poison sumac.

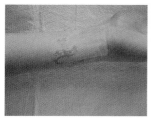

FIGURE 03-228. Typical linear "streak" pattern after the patient's arm brushed against Rhus plant leaf or vine.

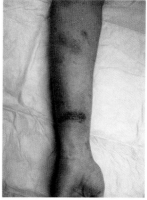

FIGURE 03-229. Pruritic, erythematous, edematous papules and vesicles occuring individually and more confluent at the distal wrist.

Physical Examination

■ Poison ivy dermatitis can present with vesicles and blisters; linear lesions (**Fig. 03-228**) (as a result of dragging of the resins over the surface of the skin by scratching) are a classic presentation (**Fig. 03-229**).

■ The involved areas are erythematous, warm to touch, swollen, and may be confused with cellulitis.

Diagnostic Tests

■ None usually necessary

DDx Differential Diagnosis

■ Impetigo
■ Lichen simplex chronicus
■ Atopic dermatitis
■ Nummular eczema
■ Seborrheic dermatitis
■ Psoriasis
■ Scabies

R Treatment

First Line

■ Removal of the irritant substance by washing the skin with plain water or mild soap within 15 min of exposure is helpful in patients with poison ivy, poison oak, or poison sumac dermatitis.

■ Cold or cool water compresses for 20 to 30 minutes five to six times a day for the initial 72 hours are effective during the acute blistering stage.

■ Oral antihistamines will control pruritus, especially at night; calamine lotion is also useful for pruritus; however, it can lead to excessive drying.

■ Colloidal oatmeal (Aveeno) baths can also provide symptomatic relief.

■ Patients with mild to moderate erythema may respond to topical steroid gels or creams.

Second Line

■ Oral corticosteroids are generally reserved for severe, widespread dermatitis.

■ Intramuscular steroids are used for severe reactions and in patients requiring oral corticosteroids but unable to tolerate them.

125. ROCKY MOUNTAIN SPOTTED FEVER

🗂 General Comments

Definition
- Rocky Mountain spotted fever (RMSF) is a life-threatening, tick-borne febrile illness caused by infection with *Rickettsia rickettsii*. The infection occurs when *R. rickettsii* in the salivary glands of a vector tick is transmitted into the dermis, spreading and replicating in the cytoplasm of endothelial cells and eliciting widespread vasculitis and end-organ damage.

Etiology
- Infectious agent: *R. rickettsii* (an intracellular bacterium)
- Vector: dog tick and wood tick (vertical transmission exists in ticks, but horizontal transmission involving rodents represents an important reservoir for the agent). In the United States, *R. rickettsii* is transmitted mainly by the American dog tick *(Dermacentor variabilis)* and the Rocky Mountain wood tick *(D. andersoni)*.

🔑 Keys to Diagnosis

Clinical Manifestation(s)
- Incubation: 3 to 12 days
- First symptoms: fever, headache, malaise, and myalgias

Physical Examination
- Rash appears during first 3 days in 50%; by day 5, 80% have it. No rash appears in 10% of patients.
- Initial appearance is blanching erythematous macules on wrists and ankles that then spread to the trunk, palms, and soles.
- Lesions may evolve into papules and eventually become nonblanching (petechiae or palpable purpura).

Diagnostic Tests
- Antibody titers to *R. rickettsii* (by indirect fluorescent antibody test). The diagnosis of RMSF requires a fourfold increase 2 weeks apart and thus is not helpful in the care of the patients despite a sensitivity and specificity of near 100%.
- The only test that can provide a timely diagnosis is the immunohistologic demonstration of *R. rickettsii* in skin biopsy specimens.

🔬 Differential Diagnosis

- Influenza A
- Enteroviral infection
- Typhoid fever
- Leptospirosis

- Infectious mononucleosis
- Viral hepatitis, sepsis
- Ehrlichiosis, gastroenteritis
- Acute abdomen
- Bronchitis
- Pneumonia
- Meningococcemia
- Disseminated gonococcal infection
- Secondary syphilis
- Bacterial endocarditis
- Toxic shock syndrome
- Scarlet fever
- Rheumatic fever
- Measles
- Rubella
- Typhus
- Rickettsialpox
- Lyme disease
- Drug hypersensitivity reactions
- Idiopathic thrombocytopenic purpura
- Thrombotic thrombocytopenic purpura
- Kawasaki syndrome
- Immune complex vasculitis
- Connective tissue disorders

℞ Treatment

First Line
- Oral or intravenous doxycycline, 200 mg/day in two divided doses

Second Line
- Oral tetracycline, 25 to 50 mg/kg/day in four divided doses

Third Line
- Chloramphenicol, 50 to 75 mg/kg/day in four divided doses; therapy continued for at least 2 days after defervescence

Clinical Pearl(s)

- Fatality rate is 1% to 4% (five times greater if treatment is initiated after day 5 of illness, which is more likely in the absence of rash and during seasonal nonpeak tick activity). Long-term sequelae seen in patients who recover from severe RMSF include paraparesis, hearing loss; peripheral neuropathy; bladder and bowel incontinence; cerebellar, vestibular, and motor dysfunction; language disorders; limb amputation; and scrotal pain after cutaneous necrosis.

126. ROSACEA

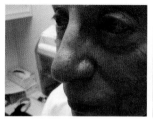

FIGURE 03-230. Persistent erythema on the cheeks and nose, often triggered by sunlight, heat, or alcohol, is a feature of rosacea.

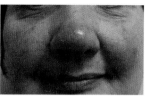

FIGURE 03-231. The facial eruption of stage 2 rosacea is characterized by erythematous papules, occasional pustules, and telangiectases; patients often present with severe facial flushing (so-called red face).

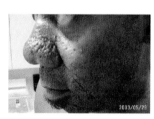

FIGURE 03-232. Enlargement of the nose with redness, telangiectasias, and prominent, open follicles (*peau d'orange* in appearance) that feel thick and rubbery on palpation.

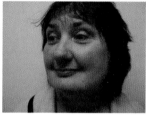

FIGURE 03-233. Marked improvement with regression of redness, telangiectasias, and pustules following a course of doxycycline and metronidazole gel.

🟠 General Comments

Definition

- Rosacea is a chronic skin disorder characterized by papules and pustules affecting the face and often associated with flushing and erythema.
- Rosacea can be classified into four major subtypes:
  1. Erythematotelengiectatic: erythema in central part of face, telangiectasia, flushing
  2. Papulopustular: presence of dome-shaped erythematous papules and small postules, in addition to facial erythema, flushing, and telengiectasia

3. Phymatous: presence of thickened skin with prominent pores that may affect the nose (rhinophyma), chin (gnathophyma), forehead (metophyma), eyelids (blepharophyma), and ears (otophyma)
4. Ocular: conjunctival injection, sensation of foreign body in the eye, telengiectasia and erythema of lid margins, scaling

Etiology

- Unknown. Hot drinks, alcohol, and sun exposure may accentuate the erythema by causing vasodilation of the skin.
- Flare-ups may also result from reactions to medications (e.g., simvastatin, ACE inhibitors, vasodilators, fluorinated corticosteroids), stress, extreme heat or cold, spicy drinks, and menstruation.

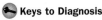 Keys to Diagnosis

Clinical Manifestation(s)

- Rosacea occurs in 1 in 20 Americans
- Onset is often between ages 30 and 50 years
- Rosacea is more common in people of Celtic origin; however, this disease may be overlooked in nonwhites because skin pigmentation results in atypical presentation.
- The female:male ratio is 3:1.
- The progression of rosacea is variable. Typical stages include the following:
  1. Facial flushing
  2. Erythema (**Fig. 03-230**) and/or edema and ocular symptoms
  3. Papules and pustules (**Fig. 03-231**)
  4. Rhinophyma (**Fig. 03-232**)

Physical Examination

- Facial erythema, presence of papules, pustules, and telangiectasia are common findings on examination.
- Excessive facial warmth and redness is the predominant presenting complaint.
- Itching is generally absent.
- Comedones are absent (unlike acne).
- Women are more likely to show symptoms on the chin and cheeks, whereas in men the nose is commonly involved.
- Ocular findings (mild dryness and irritation with blepharitis, conjunctival injection, burning, stinging, tearing, eyelid inflammation, swelling, and redness) are present in 50% of patients.

Diagnostic Tests

- Diagnosis is based on clinical findings. Distinguishing features between acne and rosacea are the presence of telangiectasia and deep diffuse erythema and absence of comedones in rosacea.

Differential Diagnosis

- Drug eruption
- Acne vulgaris
- Contact dermatitis
- SLE
- Carcinoid flush
- Idiopathic facial flushing
- Seborrheic dermatitis
- Facial sarcoidosis
- Photodermatitis
- Mastocytosis

Treatment

First Line

- Avoid alcohol, excessive sun exposure, and hot drinks of any type.
- Use of mild, nondrying soap is recommended; local skin irritants should be avoided.
- Reassure patient that rosacea is completely unrelated to poor hygiene.
- Topical therapy with metronidazole aqueous gel applied BID is effective as initial therapy for mild cases (**Fig. 03-233**) or following the use of oral antibiotics. A 1% formulation of metronidazole applied QD may improve patient compliance. Clindamycin lotion, sulfacetamide, or erythromycin 2% solution may also be effective.
- Another topical treatment modality for pustular and papular forms of rosacea is the use of azelaic acid. Azelaic cream (20%) or gel (15%). Azelaic acid is as least as effective as topical metronidazole but may be more irritating.

Second Line

- Systemic antibiotics: Doxycycline 100 mg QD tetracycline 250 mg QID until symptoms diminish, then taper off; doxycycline 100 mg BID is also effective.
- Minocycline 50 to 100 mg QD
- Oral metronidazole (200 mg QD-BID) for 4 to 6 weeks is also effective.
- Azithromycin

Third Line

- Isotretinoin 0.5 to 1 mg/kg/day in two divided doses for 15 to 20 weeks can be used for refractory papular and pustular rosacea; use of retinoids may, however, worsen erythema and telangiectasis.
- Laser treatment is an option for progressive telangiectasias or rhinophyma.
- Erythema and flushing may respond to low-dose clonidine (0.05 mg BID).
- Adapalone 0.1% at bedtime, permethrin 5% BID.

Clinical Pearl(s)

- Patients with resistant cases may have *Demodex folliculorum* mite infestation or tinea infection (diagnosis can be confirmed with potassium hydroxide examination); the role of *D. folliculorum* in rosacea is unclear. These mites can sometimes be found in large numbers in the lesions; however, their numbers do not generally decline with treatment.

- Rosacea can result in emotional and social stigmas, especially because many people associate rosacea and rhinophyma with alcohol abuse.
- Early consultation with an ophthalmologist is recommended in patients with suspected ocular involvement.

127. ROSEOLA

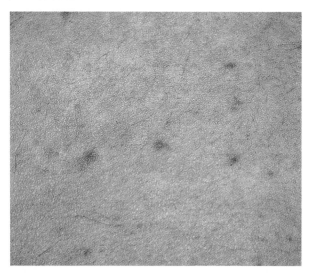

FIGURE 03-234. Roseola. As the fever breaks, multiple pale pink, 1- to 5-mm macules and papules appear and last only hours to a few days. *(From White GA, Cox NH: Diseases of the Skin: A Color Atlas and Text, ed 2, St. Louis, 2006, Mosby.)*

General Comments

Definition

- Roseola is a benign viral illness found in infants and characterized by high fevers, followed by a rash.

Etiology
- Roseola is caused by human herpesvirus 6 (HHV-6).
- The incubation period is between 5 and 15 days.

Keys to Diagnosis

Clinical Manifestation(s)
- Nearly one third of all infants develop roseola before the age of 2 years.
- More than 90% of children older than 2 years are seropositive for the virus causing roseola.
- Roseola is spread from person to person. It is not known how it is spread, but it must be very efficiently spread and presumably via the respiratory tract.
- There is no predilection for gender or time of year.

Physical Examination
- Typically the child develops a high fever, usually up to 104° F (40° C), that lasts for 3 to 5 days.
- Fever may be associated with a runny nose, irritability, and fatigue.
- A rash appears within 48 hours of defervescence, mainly on the face, neck, trunk, arms, and legs (**Fig. 03-234**). It is a faint pink maculopapular rash that blanches when palpated and usually fades away within 48 hours.
- Anorexia, seizures, and cervical adenopathy can also be seen.

Diagnostic Tests
- None necessary

DDx Differential Diagnosis

- Measles
- Rubella
- Fifth disease
- Drug eruption
- Mononucleosis
- All causes of fever (e.g., otitis media, pneumonia, and urinary tract infection)
- Meningitis

R Treatment

First Line
- Provide supportive care.
- Maintain hydration by drinking clear fluids: water, fruit juice, lemonade, and so forth.
- Sponge bathe with lukewarm water if febrile.
- Acetaminophen 10 to 15 mg/kg per dose at 4-hour intervals for fever
- Ibuprofen 5 to 10 mg/kg per dose at 6-hour intervals (maximum dose 600 mg)

🔴 Clinical Pearl(s)

■ A child with fever and rash should be excluded from daycare.
■ Human herpesvirus 6 is named accordingly because it is the sixth herpesvirus discovered, after herpes simplex virus 1 (HSV-1), HSV-2, cytomegalovirus (CMV), Epstein-Barr virus, and varicella zoster virus (VZV).

128. RUBELLA

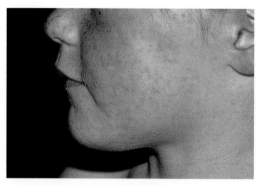

FIGURE 03-235. Rubella. The rash may be very mild in rubella; when present, it is similar to measles, with maculopapular erythema starting on the face and spreading to the trunk. The spots are 1 to 2 mm in diameter and slightly raised. In rubella there is also enlargement of the cervical and occipital lymph nodes. *(From White GA, Cox NH: Diseases of the Skin: A Color Atlas and Text, ed 2, St. Louis, 2006, Mosby.)*

🔵 General Comments

Definition

■ Rubella is a mild illness caused by the rubella virus that can lead to severe congenital problems via in vitro transmission to the fetus when a pregnant woman becomes infected.
■ Since mass vaccination began (i.e., after 1980) most cases have occurred in unimmunized people, with fewer than 1 case/100,000 person-years (acquired and congenital).
■ Currently, 10% to 20% of childbearing-age women are susceptible.

Etiology

Acquired Infection

■ Viral portal of entry is the upper respiratory tract.
■ Viral replication occurs in lymph nodes, then hematogenous dissemination occurs to many organs, including the placenta if present.
■ Immune complexes may be the cause of rash and arthritis.

Congenital Infection

■ Fetus is infected via the placenta during maternal acquired infection.
■ Cellular damage in the fetus results from cytolysis of fetal cells, mostly via a fetal vasculitis or from an immune-mediated inflammation and damage.

 Keys to Diagnosis

Clinical Manifestation(s)

Acquired Infection

■ Incubation: 14 to 21 days
■ Prodrome: 1 to 5 days; low-grade fever, headache, malaise, anorexia, mild conjunctivitis, coryza, pharyngitis, cough, and cervical, suboccipital, and postauricular lymphadenopathy
■ Occasional splenomegaly and hepatitis (during rash)
■ Complications: arthritis (15%, mostly in adult women), thrombocytopenia, myocarditis, optic neuritis, encephalitis (all less than 0.1%)

Congenital Infection

■ Deafness: 85%
■ Intrauterine growth retardation: 70%
■ Cataracts: 35%
■ Retinopathy: 35%
■ Patent ductus arteriosus: 30%
■ Pulmonary artery hypoplasia: 25%
■ In utero death: 20%
■ Mental retardation: 10% to 20%
■ Meningoencephalitis: 10% to 20%
■ Behavior disorder: 10% to 20%
■ Hepatosplenomegaly: 10% to 20%
■ Bone radiolucencies: 10% to 20%
■ Diabetes mellitus (type 1): 10% to 20% by age 35 years
■ Other congenital heart defects: 2% to 5%

Physical Examination

■ Rash: 1 to 5 days
■ Enanthema: palatal macules
■ Exanthema (rash): blotchy eruption beginning on face (**Fig. 03-235**) and neck and then spreading to trunk and limbs

Diagnostic Tests

Acquired Infection

- Serologic test (hemagglutination inhibition, neutralization tests, complement fixation tests, passive agglutination, enzyme immunoassay [EIA], ELISA)
- IgM antibodies (by EIA) detected early: second to fourth week
- IgG antibodies (by ELISA) can be measured as acute phase (7 days after rash onset) and convalescent phase (14 days later)

Congenital Infection

- Viral culture (from nasopharynx)
- Serologic studies: IgM antirubella virus detection by EIA is method of choice (after newborn is 5 months old)

DDx Differential Diagnosis

Acquired Infection

- Other viral infections by enteroviruses, adenoviruses, human parvovirus B-19, measles.
- Scarlet Fever.
- Allergic Reaction.
- Kawasaki Disease.

Congenital Infection

- Congenital syphilis, toxoplasmosis, herpes simplex, cytomegalovirus, enterovirus.

R Treatment

- There is no known effective antiviral therapy.
- Specific congenital problems should be managed as appropriate.

Clinical Pearl(s)

- The highest risk of developing long-term complications of congenital infection exists during the first trimester of gestation; both risk of congenital infection and long-term complications drop during the second trimester, and although the risk of congenital infection increases during the third trimester, there is no risk of long-term complication at that point.

129. RUBEOLA (MEASLES)

General Comments

Definition

- Measles is a childhood exanthem, caused by an RNA virus called *Morbillivirus*, belonging to the family *Paramyxoviridae*.

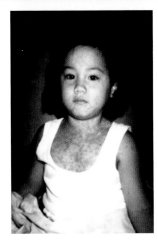

FIGURE 03-236. Rubeola classically presents as erythematous flat papules that start on the head and neck. They become confluent as they spread to the trunk and arms.

Etiology

- The measles virus is transmitted through the respiratory tract by airborne droplets.
- It initially infects the respiratory epithelium; the patient becomes viremic during the prodromal phase and the virus is disseminated to skin, respiratory tract, and other organs.
- Viral clearance is achieved via cellular immunity.

Keys to Diagnosis

Clinical Manifestation(s)

- Incubation: 10 to 14 days (up to 3 weeks in adults)
- Prodrome: 2 to 4 days; malaise, fever, rhinorrhea, conjunctivitis, cough
- Exanthem phase: 7 to 10 days
- The fever increases and peaks at 104° to 105° F together with the rash; it persists for 5 or 6 days. The patient's fever decreases over 24 hours.

Physical Examination

- Rash: Erythematous maculopapular eruption begins behind the ears, progresses to the forehead and neck (**Fig. 03-236**), then spreads to face, trunk, upper extremities, buttocks, and lower extremities in that order. After 3 days the rash fades in the same sequence by becoming copper brown and then desquamates.

- Enanthem: *Koplik* spots are white papules 1 to 2 mm in diameter on an erythematous base. They first appear on the buccal mucosa opposite the lower molar 2 days before the rash and spread over 24 hours to involve most of the buccal and lower labial mucosa. They fade after 3 days.
- Other symptoms and signs: malaise, anorexia, vomiting, diarrhea, abdominal pain, pharyngitis, lymphadenopathy, and occasional splenomegaly.

Diagnostic Tests

- ELISA for measles antibodies, which appear shortly after the onset of the rash and peak 3 to 4 weeks later

DDx Differential Diagnosis

- Other viral infections by enteroviruses, adenoviruses, human parvovirus B19, rubella
- Scarlet fever
- Allergic reaction
- Kawasaki syndrome

R Treatment

First Line

- Supportive treatment
- Vitamin A
- Ribavirin for severe measles pneumonitis

Clinical Pearl(s)

- Passive immunization: human immunoglobulin 0.25 ml/kg IM within 6 days of exposure. Double the dose for immunocompromised persons.

130. SARCOIDOSIS

General Comments

Definition

- Sarcoidosis is a systemic disease characterized by the presence of noncaseating granulomata, usually (but not invariably) affecting multiple organ systems.

Etiology

- Unknown. A cardinal feature of sarcoidosis is the presence of CD4+ T cells that interact with antigen-presenting cells to initiate the formation and maintenance of granulomas. Multiple lines of evidence suggest that sarcoidosis may result from the interaction of multiple genes with environmental exposures or infection.

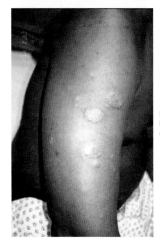

FIGURE 03-237. Several annular, violaceous lesions on the arm and trunk with central clearing and atrophy.

 Keys to Diagnosis

Clinical Manifestation(s)

- Cutaneous lesions occur (**Fig. 03-237**) in 20% to 35% of patients with systemic sarcoidosis and may be classified into nonspecific (erythema nodosum) and specific (granulomatous) subtypes.
- Cutaneous sarcoidal granulomata appear to be associated with a poorer prognosis and an increased incidence of pulmonary fibrosis and uveitis.
- Erythema nodosum occurs quite commonly in sarcoidosis (incidence 11%-30%). It presents as erythematous, tender, subcutaneous nodules, usually on the anterior tibial regions.
- A not uncommon mode of presentation is the development of a widespread, usually aymptomatic, maculopapular eruption. Individual lesions are erythematous or violaceous, 3 to 6 mm in diameter, and most commonly seen on the face.

Physical Examination

- The most characteristic skin manifestation of sarcoidosis is *lupus pernio.* This chronic violaceous plaque (**Fig. 03-237**) most often affects the nose, cheeks, and ears. It is a particularly disfiguring variant, and resolution is especially complicated by marked scarring. Lupus pernio is often associated with lesions in the upper respiratory tract and can be followed by nasal obstruction and septal perforation.

Diagnostic Tests
- Biopsy should be done on accessible tissues suspected of sarcoid involvement (conjunctiva, skin, lymph nodes); bronchoscopy with transbronchial biopsy is the procedure of choice in patients without any readily accessible site.
- Chest radiograph: adenopathy of the hilar and paratracheal nodes is a common finding.

DDx Differential Diagnosis
- TB
- Lymphoma
- Hodgkin's disease
- Metastases
- Pneumoconioses
- Enlarged pulmonary arteries
- Infectious mononucleosis
- Lymphangitic carcinomatosis
- Idiopathic hemosiderosis
- Alveolar cell carcinoma
- Pulmonary eosinophilia
- Hypersensitivity pneumonitis
- Fibrosing alveolitis
- Collagen disorders
- Parasitic infection

R Treatment

First Line
- Many patients with sarcoidosis will not require any treatment. Generally treatment should be instituted when organ function is threatened. Corticosteroids remain the mainstay of therapy when treatment is required (e.g., prednisone 40 mg QD for 8-12 weeks with gradual tapering of the dose to 10 mg QOD over 8-12 months); corticosteroids should be considered in patients with severe symptoms (e.g., dyspnea, chest pain); hypercalcemia; ocular, CNS, or cardiac involvement; and progressive pulmonary disease. Patients with interstitial lung disease benefit from oral steroid therapy for 6 to 24 months.
- Hydroxychloroquine is effective for chronic disfiguring skin lesions, hypercalcemia, and neurologic involvement.
- NSAIDs are useful for musculoskeletal symptoms and erythema nodosum.

Second Line
- Patients with progressive disease refractory to corticosteroids may be treated with methotrexate 7.5 to 15 mg once/week.

Third Line
- Azathioprine, UVA, excision, laser

Clinical Pearl(s)

■ Approximately 15% to 20% of patients with lung involvement advance to irreversible lung impairment (bronchiectasis, cavitation, progressive fibrosis, pneumothorax, and respiratory failure). Death from pulmonary failure occurs in 5% to 7% of patients with sarcoidosis.

131. SCABIES

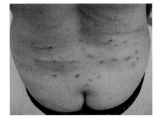

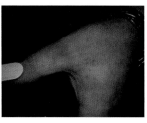

FIGURE 03-238. Scattered, inflamed, excoriated vesicles and papules over the back and buttocks associated with intense itching and uncontrollable scratching. Her bed partner also had scabies.

FIGURE 03-239. Scabies is often found on the hands and in the webs of fingers with evidence of telltale tracks or burrows.

 General Comments

Definition

■ Scabies is a contagious disease caused by the mite *Sarcoptes scabiei*. It is generally acquired by sleeping with or in the bedding of infested individuals. Scabies is generally associated with poor living conditions and is also common in hospitals and nursing homes.

Etiology

■ Human scabies is caused by the mite *S. scabiei*, var. *hominis*.

 Keys to Diagnosis

Clinical Manifestation(s)

■ Primary lesions are caused when the female mite burrows within the stratum corneum, laying eggs within the tract she leaves behind; burrows (linear or serpiginous tracts) end with a minute papule or vesicle.
■ Primary lesions are most commonly found in the web spaces of the hands, wrists, buttocks (**Fig. 03-238**), scrotum, penis, breasts, axillae, and knees.

- Secondary lesions result from scratching or infection.
- Intense pruritus, especially nocturnal, is common; it is caused by an acquired sensitivity to the mite or fecal pellets and is usually noted 1 to 4 weeks after the primary infestation.
- Widespread and crusted lesions (Norwegian or crusted scabies) may be seen in elderly and immunocompromised patients.

Physical Examination

- Examination of the skin may reveal burrows, tiny vesicles, excoriations (**Fig. 03-239**), and inflammatory papules.

Diagnostic Tests

- Microscopic demonstration of the organism, feces, or eggs: A drop of mineral oil may be placed over the suspected lesion before removal; the scrapings are transferred directly to a glass slide; a drop of potassium hydroxide is added and a cover slip is applied.
- Skin biopsy is rarely necessary to make the diagnosis.

DDx Differential Diagnosis

- Pediculosis
- Atopic dermatitis
- Flea bites
- Seborrheic dermatitis
- Dermatitis herpetiformis
- Contact dermatitis
- Nummular eczema
- Syphilis
- Other insect infestation

R Treatment

First Line

- Clothing, underwear, and towels used in the 48 hours before treatment must be laundered.
- Following a warm bath or shower, lindane lotion should be applied to all skin surfaces below the neck (can be applied to the face if area is infested); it should be washed off 8 to 12 hours after application. Repeat application 1 week later is usually sufficient to eradicate infestation.
- Pruritus generally abates 24 to 48 hours after treatment, but it can last up to 2 weeks; oral antihistamines are effective in decreasing postscabietic pruritus.
- Topical corticosteroid creams may hasten the resolution of secondary eczematous dermatitis.
- If the patient is a resident of an extended care facility, it is important to educate the patients, staff, family, and frequent visitors about scabies and the need to

have full cooperation in treatment. Scabicide should be applied to all patients, staff, and frequent visitors, whether symptomatic or not; symptomatic family members of staff and visitors should also receive treatment.

Second Line
- Permethrin 5% cream is also effective with usually one treatment; it should be massaged into the skin from head to soles of feet; remove 8 to 14 hours later by washing. If living mites are present after 14 days, treat again.

Third Line
- A single dose (150-200 mcg/kg in 6-mg tablets) of ivermectin, an antihelminthic agent, is as effective as topical lindane for the treatment of scabies. It is the best treatment for generalized crusted scabies.

🗣 Clinical Pearl(s)
- Lindane is potentially neurotoxic and should not be used for infants and pregnant women (permethrin is safe and effective in these situations).
- Sexual partners should be notified and treated.

132. SCARLET FEVER

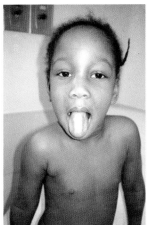

FIGURE 03-240. White strawberry tongue, which appears early in the course of scarlet fever and has scattered, hypertrophied papillae on its surface.

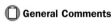 General Comments

Definition
- Scarlet fever is a rash involving the skin and tongue and complicating a streptococcal group A pharyngitis.

Etiology
- Scarlet fever is caused by group A beta-hemolytic *Streptococcus* infection, which produces one of three erythrogenic toxins. (NOTE: Some streptococcal species have the ability to cause both scarlet fever and rheumatic fever.)

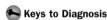 Keys to Diagnosis

Clinical Manifestation(s)
- Rash lasts about 1 week and then desquamates.
- Febrile illness with headache, malaise, anorexia, and pharyngitis begins after a 2- to 4-day incubation period.
- Scarlatinal rash begins 1 or 2 days after the onset of pharyngitis.

Physical Examination
- Diffuse erythema begins on the face and spreads to the neck, back, chest, rest of trunk, and extremities. It is most intense on the inner aspects of the arms and thighs.
- Erythema blanches, but nonblanching petechiae may be present or produced by a tourniquet.
- Strawberry or raspberry tongue is seen (**Fig. 03-240**).

Diagnostic Tests
- Identification of group A *Streptococcus* by throat culture
- Antistreptolysin O (SLO) antibody titers

DDx Differential Diagnosis

- Viral exanthems
- Kawasaki syndrome
- Toxic shock syndrome
- Drug rashes

R Treatment

First Line
- Penicillin 250 mg PO QID for 10 days or erythromycin 250 mg PO QID for 10 days in penicillin-allergic patients; clinical response can be expected in 24 to 48 hours
- Benzathine penicillin 1 to 2 million U IM once; may be used for a patient who cannot swallow pills

Clinical Pearl(s)

- Patients with antibodies against the toxin are spared the rash but still develop other symptoms of the infection (e.g., sore throat).

133. SCLERODERMA

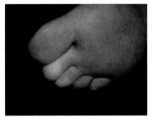

FIGURE 03-241. Persistent, progressive tricolor changes of the foot with exposure to cold is an early sign of scleroderma.

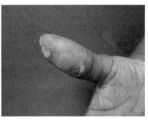

FIGURE 03-242. Painful ulcerations of the thumb, often referred to as "rat bite necrosis."

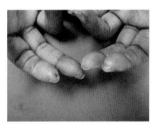

FIGURE 03-243. Progressive edema of the hand and painful digital ulcerations occur early in the course of scleroderma.

General Comments

Definition

- Scleroderma is a connective tissue disorder characterized by thickening and fibrosis of the skin and variably severe involvement of diverse internal organs.

Etiology

- Etiology is unknown. Stimulatory autoantibodies against platelet-derived growth factor (PDGF) appear to be a specific hallmark of scleroderma. Their biologic activity on fibroblasts suggests that they have a causal role in the pathogenesis of the disease.

Keys to Diagnosis

Clinical Manifestation(s)

- Raynaud's phenomenon (**Fig. 03-241**): initial complaint in 70% of patients. (Note: The prevalence of Raynaud's is 5% to 10% of the general population; most do not progress to scleroderma.)
- Finger or hand swelling, sometimes associated with carpal tunnel syndrome
- Arthralgias/arthritis
- Internal organ involvement

Physical Examination

Skin

- Scleroderma begins on the hands (**Fig. 03-242**), then moves to the face; skin is shiny, taut, and sometimes red, with loss of creases and hair.
- Later skin tightening may limit movement. Progressive edema of the hand and painful digital ulcerations occur early in the course of scleroderma (**Fig. 03-243**).
- Pigmentary changes occur.
- Skin atrophy occurs in late stages.

Diagnostic Tests

- Antinuclear antibodies (homogeneous, speckled, or nucleolar patterns)
- Anticentromere antibodies in fewer than 10% with systemic illness and in 50% to 95% with limited scleroderma (i.e., good prognosis if positive)
- Skin biopsy

DDx Differential Diagnosis

- Mycosis fungoides
- Amyloidosis
- Porphyria cutanea tarda
- Eosinophilic fasciitis
- Reflex sympathetic dystrophy

R Treatment

First Line

- Calcium channel blockers (nifedipine, amlodipine)
- D-penicillamine

Second Line

- Cochicine
- Methotrexate
- Losartan

Third Line
■ Cyclosporine

 Clinical Pearl(s)

■ CREST syndrome is calcinosis, Raynaud's phenomenon, esophageal dysmotility, sclerodactyly, and telangiectasias (in CREST, scleroderma is limited to the distal extremities).

134. SEBORRHEIC DERMATITIS

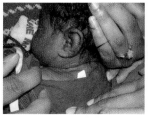

FIGURE 03-244. Redness and thick scale cover this child's scalp, face, and shoulders.

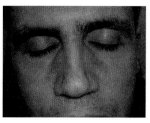

FIGURE 03-245. Erythematous, scaling papules and plaques involving the paranasal area and forehead.

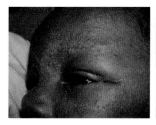

FIGURE 03-246. Confluent red papules with heavy scale over the forehead and eyebrows of this infant.

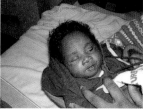

FIGURE 03-247. Facial and periorbital edema, with redness and moist scale most intense over the forehead and extending to the scalp (referred to as "cradle cap").

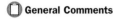 General Comments

Definition

- Seborrheic dermatitis is a common relapsing inflammatory dermatosis affecting up to 2% of the population, with a predilection for areas rich in sebaceous glands and consisting of erythematous patches often covered in a greasy scale (**Fig. 03-244**).

Etiology

- Unknown. It has been reported to be associated with parkinsonism and familial amyloidosis with polyneuropathy and exacerbated by stress.

Keys to Diagnosis

Clinical Manifestation(s)

- It particularly affects areas where sebaceous glands are most numerous (scalp, forehead [**Fig. 03-245**], eyebrows [**Fig. 03-246**], eyelids, ears, cheeks, and presternal and interscapular areas)
- The lesions are often easily confused with psoriasis.
- Dandruff and cradle cap (**Fig. 03-247**) are also sometimes included in the spectrum of seborrheic dermatitis.

Physical Examination

- The lesions are sharply marginated, dull red, or yellowish and covered with a greasy scale.

Diagnostic Tests

- HIV

Differential Diagnosis

- Psoriasis
- Tinea capitis
- Contact dermatitis
- Atopic dermatitis
- Rosacea
- Erythrasma
- Xerotic eczema
- Candidiasis

Treatment

First Line

- Topical ketoconazole
- Topical corticosteroids

Second Line
- Miconazole nitrate, topical lithium salts (lithium succinate, lithium gluconate), and selenium sulfide

Third Line
- Calcineurin inhibitors (pimecrolimus), phototherapy, oral itraconazole

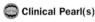 Clinical Pearl(s)

- Seborrheic dermatitis is one of the most common dermatoses seen in AIDS. It has also been associated with stress and neurologic disorders, including Parkinson's disease.

135. SEBORRHEIC KERATOSIS

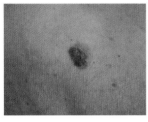

FIGURE 03-248. Velvety brown seborrheic keratosis on a tan, round base can be confused with nodular melanoma. The lighter areas of the keratosis could be confused with an area of tumor regression as occurs in melanoma.

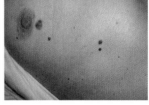

FIGURE 03-249. Round-to-oval verrucous, raised lesion just below the breast appearing to be "stuck-on." Also note several cherry angiomas of varying sizes.

General Comments

Definition
- Seborrheic keratosis are exophytic, lightly pigmented, wart-like growths common in the middle aged and elderly (**Fig. 03-248**).

Etiology
- Unknown

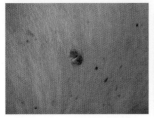

FIGURE 03-250. Brown, polypoid lesion with a smooth surface and sharply demarcated borders that tended to crumble when scraped.

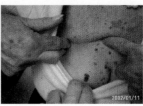

FIGURE 03-251. Multiple raised brown lesions that characteristically appear on the anterior chest and around the breasts. These are caused by chafing and irritation from clothing.

 Keys to Diagnosis

Clinical Manifestation(s)
- Although they may be found anywhere on the body (except palms and soles), growths are particularly common on the face, chest (**Fig. 03-249**), and back.

Physical Examination
- Seborrheic keratosis appears as sharply delineated, round or oval, flesh-colored or brown-black warty (**Fig. 03-250**) plaques with a rather greasy texture (**Fig. 03-251**).

Diagnostic Tests
- Skin biopsy

 Differential Diagnosis
- Actinic keratosis
- Melanoma
- Wart
- Lentigo
- Skin tag

 Treatment

First Line
- Curettage and cautery

Second Line
- Cryotherapy
- Chemical peels, lasers

Third Line
- 5-Fluorouracil

Clinical Pearl(s)

- Sudden onset of numerous seborrheic keratoses *(Leser-Trelat sign)* has been reported in association with internal malignancy, most commonly adenocarcinoma of the stomach. It has also been described after treatment with chemotherapy.

136. SJÖGREN'S SYNDROME

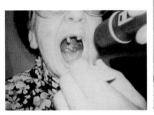

FIGURE 03-252. Dry mouth, hyperemic oral mucosa, and poor dentition in this patient with Sjogren's syndrome and underlying lymphoma.

FIGURE 03-253. Enlargement of right parotid gland secondary to autoimmune damage that occurs in Sjogren's syndrome.

General Comments

Definition

Sjögren's syndrome (SS) is an autoimmune disorder characterized by lymphocytic and plasma cell infiltration and destruction of salivary and lacrimal glands with subsequent diminished lacrimal and salivary gland secretions.
- *Primary:* dry mouth (xerostomia) and dry eyes (xerophthalmia) develop as isolated entities.
- *Secondary:* associated with other disorders.

Etiology

- Autoimmune disorder. It is one of the 3 most common systemic autoimmune diseases (prevalence between 0.05 and 4.8% of population in the USA)

Keys to Diagnosis

Clinical Manifestation(s)

- Evidence of associated conditions (e.g., rheumatoid arthritis [RA] or other connective tissue disease, lymphoma, hypothyroidism, chronic obstructive pulmonary disease [COPD], trigeminal neuropathy, chronic liver disease, polymyopathy)

Physical Examination
- Dry mouth (**Fig. 03-252**) with dry lips (cheilosis), erythema of tongue and other mucosal surfaces, carious teeth
- Dry eyes (conjunctival injection, decreased luster, and irregularity of the corneal light reflex)
- Possible salivary gland enlargement (**Fig. 03-253**) and dysfunction with subsequent difficulty in chewing and swallowing food and in speaking without frequent water intake
- Possible purpura (nonthrombocytopenic, hyperglobulinemic, vasculitic)

Diagnostic Tests
- Symptoms and objective signs of ocular dryness:
  - Schirmer's test: less than 8 mm wetting per 5 minutes
  - Positive rose bengal or fluorescein staining of cornea and conjunctiva to demonstrate keratoconjunctivitis sicca
- Symptoms and objective signs of dry mouth:
  - Decreased parotid flow using Lashley cups or other methods
  - Abnormal biopsy result of minor salivary gland (focus score > 2 based on average of four assessable lobules)
- Evidence of systemic autoimmune disorder:
  - Elevated titer of rheumatoid factor greater than 1:320
  - Elevated titer of ANA greater than 1:320
  - Presence of anti-SS A (Ro) or anti-SS B (La) antibodies
  Secondary:
- Characteristic signs and symptoms of SS
- Clinical features sufficient to allow a diagnosis of RA, SLE, polymyositis, or scleroderma

DDx Differential Diagnosis
- Medication-related dryness (e.g., anticholinergics)
- Age-related exocrine gland dysfunction
- Mouth breathing
- Anxiety
- Other: sarcoidosis, primary salivary hypofunction, radiation injury, amyloidosis

Rx Treatment
First Line
- Adequate fluid replacement is necessary. Ameliorate skin dryness by gently blotting dry after bathing, leaving a small amount of moisture, and then applying a moisturizer.
- Ensure proper oral hygiene to reduce the incidence of caries.
- Use artificial tears frequently.

- Pilocarpine 5 mg PO QID is useful to improve dryness. A cyclosporine 0.05% ophthalmic emulsion may also be useful for dry eyes. Recommended dose is 1 drop BID in both eyes.

Second Line

- Pilocarpine 5 mg PO QID is useful to improve dryness. A cyclosporine 0.05% ophthalmic emulsion may also be useful for dry eyes. Recommended dose is 1 drop BID in both eyes.
- Cevimeline, a cholinergic agent with muscarinic agonist activity, 30 mg PO TID, is effective for the treatment of dry mouth in patients with Sjögren's syndrome.

Third Line

- Hydroxchloroquine may be useful for treating Arthralgias and fatigue.
- Rhuximab may be beneficial for treating severe inflammatory manifestations.

 Clinical Pearl(s)

- Periodic dental and ophthalmology evaluations are mandatory to screen for complications.

137. SPIDER ANGIOMA

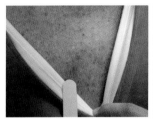
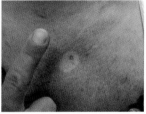

FIGURE 03-254. Dilated red capillaries resembling the spindly legs of a spider emanating from a central feeding arteriole in a cirrhotic patient. This painless lesion compresses easily on direct pressure.

FIGURE 03-255. Refilling of a spider angioma following release of applied pressure.

 General Comments

Definition

- A spider nevus is a skin lesion consisting solely of a dilated dermal arteriole that communicates with a network of ecstatic superficial capillaries.

Etiology
- Unknown

 Keys to Diagnosis

Clinical Manifestation(s)
- These lesions are extremely common and of little clinical significance.

Physical Examination
- The lesions manifest as pinhead-sized deep red puncta from which tiny tortuous vessels radiate (**Fig. 03-254**).
- Following release of applied pressure there is initial blanching and then refilling (**Fig. 03-255**).

Diagnostic Tests
- None necessary

 Differential Diagnosis
- Cherry angioma
- Telengiectasia
- Insect bite

 Treatment
First Line
- Electrodesiccation

Second Line
- Laser ablation

 Clinical Pearl(s)
- An increased frequency of these lesions is seen with chronic liver disease, thyrotoxicosis, and pregnancy.

138. SPOROTRICHOSIS

 General Comments

Definition
- Sporotrichosis is a granulomatous disease caused by *Sporothrix schenckii*.

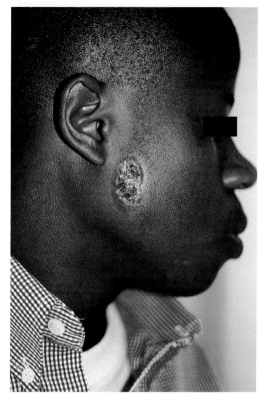

FIGURE 03-256. Sporotrichosis. Localized variant presenting as an ulcerated plaque. *(Courtesy N. C. Dlova, MD, Nelson R. Mandela School of Medicine, University of KwaZulu- Natal, South Africa. From McKee PH, Calonje JE, Granter SR: Pathology of the Skin, ed 3, St. Louis, 2005, Mosby.)*

Etiology

- *Sporothrix schenckii*
  - Global in distribution
  - Often isolated from soil, plants, and plant products
  - Majority of case reports from tropical and subtropical regions of the Americas

 Keys to Diagnosis

Clinical Manifestation(s)

Physical Examination

- Cutaneous disease
  - Arises at the site of inoculation
  - Initial lesion usually located on the distal part of an extremity, although any area may be affected, including the face
  - Variable incubation period of approximately 3 weeks once introduced into the skin
  - Granulomatous reaction provoked
  - Lesion becomes papulonodular, erythematous, elastic, variable in size
  - Subsequently, nodule becomes fluctuant, undergoes central necrosis, breaks down, discharges mucoid pus from which fungus may be isolated (**Fig. 03-256**)
  - Indolent ulcer with raised erythematous or violaceous borders
  - Secondary lesions:
    Develop along superficial lymphatic channels
    Evolve in the same manner as the primary lesion, with subsequent inflammation, induration, and suppuration
- Fixed, or plaque form
  - Erythematous verrucous, ulcerated, or crusted lesions
  - Does not spread locally
  - Does not involve lymphatic vessels
  - Rarely undergoes spontaneous resolution
  - More often persists for years without systemic symptoms and within a setting of normal laboratory examinations

Diagnostic Tests

- The diagnosis should be considered in individuals who are occupationally exposed to soil, decaying plant matter, and thorny plants (gardeners, horticulturists, farmers) who present with chronic nonhealing ulcers or lesions with or without associated arthritis or pulmonary symptoms.
- Skin biopsy should be performed. Biopsy specimens are diagnostic if characteristic cigar-shaped, round, oval, or budding yeast forms are seen.
- Despite special staining, the yeast may remain difficult to detect unless multiple sections are examined.
- Isolation of the fungus from any site is considered diagnostic of infection.

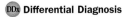 **Differential Diagnosis**

- Fixed, or plaque, sporotrichosis
- Bacterial pyoderma
- Foreign body granuloma
- Tularemia
- Anthrax
- Other mycoses: blastomycosis, chromoblastomycosis

 Treatment

First Line

- Itraconazole at doses of 100 to 200 mg/day is the drug of choice and should be given for 3 to 6 months.
- Use saturated solution of potassium iodide (SSKI) 5 to 10 drops PO TID or 1.5 mL PO TID, gradually increasing to 40 to 50 drops PO TID or 3 mL PO TID after meals.
- Maximum tolerated dose should be continued until cutaneous lesions have resolved, approximately 6 to 12 weeks.

Second Line

- For lymphocutaneous and visceral disease, therapy with itraconazole 200 mg/day for periods of 24 months or longer; newer agents such as voriconazole and posaconazole might be useful in refractory to standard therapy, but existing data for these new agents are very limited at present.

Third Line

- Parenteral amphotericin B.

 Clinical Pearl(s)

- In patients with underlying immunosuppression (e.g., hematologic malignancy or infection with HIV), progression of the initial infection may develop into multifocal extracutaneous sporotrichosis.
- In this subset of patients, dissemination of cutaneous lesions is accompanied by hematogenous spread to lungs, bone, mucous membranes, and CNS.

139. SQUAMOUS CELL CARCINOMA (SCC)

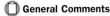 **General Comments**

Definition

- Squamous cell carcinoma (SCC) is a malignant tumor of the skin arising in the epithelium.
- SCC is the second most common cutaneous malignancy, comprising 20% of all cases of nonmelanoma skin cancer.

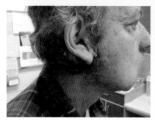

FIGURE 03-257. Necrotic, crusted, large nodular squamous cell carcinoma posterior to the right ear. Also note loss of muscle tone with flattening of the right face secondary to facial nerve compression from the tumor.

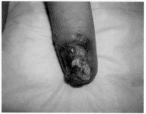

FIGURE 03-258. Oozing, red, nodular lesion involving the nail bed of the index finger previously damaged by a chronic human papillomavirus infection in this HIV-infected male. Note hyperkeratosis and destruction of the nail.

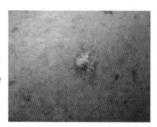

FIGURE 03-259. Hyperkeratotic, scaling actinic keratosis covering an underlying pink lesion diagnosed as squamous cell carcinoma in situ on biopsy. This appeared on the back of an elderly patient who was exposed to excessive amounts of ultraviolet radiation.

- Incidence is highest in lower latitudes (e.g., southern United States, Australia).
- The male:female ratio is 2:1.
- Incidence increases with age and sun exposure.
- Average age at diagnosis is 66 years.

Etiology
- Risk factors include UVB radiation and immunosuppression (renal transplant recipients have a threefold increased risk).

Keys to Diagnosis

Clinical Manifestation(s)
- SCC commonly affects scalp, neck region, back of hands, superior surface of the pinna (**Fig. 03-257**), and the lip.
- Most SCCs present as exophytic lesions (**Fig. 03-258**) that grow over a period of months.

Physical Examination
- The lesion may have a scaly, erythematous macule or plaque (**Fig. 03-259**).
- Telangiectasia and central ulceration may also be present.

Diagnostic Tests
- Diagnosis is made with full-thickness skin biopsy (incisional or excisional).

DDx Differential Diagnosis

- Keratoacanthomas
- Actinic keratosis
- Amelanotic melanoma
- Basal cell carcinoma
- Benign tumors
- Healing traumatic wounds
- Spindle cell tumors
- Warts

R Treatment

First Line
- Electrodesiccation and curettage can be done for small SCCs (<2 cm in diameter), superficial tumors, and lesions located on the extremities and trunk.
- Tumors thinner than 4 mm can be managed by simple local removal.
- Lesions between 4 and 8 mm thick or those with deep dermal invasion should be excised.
- Tumors penetrating the dermis can be treated with several modalities, including excision and Mohs' surgery, radiation therapy, and chemotherapy.
- Metastatic SCC can be treated with cryotherapy and combination of chemotherapy using 13-*cis*-retinoic acid and interferon alfa-2A.

Second Line
- Intralesional 5-fluorouracil, interferon alfa

Third Line
- Photodynamic therapy, systemic retinoids, systemic interferon alfa

Clinical Pearl(s)

- Survival is related to size, location, degree of differentiation of lesions; immunologic status of the patient; depth of invasion; and presence of metastases. Risk factors for metastasis include lesions on the lip or ear, increasing lesion depth, and poor cell differentiation.
- Patients whose tumors penetrate through the dermis or exceed 8 mm in thickness are at risk of tumor recurrence.

- The most common metastatic locations are regional lymph nodes, liver, and lung.
- Tumors on the scalp, forehead, ears, nose, and lips also carry a higher risk.
- SCCs originating in the lip and pinna metastasize in 10% to 20% of cases.

140. STAPHYLOCOCCAL SCALDED SKIN SYNDROME (SSSS)

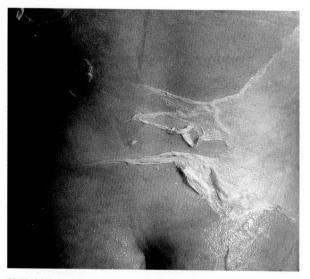

FIGURE 03-260. Staphylococcal scalded skin syndrome. Note the very extensive blistering. (Courtesy A. du Vivier, MD, King's College Hospital, London, UK. From McKee PH, Calonje JE, Granter SR: Pathology of the Skin, ed 3, St. Louis, 2005, Mosby, Fig. 17.101.)

🗋 General Comments

Definition
- Staphylococcal scalded skin syndrome is a blistering skin disease usually occurring in association with a staphylococcal infection.

Etiology
- SSSS is due to exfoliative toxins of certain strains of *S. aureus*.

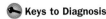 Keys to Diagnosis

Clinical Manifestation(s)

- It is often associated with fever, irritability, and skin tenderness.
- The condition is usually seen in neonates and young children, who develop first a macular scarlatiniform eruption. The eruption spreads from its usual original sites on the face, axillae, and groins to involve large areas of skin surface.
- Conjunctivitis is often also present.
- Mucous membranes are not affected.

Physical Examination

- Traction pressure on intact skin causes bullae formation (Nikolsky's sign). At the same time the skin becomes edematous and the surface fragile so that it can be sheared off in thin wrinkled sheets, likened to peeling wet wallpaper, leaving a glistening red surface, and the child becomes sick and feverish (**Fig. 03-260**).

Diagnostic Tests

- CBC
- Blood cultures, nose and throat swabs
- Histologic examination of frozen section of blister roof
- Skin biopsy

Differential Diagnosis

- Erythema multiforme
- Scarlet fever
- Kawasaki syndrome
- Toxic epidermal necrolysis
- Graft-versus-host disease

℞ Treatment

First Line

- Intravenous nafcillin or oxacillin

Second Line

- Intravenous vancomycin

Third Line

- Intravenous linezolid

Clinical Pearl(s)

- SSSS in adults tends to occur in immunocompromised and debilitated patients and therefore carries a much worse prognosis.

141. STASIS DERMATITIS

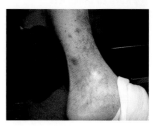

FIGURE 03-261. Chronic venous stasis with eczematoid dermatitis, brown hyperpigmentation secondary to hemosiderin deposition, and multiple dilated varicose veins. An incipient shallow ulcer is just starting to form above the medial malleolus—a common complication of stasis dermatitis.

General Comments

Definition

■ Stasis dermatitis is an inflammatory skin disease of the lower extremities, commonly seen in patients with chronic venous insufficiency.

Etiology

■ Stasis dermatitis is thought to occur as a direct result of any insult or injury of the lower extremity venous system leading to venous insufficiency, including:
  ● Deep vein thrombosis
  ● Trauma
  ● Pregnancy
  ● Vein stripping
  ● Vein harvesting in patients requiring coronary artery bypass grafting (CABG)
■ Venous insufficiency subsequently results in venous hypertension, causing skin inflammation and the aforementioned physical findings and clinical presentation.

Keys to Diagnosis

Clinical Manifestation(s)

■ Stasis dermatitis occurs more commonly in the elderly.
■ It is rarely seen before the age of 50 years and is estimated to occur in up to 6% to 7% of the patients older than 50 years.
■ It occurs in woman more often than men, perhaps related to lower-extremity venous impairment aggravated through pregnancy.
■ Onset is insidious.
■ Pruritus is present.
■ Progressive pigment changes can occur as a result of extravasation of red blood cells and hemosiderin deposition within the cutaneous tissue (**Fig. 03-261**).

Physical Examination

■ Chronic edema usually described as "brawny" edema, as stasis dermatitis pathologically is associated with dermal fibrosis.

- Erythema
- Scaly
- Eczematous patches
- Commonly located over the medial malleolus

Diagnostic Tests
- The diagnosis of stasis dermatitis is primarily made by a detailed history and physical examination.

DDx Differential Diagnosis

- Contact dermatitis
- Atopic dermatitis
- Cellulitis
- Tinea dermatophyte infection
- Pretibial myxedema
- Nummular eczema
- Lichen simplex chronicus
- Xerosis
- Asteatotic eczema
- Deep vein thrombosis

R Treatment

First Line
- Elevate the leg above heart level for 30 minutes three to four times a day (avoid in arterial occlusive diseases).
- Use a compression stocking with a gradient of at least 30 to 40 mm Hg. In obese patients, an intermittent pneumatic compression pump is recommended.
- For weeping skin lesions, wet to dry dressing changes are helpful.
- The mainstay of treatment of stasis dermatitis is to control leg edema and prevent venous stasis ulcers from developing.
- In patients with acute stasis dermatitis, a compression (Unna) boot can be applied.
- Topical corticosteroid creams or ointments (e.g., triamcinolone 0.1% BID) are used often to help reduce inflammation and itching.
- Secondary infections should be treated with appropriate antibiotics. Most secondary infections are the result of *Staphylococcus* or *Streptococcus* organisms.
- Diuretics may be helpful in controlling edema.
- Aspirin (300-325 mg) promotes healing of chronic venous ulcers.

Second Line
- Patients with chronic stasis dermatitis can be treated with topical emollients (e.g., white petrolatum, lanolin, Eucerin).
- Topical dressings (e.g., DuoDerm) are effective in the treatment of chronic venous stasis ulcers.

Third Line
- Surgical therapy:
  - Venous stripping
  - Superficial and deep perforator vein ligation
  - Endovenous stenting

Clinical Pearl(s)

- Inflammatory skin changes from stasis dermatitis are thought to result from poor oxygen perfusion to the lower-extremity skin tissue.

142. STEVENS-JOHNSON SYNDROME

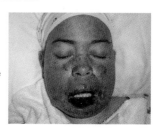

FIGURE 03-262. Edema, erythema, blister formation (lower right cheek), blister rupture with erosions (Nikolsky's sign), and hemorrhagic crusts and swelling of the lips. Stevens-Johnson syndrome developed in this patient soon after hydantoin therapy had been started for seizures.

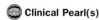 General Comments

Definition
- Stevens-Johnson syndrome (SJS) is a severe vesiculobullous form of erythema multiforme affecting skin, mouth, eyes, and genitalia.

Etiology
- Drugs (e.g., phenytoin, penicillins, phenobarbital, sulfonamides) are the most common cause.
- Upper respiratory tract infections (e.g., *Mycoplasma pneumoniae*) and herpes simplex viral infections have also been implicated in SJS.

Keys to Diagnosis

Clinical Manifestation(s)
- The cutaneous eruption is generally preceded by vague, nonspecific symptoms of low-grade fever and fatigue occurring 1 to 14 days before the skin lesions. Cough is often present. Fever may be high during the active stages.
- Corneal ulcerations may result in blindness.

- Ulcerative stomatitis results in hemorrhagic crusting.
- The pain from oral lesions may compromise fluid intake and result in dehydration.
- Thick, mucopurulent sputum and oral lesions may interfere with breathing.

Physical Examination

- Bullae generally occur on the conjunctiva, mucous membranes of the mouth (**Fig. 03-262**), nares, and genital regions.
- Flat, atypical target lesions or purpuric maculae may be distributed on the trunk or be widespread.

Diagnostic Tests

- Diagnosis is generally based on clinical presentation and characteristic appearance of the lesions.
- Skin biopsy is generally reserved for when classic lesions are absent and diagnosis is uncertain.

DDx Differential Diagnosis

- Toxic erythema (drugs or infection)
- Pemphigus
- Pemphigoid
- Urticaria
- Hemorrhagic fevers
- Serum sickness
- Staphylococcal scalded skin syndrome
- Behçet's syndrome

Rx Treatment

First Line

- Withdraw any potential drug precipitants.
- Carefully nurse skin to prevent secondary infection.
- Treat associated conditions (e.g., acyclovir for herpes simplex virus infection, erythromycin for *Mycoplasma* infection).
- Antihistamines can be helpful for pruritus.
- Treat the cutaneous blisters with cool, wet Burow's compresses.
- Relieve oral symptoms by frequent rinsing with lidocaine (Xylocaine Viscous).
- A liquid or soft diet with plenty of fluids will ensure proper hydration.
- Treat secondary infections with antibiotics.
- Topical steroids may be used to treat papules and plaques; however, they should not be applied to eroded areas.
- Vitamin A may be used for lacrimal hyposecretion.

Second Line

- Corticosteroids use remains controversial; when used, prednisone 20 to 30 mg BID may be given until new lesions no longer appear, then rapidly tapered.

Third Line
- Cyclosporine, cyclophosphamide, plasmapheresis

🔵 Clinical Pearl(s)

- Prognosis varies with severity of disease. It is generally good in patients with limited disease; however, mortality may approach 10% in patients with extensive involvement.
- Oral lesions may continue for several months.
- Scarring and corneal abnormalities may occur in 20% of patients.
- Risk of recurrence of SJS is 30% to 40%.

143. STRIAE (STRETCH MARKS)

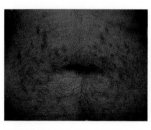

FIGURE 03-263. Purple striae developed during long-term steroid therapy for Crohn's disease.

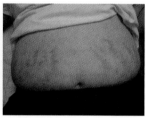

FIGURE 03-264. Linear, flesh-colored abdominal striae developed during pregnancy.

📋 General Comments

Definition
- Streaklike skin lesion caused by changes in dermal collagen.

Etiology
- Rapid growth in adolescence
- Pregnancy
- Cushing's syndrome, prolonged corticosteroid use (**Fig. 03-263**)
- Overuse of topical steroids

- Rapid weight gain
- Exercise, use of anabolic steroids

Keys to Diagnosis

Clinical Manifestation(s)
- Striae are most often found on the abdomen (**Fig. 03-264**), breasts, lumbosacral area, thighs, buttocks, and junction between arms and shoulders.

Physical Examination
- Linear pink or purple lesions are seen that eventually become atrophic and silvery-white in appearance.

Diagnostic Tests
- Usually none necessary
- Overnight dexamethasone suppression test in suspected Cushing's syndrome

DDx Differential Diagnosis

- Cushing's disease
- Linear focal elastosis
- Trauma
- Anetoderma
- Cutis laxa
- Focal dermal hypolasia

R Treatment

First Line
- Pulse dye laser ablation

Second Line
- Topical tretinoin (avoid during pregnancy)

Third Line
- Tacrolimus ointment

Clinical Pearl(s)

- Horizontal striae in the lumbosacral area of adolescents due to rapid vertical growth may be confused with signs of child abuse.

144. SYPHILIS

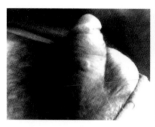

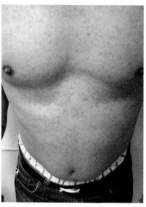

FIGURE 03-265. Painless "hard" chancre (like a "coin under the skin") associated with nontender regional lymphadenopathy marks the site of entry of the primary syphilis infection.

FIGURE 03-266. Erythematous, nonpruritic, round to oval macules and papules on the trunk, palms, and soles appearing 6 to 8 weeks after the genital chancre has healed.

General Comments

Definition
■ Syphilis is a sexually transmitted treponemal disease, acute and chronic, characterized by primary skin lesion, secondary eruption involving skin and mucous membranes, long periods of latency, and late lesions of skin, bone, viscera, CNS, and cardiovascular system.

Etiology
■ Syphilis is caused by *Treponema pallidum*, a spirochete, and is spread by sexual intercourse or by intrauterine transfer.

Keys to Diagnosis

Clinical Manifestation(s)
■ Primary syphilis: The characteristic lesion is a painless chancre on genitalia, mouth, or anus; atypical primary lesions may occur. The lesion usually appears 3 weeks after exposure and may spontaneously involute.

- Secondary syphilis: Localized or diffuse mucocutaneous lesions and generalized lymphadenopathy are seen. It is common to have constitutional, flulike symptoms. Symptoms may begin about 4 to 6 weeks after appearance of the primary lesion. Manifestations may resolve in 1 week to 12 months.
- Approximately 60% to 80% of patients have maculopapular lesions on their palms and soles.
- Condylomata lata intertriginous papules form at areas of friction and moisture, such as the vulva.
- Approximately 21% to 58% have mucocutaneous or mucosal lesions (pharyngitis, tonsillitis, "mucous patch" lesion on oral and genital mucosa).
- Early latent syphilis (<1 year) is generally asymptomatic.
- Late latent syphilis (>1 year) is characterized by gummas (nodular, ulcerative lesions) that can involve the skin, mucous membranes, skeletal system, and viscera.
- Manifestations of cardiovascular syphilis include aortitis, aneurysm, or aortic regurgitation.
- Neurosyphilis may be asymptomatic or symptomatic. Tabes dorsalis, meningovascular syphilis, general paralysis, or insanity may occur. Iritis, choroidoretinitis, and leukoplakia may also occur.

Physical Examination
- Primary syphilis: characteristic lesion is a painless chancre on genitalia (**Fig. 03-265**), mouth, or anus
- Secondary syphilis: localized or diffuse mucocutaneous lesions (**Fig. 03-266**) and generalized lymphadenopathy

Diagnostic Tests
- Dark-field microscopy of fluid from lesion to look for treponeme
- Serologic testing, both nontreponemal (VDRL, RPR) and treponemal (FTA, MHA)

DDx Differential Diagnosis
- Herpes
- Chancroid
- Lymphogranuloma venereum (LVG)
- Granuloma inguinale

R Treatment
First Line
- Early (primary, secondary, early latent): penicillin G benzathine 2.4 million U IM for 1 day or doxycycline 100 mg PO BID for 14 days
- Late (late latent, cardiovascular, gumma): penicillin G benzathine 2.4 million U IM QWK for 3 weeks or doxycycline 100 mg PO BID for 4 weeks
- Neurosyphilis: aqueous crystalline penicillin G 18 to 24 million U/day, administered as 3 to 4 million U IV Q4H for 10 to 14 days, or procaine penicillin 2.4 million U IM/day plus probenecid 500 mg PO QID, both for 10 to 14 days

■ Congenital syphilis: aqueous crystalline penicillin G 50,000 U/kg/dose IV Q12H for first 7 days of life and q8h after that for total of 10 days or procaine penicillin G 50,000 U/kg/dose IM/day for 10 days

Second Line
■ Early (primary, secondary, early latent): doxycycline 100 mg PO BID for 14 days
■ Late (late latent, cardiovascular, gumma): doxycycline 100 mg PO BID for 4 weeks

Third Line
■ Ceftriaxone 1 g Q24H for 8 to 10 days or azithromycin 2 g PO

🗨 Clinical Pearl(s)

■ Jarisch-Herxheimer reaction (fever, myalgia, tachycardia, hypotension) may occur within 24 hours of treatment.
■ One third of untreated patients develop CNS and/or cardiovascular sequelae.
■ Up to 80% of those treated during late stages remain seropositive indefinitely.
■ Treponemal tests remain positive even after adequate therapy.
■ Male circumcision significantly reduces the incidence of syphilis.

145. SYSTEMIC LUPUS ERYTHEMATOSUS (SLE, LUPUS)

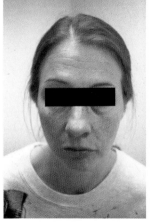

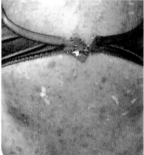

FIGURE 03-267. Malar erythematous butterfly rash with mild scaling.

FIGURE 03-268. Scaly erythematous plaques with areas of chronic hyperpigmentation and hypopigmention due to systemic lupus erthymatosus.

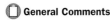 General Comments

Definition

- Systemic lupus erythematosus is a chronic multisystemic disease characterized by production of autoantibodies and protean clinical manifestations.

Etiology

- Unknown. Autoantibodies are typically present many years before the diagnosis of SLE. A haplotype of STAT4 is associated with increased risk for both rheumatoid arthritis and SLE, suggesting a shared pathway for these illnesses. Genetic susceptibility to lupus is inherited as a complex trait. An interval on the long arm of chromosome 1, 1q23-24 has been linked with SLE in many populations.

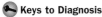 Keys to Diagnosis

Clinical Manifestation(s)

- Butterfly rash
- Discoid rash
- Photosensitivity (particularly leg ulcerations)
- Oral ulcers
- Arthritis
- Serositis (pleuritis, pericarditis)
- Neurologic disorder (seizures, psychosis [in absence of offending drugs or metabolic derangement])

Physical Examination

- Skin: erythematous rash over the malar eminences (**Fig. 03-267**) generally with sparing of the nasolabial folds (butterfly rash); alopecia; raised erythematous patches with subsequent edematous plaques (**Fig. 03-268**) and adherent scales (discoid lupus); leg, nasal, or oropharyngeal ulcerations; livedo reticularis; pallor (from anemia); petechiae (from thrombocytopenia)

Diagnostic Tests

- ANA, anti-DNA (presence of antibody to native DNA in abnormal titer), anti-Sm (presence of antibody to Smith nuclear antigen)
- CBC (hemolytic anemia with reticulocytosis, leukopenia, lymphopenia, thrombocytopenia)
- Urinalysis (persistent proteinuria > 0.5 g/day or 3 if quantitation not performed, cellular casts)

DDx Differential Diagnosis

- Other connective tissue disorders (e.g., rheumatoid arthritis (RA), mixed connective tissue disease (MCTD), progressive systemic sclerosis)
- Metastatic neoplasm
- Infection

Treatment

First Line

- Patients with photosensitivity should avoid sunlight and use high-factor sunscreen.
- Cutaneous manifestations are treated with the following:
  - Topical corticosteroids; intradermal corticosteroids for individual discoid lesions, especially in the scalp
  - Antimalarials (e.g., hydroxychloroquine and quinacrine)
  - Sunscreens that block UVA and UVB radiation

Second Line

- Immunosuppressive drugs (methotrexate or azathioprine) are used as steroid-sparing drugs.

Third Line

- Newer treatment modalities include the use of rituximab (a chimeric human-murine monoclonal antibody directed against CD20 on B cells and their precursors) to induce substantial remissions in patients previously unresponsive to conventional agents. Intravenous immunoglobulins are also increasingly being used in the treatment of patients with resistant lupus.

Clinical Pearl(s)

- Antiphospholipid syndrome with thrombotic manifestations is a major predictor of irreversible organ damage and death in patients with SLE.

146. TELOGEN EFFLUVIUM

General Comments

Definition

- Telogen effluvium is a disorder characterized by an early end to anagen stage with progression of many hairs to catagen and subsequently telogen.

Etiology

- Several medications have also been implicated (lipid-lowering agents, anticoagulants, beta blockers, oral contraceptives).

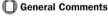 Keys to Diagnosis

Clinical Manifestation(s)

- The loss of hair begins approximately 3 to 4 months after the precipitating event. Baldness, however, is never observed.

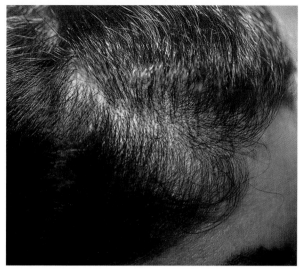

FIGURE 03-269. Telogen effluvium. There is diffuse hair loss without inflammation. *(Reproduced with permission from Hordinsky ME, Sawaya ME, Scher RK [eds], Atlas of Hair and Nails, Philadelphia, 2000, Saunders.)*

Physical Examination

■ Patients show diffuse noninflammatory hair loss involving the entire scalp (**Fig. 03-269**).

Diagnostic Tests

■ None necessary. Histologically the only finding is an increase in the number of telogen hair follicles and follicular stellae in the deep layers.

DDx Differential Diagnosis

■ Androgenic alopecia
■ Alopecia areata
■ Tinea capitis
■ Trichotillomania
■ Anagen effluvium

$\mathbb{R}$ Treatment

First Line
- Elimination of contributing factors

Second Line
- Topical minoxidil

Clinical Pearl(s)

- Telogen effluvium may be precipitated by physiologic processes such as severe psychologic stress, postpartum period, or crash diets or by pathologic events such as spinal cord injury, major surgery, hypothyroidism, HIV infection, septicemia, and Hodgkin's lymphoma.

147. THROMBOPHLEBITIS, SUPERFICIAL

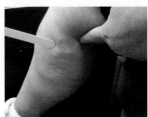

FIGURE 03-270. Erythema, tenderness, and palpable cord in a superficial varicose calf vein consistent with superficial thrombophlebitis. This was confirmed by ultrasound in this obese patient with uterine cancer.

General Comments

Definition
- Superficial thrombophlebitis is inflammatory thrombosis in subcutaneous veins. Superficial suppurative thrombophlebitis is an inflammation of the vein wall due to the presence of microorganisms occurring as a complication of either dermal infection or use of an indwelling intravenous catheter.

Etiology
- Trauma to preexisting varices.
- Intravenous cannulation of veins (most common cause)
- Abdominal cancer (e.g., carcinoma of pancreas)
- Infection: *S. aureus* was the most common pathogen, found in 65% to 78% of the cases of superficial suppurative thrombophlebitis before 1970; now most cases are due to *Enterobacteriaceae*, especially *Klebsiella-Enterobacter* spp. These agents are acquired nosocomially and are often resistant to multiple antibiotics.

Infection with fungi or gram-negative aerobic bacilli is often seen in patients who are receiving broad-spectrum antibiotics at the time of the superficial suppurative phlebitis.

- Hypercoagulable state
- DVT

Keys to Diagnosis

Clinical Manifestation(s)

- Low-grade fever, tenderness localized along the course of the vein

Physical Examination

- The subcutaneous vein is palpable, tender; a tender cord is present with erythema and edema of the overlying skin and subcutaneous tissue.
- Induration, redness, and tenderness are localized along the course of the vein (**Fig. 03-270**). This linear appearance rather than circular appearance is useful to distinguish thrombophlebitis from other conditions (cellulitis, erythema nodosum).

Diagnostic Tests

- CBC with differential, blood cultures, culture of intravenous catheter tip (when secondary to intravenous cannulation). Bacteremia occurs in 80% to 90% of the cases of superficial suppurative thrombophlebitis.
- Culture of the catheter may be misleading because even though bacteria are isolated in 60% of the cases, a positive culture does not correlate with inflammation.
- Serial ultrasound and plasma D-dimer measurement in patients with suspected DVT
- CT scan of abdomen in patients with suspected malignancy (*Trousseau's syndrome:* recurrent migratory thrombophlebitis)

DDx Differential Diagnosis

- Lymphangitis
- Cellulitis
- Erythema nodosum
- Panniculitis
- Kaposi's sarcoma

Treatment

First Line

- NSAIDs to relieve symptoms
- Treatment of septic thrombophlebitis with antibiotics with adequate coverage of *Enterobacteriaceae* and *Staphylococcus;* initial empirical treatment with a semisynthetic penicillin (intravenous nafcillin 2 g Q4-6H plus either an aminoglycoside

[gentamicin 1 mk/kg IV q8h] or a third-generation cephalosporin [cefotaxime] or a quinolone [ciprofloxacin]).

Second Line
■ Ligation and division of the superficial vein at the junction to avoid propagation of the clot in the deep venous system when the thrombophlebitis progresses toward the junction of the involved superficial vein with deep veins

Third Line
■ The role of antifungal therapy for superficial suppurative thrombophlebitis due to *C. albicans* is controversial. Most of these infections can be cured by vein excision. Because of the propensity of these infections for hematogenous spread, a 10- to 14-day course of amphotericin B or fluconazole is advisable.

Clinical Pearl(s)
■ Patients with positive cultures should be evaluated and treated for endocarditis.
■ Suppurative thrombophlebitis is a particular problem in burned patients, for whom it represents a common cause of death due to infection.
■ Septic thrombophlebitis is more common in intravenous drug addicts.

148. TINEA BARBAE (TINEA OF THE BEARD) AND TINEA FACIE (TINEA OF THE FACE)

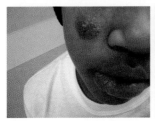 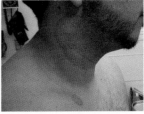

FIGURE 03-271. Annular, erythematous, hyperpigmented lesion with overlying scale. Scrapings of the latter were positive for hyphae on KOH preparation.

FIGURE 03-272. Red, circular patch with a distinct border presenting on the anterior neck and extending to the chin and beard area. Some of the hair follicles within the affected beard have been broken off at the surface.

General Comments

Definition
- Tinea barbae is a dermatophyte infection of the beard area. When the facial infection is outside the beard area it is called tinea facie (**Fig. 03-271**).

Etiology
- Most common causes of tinea barbae are trichophytoin mentagrophyytes and trichophytoin verrucosum.
- Tinea faciae usually results from direct inoculation or by extension of tinea from beard, scalp, or body.

Keys to Diagnosis

Clinical Manifestation(s)
- Onset is generally insidious. It may evolve into a ringworm pattern or follicular pattern (appearance similar to bacterial folliculitis).
- Pruritus is often present. Pain and swelling can occur with infections of the hair follicles.

Physical Examination
- Annular red scaly plaques with some crusting (ringworm pattern) (**Fig. 03-272**)
- Pustules, draining nodules (follicular pattern)

Diagnostic Tests
- Potassium hydroxide examination of the plucked hair and skin scales

DDx Differential Diagnosis
- Folliculitis
- Furunculosis
- Actinomycosis
- Acne

R Treatment

First Line
- Terbinafine 250 mg PO QD for 3 to 4 weeks

Second Line
- Fluconazole

Third Line
- Griseofulvin
- Sporonox

Clinical Pearl(s)

■ Tinea barbae is most common in farmworkers who handle cattle and athletes (wrestlers).

149. TINEA CAPITIS

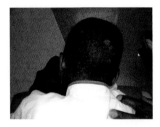

FIGURE 03-273. Several well-circumscribed patches of alopecia with minimal inflammation and fine scaling.

 General Comments

Definition

■ Tinea capitis is a dermatophyte infection of the scalp. It is the most common dermatophytosis of childhood, primarily affecting children between 3 and 7 years. About 3% to 8% of American children are affected, and 34% of household contacts are asymptomatic carriers.

Etiology

■ Tinea capitis is most commonly caused by the *Trichophyton* (>90% of the cases in the United States) or *Microsporum* genera (5%). Most common causative species for black dot tinea capitis is *Trichophyton tonsurans* and for gray patch tinea capitis are *Microsporum andouinii* and *Microsporum canis*. Transmission occurs via infected persons or asymptomatic carriers, fallen infected hairs, animal vectors, and fomites. *M. audouinii* is commonly spread by dogs and cats. Infectious fungal particles may remain viable for many months.

 Keys to Diagnosis

Clinical Manifestation(s)

■ The triad of scalp scaling, alopecia, and cervical adenopathy is a common manifestation.
■ Primary lesions include plaques, papules, pustules, or nodules on the scalp (usually occipital region).
■ Secondary lesions include scales, alopecia (usually reversible), erythema, exudates, and edema.

- Scalp pruritus may be present.
- Fever, pain, and lymphadenopathy (commonly postcervical) are present with inflammatory lesions.

Physical Examination
- Two distinctly different forms are seen:
  - Gray patch: Several scaly, well-demarcated lesions are present (**Fig. 03-273**). The hairs within the patch break off a few millimeters above the scalp. One or several lesions may be present; sometimes the lesions join to form larger ones.
  - Black dot: Early lesions with erythema and scaling patch are easily overlooked until areas of alopecia develop. Hairs within the patches break at the surface of the scalp, leaving behind a pattern of swollen black dots.
- Kerion: Inflamed, exudative, pustular, boggy, tender nodules exhibit marked edema, and hair loss is seen in severe tinea capitis. Caused by an immune response to the fungus, this may lead to some scarring.
- Favus: Production of scutula (hair matted together with dermatophyte hyphae and keratin debris) is seen, characterized by yellow cup-shaped crusts around hair shafts. A fetid odor may be present.

Diagnostic Tests
- KOH testing should be done on hair shaft extracted from the lesion, not the scale, because the *T. tonsurans* spores attach to or reside inside hair shafts and will rarely be found in the scales.
- Wood's ultraviolet light fluoresces blue-green on hair shafts for *Microsporum* infections but will fail to identify *T. tonsurans*.
- Fungal culture of hairs and scales on fungal medium such as Sabouraud's agar may be used to confirm the diagnosis, especially if uncertain.
- Histology of biopsy specimens with fungal staining may be done in cases where mycology tests are negative because of treatment initiation.

DDx Differential Diagnosis

- Alopecia areata
- Impetigo
- Pediculosis
- Trichotillomania
- Traction alopecia
- Folliculitis
- Pseudopelade
- Seborrhea/atopic
- Dermatitis
- Psoriasis
- Carbuncles
- Pyoderma

- Lichen ruber planus
- Lupus erythematosus

 Treatment

First Line
- Oral terbinafine
- Itraconazole
- Fluconazole
- The adjuvant use of antifungal shampoos is recommended for all patients and household contacts. Shampoo like selenium sulfide 2.5% used on scalp for at least 5 minutes 2 to 3 times/week can help prevent infection or eradicate asymptomatic carrier state by inhibiting fungal growth.
- Patients and their families should look for sources of infections and disinfect contaminated objects such as combs, brushes, towels, and headgear. Avoid sharing personal hygiene utensils.
- Culture of hairs and scalp dander facilitates carrier identification and prevention.
- Pets that are infected or asymptomatic carriers should be treated.
- Recommend follow-up visits every 2 to 4 weeks using Wood's light, microscopic study, and fungal culture. A mycologically documented cure is the goal of treatment.

Second Line
- Griseofulvin

Third Line
- Severe inflammatory kerion can be managed with additional prednisone 1 mg/kg/day and erythromycin.

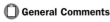 **Clinical Pearl(s)**

- Confirming the diagnosis of tinea capitis with a laboratory specimen is important because misdiagnosis will result in delay or improper treatment.

150. TINEA CORPORIS

General Comments

Definition
- Tinea corporis, also known as "ringworm," is a dermatophyte fungal infection caused by the genera *Trichophyton* or *Microsporum*.

Etiology
- *T. rubrum* is the most common pathogen.

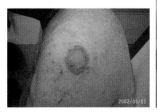

FIGURE 03-274. Round, rapidly expanding red plaque with moderate scaling, a raised border, and central clearing. Because it was zoophilic in origin (contracted from his cat), this lesion was relatively more inflammatory.

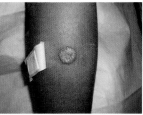

FIGURE 03-275. This tinea corporis infection, which was initially covered with a bandage, developed marked vesiculation because of increased moisture.

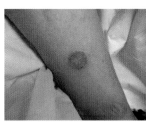

FIGURE 03-276. Annular lesion with a raised, scaly border on the forearm.

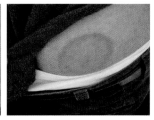

FIGURE 03-277. The borders of tinea corporis can extend at variable rates, causing a lesion that is more ovoid than annular.

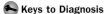 Keys to Diagnosis

Clinical Manifestation(s)

■ The disease typically begins as an isolated lesion with subsequent development of satellite lesions (**Fig. 03-274**). Vesciculation may develop if the lesion is covered (**Fig. 03-275**).

Physical Examination

■ Annular red scaly plaques with active border are seen with some crusting and central clearing (**Fig. 03-276**).

■ In some cases the borders of tinea corporis can extend at variable rates, producing a lesion that is more ovoid than annular (**Fig. 03-277**).

Diagnostic Tests

- Diagnosis is usually made on clinical grounds. It can be confirmed by direct visualization under the microscope of a small fragment of the scale using wet mount preparation and potassium hydroxide solution; dermatophytes appear as translucent branching filaments (hyphae) with lines of separation appearing at irregular intervals.
- Biopsy is indicated only when the diagnosis is uncertain and the patient has failed to respond to treatment.

 Differential Diagnosis

- Pityriasis rosea
- Erythema multiforme
- Psoriasis
- Cutaneous SLE
- Secondary syphilis
- Nummular eczema
- Eczema
- Granuloma annulare
- Lyme disease
- Tinea versicolor
- Contact dermatitis

℞ **Treatment**

First Line

- Various creams are effective; the application area should include normal skin about 2 cm beyond the affected area:
  - Betenafine cream, applied QD for 14 days
  - Terbinafine cream applied BID for 14 days

Second Line

- Systemic therapy is reserved for severe cases and is usually given up to 4 weeks; commonly used agents include the following:
  - Fluconazole 200 mg QD
  - Terbinafine 250 mg QD

😀 **Clinical Pearl(s)**

- The majority of cases resolve without sequelae within 3 to 4 weeks of therapy.

151. TINEA CRURIS

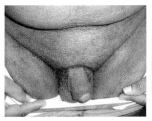

FIGURE 03-278. Extensive tinea cruris with well-demarcated border in this HIV-positive patient. Note marked hyperpigmentation and scaling involving the groin and suprapubic areas. A Wood's lamp examination ruled out erythrasma.

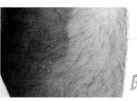

FIGURE 03-279. Well-defined, scaly, raised border positive for dermatophyte hyphae on KOH prep. This affected the crural folds and medial thighs.

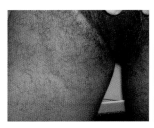

FIGURE 03-280. An erythematous, well-demarcated, scaly rash in the crural folds that does not affect the scrotum is characteristic for tinea cruris.

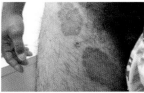

FIGURE 03-281. Tinea cruris may appear in a ringworm pattern with erythematous patches and raised, scaly borders.

General Comments

Definition
■ Tinea cruris (jock itch, ringworm) is a dermatophyte infection of the groin (**Fig. 03-278**).

Etiology
■ Dermatophytes of the genera *Trichophyton, Epidermophyton,* and *Microsporum. T. rubrum* and *Epidermophyton floccosum* are the most common causes.

- Transmission is from direct contact (e.g., infected persons, animals). The patient's feet should be evaluated as a source of infection because tinea cruris is often associated with tinea pedis.

Keys to Diagnosis

Clinical Manifestation(s)

- Tinea cruris is most common during the summer in adolescent and young adult men.
- Men are affected more often than women; however, it has become more common in postpubertal females who are overweight or who often wear tight jeans or pantyhose.
- The infection often coexists with tinea pedis.

Physical Examination

- Erythematous plaques have a half-moon shape and a scaling border (**Fig. 03-279**).
- The acute inflammation tends to move down the inner thigh and usually spares the scrotum (**Fig. 03-280**); in severe cases the fungus may spread onto the buttocks.
- Itching may be severe.
- Red papules and pustules may be present.
- Tinea cruris may appear in a ringworm pattern with erythematous patches and raised, scaly borders (**Fig. 03-281**).

Diagnostic Tests

- Diagnosis is based on clinical presentation and microscopic demonstration of hyphae using potassium hydroxide.

Differential Diagnosis

- Candidal intertrigo
- Psoriasis
- Seborrheic dermatitis
- Erythrasma
- Contact dermatitis
- Tinea versicolor

℞ Treatment

First Line

- Keep the infected area clean and dry.
- Use of boxer shorts is preferred to regular underwear.
- Various topical antifungal agents are available:
  - Betenafine cream, applied QD for 14 days.
  - Terbinafine cream applied BID for 14 days

- Drying powders (e.g., miconazole nitrate) may be useful in patients with excessive perspiration.

Second Line
- Oral antifungal therapy is generally reserved for cases unresponsive to topical agents. Effective medications are fluconazole 200 mg QD and terbinafine 250 mg QD for 10–14 days.

🟤 Clinical Pearl(s)

- An important diagnostic sign is the advancing well-defined border with a tendency toward central clearing.

152. TINEA PEDIS

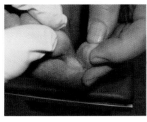
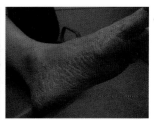

FIGURE 03-282. Interdigital tinea pedia characterized by white, macerated, peeling skin typically found in the fourth interdigital web space.

FIGURE 03-283. Erythematous, scaly skin involving the entire plantar surface of the foot and extending just to the medial border. Involvement includes the area typically covered by a moccasin or ballet slipper.

🔘 General Comments

Definition
- Tinea pedis (athlete's foot) is a dermatophyte infection of the feet.

Etiology
- Dermatophyte infection caused by *T. rubrum, T. mentagrophytes,* or, less commonly, *E. floccosum*

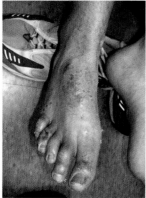

FIGURE 03-284. Ulcerative type, extending from interdigital tinea to the dorsum of the foot, with acute vesicular/bullous formation and erosive inflammation.

FIGURE 03-285. Erosion and redness of toes from rupture of vesicles and bullae. Also note extensive dry, white scale distributed in a moccasin-type pattern on the plantar surface of the foot.

Keys to Diagnosis

Clinical Manifestation(s)

- The infection usually starts in the interdigital spaces of the foot. Most infections are found in the toe webs (**Fig. 03-282**) or in the soles.
- Fourth or fifth toes are most commonly involved.
- Pruritus is common and is most intense following removal of shoes and socks (**Fig. 03-283**).
- Infection with *T. rubrum* often manifests with a moccasin distribution affecting the soles and lateral feet.

Physical Examination

- Typical presentation is variable and ranges from erythematous scaling plaques and isolated blisters to interdigital maceration (**Fig. 03-284**). Erosion and redness of toes from rupture of vesicles and bullae may be present (**Fig. 03-285**).

Diagnostic Tests

- Diagnosis is usually made by clinical observation.
- Laboratory testing, when performed, generally consists of a simple potassium hydroxide (KOH) preparation with mycologic examination under a light microscope to confirm the presence of dermatophytes.

- Mycologic culture is rarely indicated in the diagnosis of tinea pedis.
- Biopsy is reserved for when the diagnosis remains in question after testing or failure to respond to treatment.

DDx Differential Diagnosis

- Contact dermatitis
- Toe web infection (bacterial or candidal infection)
- Eczema
- Psoriasis
- Keratolysis exfoliativa
- Juvenile plantar dermatosis

℞ Treatment

First Line

- Keep the infected area clean and dry. Aerate feet by using sandals when possible.
- Use 100% cotton socks rather than nylon socks to reduce moisture.
- Areas likely to become infected should be dried completely before being covered with clothes.
- Butenafine Hcl 1% cream applied BID for 1 week or QD for 4 week is effective in interdigital tinea pedis.
- Terbinafine cream may be applied BID for 14 days.
- Ciclopirox 0.77% cream applied BID for 4 weeks is also effective.
- Clotrimazole 1% cream is an over-the-counter (OTC) treatment. It should be applied to affected and surrounding area BID for up to 4 weeks.
- Naftifine 1% cream applied QD or gel applied BID for 4 weeks also produces a significantly high cure rate.
- When using topical preparations, the application area should include normal skin about 2 cm beyond the affected area.
- Areas of maceration can be treated with Burow's solution soaks for 10 to 20 min BID followed by foot elevation.

Second Line

- Oral agents (fluconazole 150 mg once/week for 4 weeks) can be used in combination with topical agents in resistant cases.

Clinical Pearl(s)

- This is the most common dermatophyte infection.
- There is an increased incidence in hot humid weather. Occlusive footwear is a contributing factor.
- Occurrence is rare before adolescence.
- It is more common in adult males.

- Combination therapy of antifungal and corticosteroid (clotrimazole/betamethasone) should only be used when the diagnosis of fungal infection is confirmed and inflammation is a significant issue.

153. TINEA VERSICOLOR (PITYRIASIS VERSICOLOR)

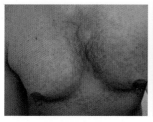

FIGURE 03-286. Numerous circular, salmon-colored, well-defined macules in this untanned individual.

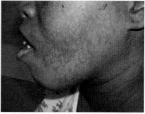

FIGURE 03-287. Circular, hypopigmented areas can also occur in dark-skinned individuals, as on the face of this African-American woman.

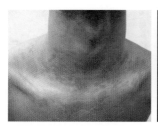

FIGURE 03-288. Tinea versicolor can appear as brown, hyperpigmented macules in dark-skinned individuals.

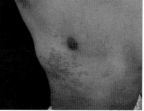

FIGURE 03-289. Rapidly expanding brown, scaly macules of tinea versicolor are well dermacated and coalescing into patches.

General Comments

Definition

- Tinea versicolor is a fungal infection of the skin caused by the yeast *Pityrosporum orbiculare (Malassezia furfur)*.

Etiology

- The infection is caused by the lipophilic yeast *Pityrosporum orbiculare* (round form) and *Pityrosporum ovale* (oval form); these organisms are normal inhabitants of the skin flora; factors that favor their proliferation are pregnancy, malnutrition, immunosuppression, oral contraceptives, and excess heat and humidity.

Keys to Diagnosis

Clinical Manifestation(s)

- There is an increased incidence in adolescence and young adulthood.
- Tinea versicolor is more common during the summer (hypopigmented lesions are more evident when the skin is tanned).
- Most patients become aware of the eruption when the involved areas do not tan.
- Eruption is generally of insidious onset and asymptomatic.

Physical Examination

- Most lesions begin as multiple small, circular macules of various colors.
- The macules may be darker or lighter than the surrounding normal skin (**Fig. 03-286**) and will scale with scraping.
- The most common site of distribution is the trunk.
- Facial lesions are more common in children (forehead is most common facial site).
- Lesions may be hypopigmented in African Americans (**Fig. 03-287**) or may be hyperpigmented in other dark-skinned individuals (**Fig. 03-288**).
- Lesions may be inconspicuous in fair-complexioned individuals, especially during the winter.
- Rapidly expanding brown, scaly macules of tinea versicolor may be well demarcated and coalescing into patches (**Fig. 03-289**).

Diagnostic Tests

- Diagnosis is based on clinical appearance; identification of hyphae and budding spores (spaghetti and meatballs appearance) with microscopy confirms diagnosis.
- Microscopic examination using potassium hydroxide confirms diagnosis when in doubt.

DDx Differential Diagnosis

- Vitiligo
- Pityriasis alba
- Secondary syphilis
- Pityriasis rosea
- Seborrheic dermatitis

Treatment

First Line

- Antifungal topical agents (e.g., miconazole, ciclopirox, clotrimazole)

Second Line

- Oral treatment is generally reserved for resistant cases. Effective agents are ketoconazole 200 mg QD for 5 days, or single 400-mg dose (cure rate >80%), fluconazole 400 mg given as a single dose (cure rate >70% at 3 weeks after treatment), or itraconazole 200 mg/day for 5 days.

Third Line

- Topical treatment: selenium sulfide 2.5% suspension applied daily for 10 minutes for 7 consecutive days results in a cure rate of 80% to 90%.

 Clinical Pearl(s)

- Sunlight accelerates repigmentation of hypopigmented areas.
- Patients should be informed that the hypopigmented areas will not disappear immediately after treatment and that several months may be necessary for the hypopigmented areas to regain their pigmentation.

154. TOXIC EPIDERMAL NECROLYSIS

 General Comments

Definition

- Toxic epidermal necrolysis (TEN, Lyell's syndrome) and Stevens-Johnson syndrome are part of a spectrum of potentially life-threatening conditions manifesting with widespread epidermal loss and significant involvement of mucous membranes. They represent severe drug hypersensitivity reactions.
- Classification of these disorders is based upon the extent of detachable skin at the worst stage of illness.
- In TEN, 30% or more of the skin is involved, whereas in SJS less than 10% is affected.
- An intermediate category where 10% to 30% of the skin is involved has also been recognized.

Etiology

- Drugs (e.g., phenytoin, penicillins, phenobarbital, sulfonamides) are the most common cause.

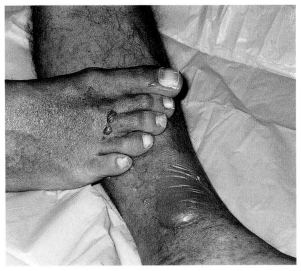

FIGURE 03-290. Toxic epidermal necrolysis. Early stage showing a large, fluid-filled blister. *(Courtesy R. Reynolds, MD, Harvard Medial School, Boston. From McKee PH, Calonje JE, Granter SR: Pathology of the Skin, ed 3, St. Louis, 2005, Mosby.)*

Keys to Diagnosis

Clinical Manifestation(s)

■ The cutaneous eruption is generally preceded by vague, nonspecific symptoms of low-grade fever and fatigue occurring 1 to 14 days before the skin lesions. Cough is often present. Fever may be high during the active stages.

Physical Examination

■ There is widespread epidermal loss with involvement of mucous membranes. Bullae generally occur on the conjunctiva, mucous membranes of the mouth, nares, and genital regions (**Fig. 03-290**).

Diagnostic Tests

■ Diagnosis is generally based on clinical presentation and characteristic appearance of the lesions.

- Skin biopsy is generally reserved for when classic lesions are absent and diagnosis is uncertain.

 Differential Diagnosis

- Toxic erythema (drugs or infection)
- Pemphigus
- Pemphigoid
- Urticaria
- Hemorrhagic fevers
- Serum sickness
- Staphylococcal scalded skin syndrome
- Behçet's syndrome

Ⓡ **Treatment**

First Line

- Withdrawal of any potential drug precipitants
- Careful skin nursing to prevent secondary infection
- Antihistamines for pruritus
- Treatment of the cutaneous blisters with cool, wet Burow's compresses
- Relief of oral symptoms by frequent rinsing with lidocaine (Xylocaine Viscous)
- Liquid or soft diet with plenty of fluids to ensure proper hydration
- Treatment of secondary infections with antibiotics
- Topical steroids: may use to treat papules and plaques; however, should not be applied to eroded areas
- Vitamin A: may be used for lacrimal hyposecretion

Second Line

- Corticosteroids: use remains controversial; when used, prednisone 20 to 30 mg BID until new lesions no longer appear, then rapidly tapered

Third Line

- Cyclosporine, cyclophosphamide, plasmapheresis

👄 **Clinical Pearl(s)**

- Prognosis varies with severity of disease. It is generally good in patients with limited disease; however, mortality may approach 10% in patients with extensive involvement.

155. TRICHOTILLOMANIA

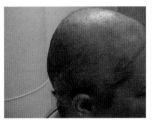

FIGURE 03-291. Compulsive hair pulling typically involving the readily reachable frontoparietal area. The remaining hair is short and of variable length. Her scalp is not entirely smooth and bald as in female pattern hair loss.

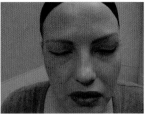

FIGURE 03-292. Careful application of cosmetics hid the fact that both eyebrows and upper lid eyelashes had also been plucked free of hair by this patient who was under psychologic stress. Lower lid eyelashes are embedded into the lid and cannot be forcibly pulled out.

General Comments

Definition
■ Traumatic alopecia due to traction and pulling of hair (**Fig. 03-291**). Patients experience an irresistible urge to pull out their hair.

Etiology
■ Trichotillomania represents a chronic mental illness of variable intensity and presentation. In the most severe cases it can be associated with trichophagia and trichobezoar.

Keys to Diagnosis

Clinical Manifestation(s)
■ Although some patients admit to pulling the hair, the majority deny it.
■ Trichotillomania affects mainly young women.
■ Occasionally the compulsion to pull hair is not limited to the scalp but can involve other body sites including the pubis, the eyebrows (**Fig. 03-292**), the eyelashes, and even the nostrils.

Physical Examination
■ Excoriations may be evident upon examination of the affected areas.

Diagnostic Tests
■ Hair microscopy; histologically, the most important feature is the very high percentage of catagen or telogen follicles

- Scalp biopsy
- CBC, ferritin

DDx Differential Diagnosis

- Iron deficiency
- Malnutrition
- Hypothyroidism
- Telogen effluvium
- Traction alopecia
- Alopecia areata
- Anagen effluvium
- Tinea capitis

R Treatment

First Line
- Psychotherapy, behavioral therapy

Second Line
- SSRIs

Third Line
- Neuroleptics
- Hypnotherapy

Clinical Pearl(s)

- Most patients with trichotillomania have depressive illnesses. Identification and treatment of these are essential for proper treatment of this disorder.

156. URTICARIA (HIVES)

General Comments

Definition
- Urticaria (hives, wheals) is a pruritic rash involving the epidermis and the upper portions of the dermis (**Fig. 03-293**), resulting from localized capillary vasodilation and followed by transudation of protein-rich fluid in the surrounding tissue and manifesting clinically with the presence of hives. Urticaria is classified according to its chronicity into acute (<6 weeks duration) and chronic (>6 weeks duration).

Etiology
- Foods (e.g., shellfish, eggs, strawberries, nuts)
- Drugs (e.g., penicillin, aspirin, sulfonamides)

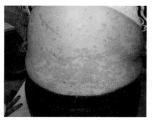

FIGURE 03-293. Confluent red plaques on the torso of this patient following a bee sting. The linear configuration of some of the hives caused by scratching is suggestive of dermographism.

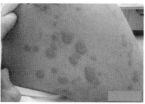

FIGURE 03-294. Well-circumscribed, round, intensely pruritic pink plaques after ingesting shellfish.

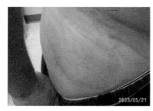

FIGURE 03-295. Giant flesh-colored, edematous hive with more intense red border. This could be mistaken for erythema migrans, but the appearance of other typical hives in this patient confirmed the diagnosis of acute urticaria.

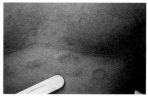

FIGURE 03-296. Edematous, pruritic plaques that are confluent in some areas with clear centers resembling a targetoid lesion. These alone could be confused with erythema multiforme.

- Systemic diseases (e.g., SLE, serum sickness, autoimmune thyroid disease, polycythemia vera)
- Food additives (e.g., salicylates, benzoates, sulfites)
- Infections (e.g., viral infections, fungal infections, chronic bacterial infections)
- Physical stimuli (e.g., pressure urticaria, exercise induced, solar urticaria, cold urticaria)
- Inhalants (e.g., mold spores, animal danders, pollens)
- Contact (nonimmunologic) urticaria (e.g., caterpillars, plants)
- Other: hereditary angioedema, urticaria pigmentosa, pregnancy, cryoglobulinemia, hair bleaches, chemicals, saliva, cosmetics, perfumes, pemphigoid, emotional stress, malignancy (lymphomas, endocrine tumors)

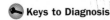 Keys to Diagnosis

Clinical Manifestation(s)

- Urticaria manifests with the presence of short-lived pruritic raised wheals (**Fig. 03-294**) following exposure to triggering agent.

Physical Examination

- Urticaria is marked by the presence of elevated, erythematous, or white nonpitting plaques that change in size and shape over time (**Fig. 03-295**); they generally last a few hours and disappear without a trace.
- Skin lesions have an annular configuration with central pallor (**Fig. 03-296**).

Diagnostic Tests

- CBC with differential
- Stool for ova and parasites in patients with suspected parasitic infestations
- Skin biopsy is helpful in patients with fever, arthralgias, and elevated ESR. Histologic evidence of leukocytoclasia (neutrophilic infiltration with fragmentation of nuclei) is indicative of urticarial vasculitis.
- When suspecting food allergy in acute urticaria, testing can be performed using skin prick, immunoCAP, and radioallergosorbent testing (RAST).

Differential Diagnosis

- Erythema multiforme
- Erythema marginatum
- Erythema infectiosum
- Urticarial vasculitis
- Herpes gestationis
- Drug eruption
- Multiple insect bites
- Bullous pemphigoid

℞ Treatment

First Line

- Remove suspected etiologic agents (e.g., stop aspirin and all nonessential drugs), restrict diet (e.g., elimination of tomatoes, nuts, eggs, shellfish).
- Elimination of yeast should be attempted in patients with chronic urticaria (*C. albicans* sensitivity may be a factor in patients with chronic urticaria).
- Oral antihistamines: use of nonsedating antihistamines (e.g., loratadine 10 mg QD, cetirizine 10 mg QD, fexofenadine 180 mg QD, levocetirizine 5 mg QD) is preferred over first-generation antihistamines (e.g., hydroxyzine, diphenhydramine).

Second Line

- Oral corticosteroids should be reserved for refractory cases (e.g., prednisone 20 mg QD or 20 mg BID).

- H2 receptor antagonists (cimetidine, ranitidine, famotidine) can be added to H1 antagonists in refractory cases.

Third Line

- Doxepin (a tricyclic antidepressant that blocks both H1 and H2 receptors) 25 to 75 mg QHS may be effective in patients with chronic urticaria.
- Low dose of the immunosuppressant cyclosporine (2.5-3 mg/kg body weight/day) has been shown to be effective and corticosteroid sparing in chronic urticaria.

Clinical Pearl(s)

- Approximately 12% to 24% of the population will have one episode of hives during their lifetime.
- Incidence is increased in atopic patients.
- The etiology of chronic urticaria (hives lasting longer than 6 weeks) is determined in only 5% to 20% of cases.

157. VARICELLA (CHICKENPOX)

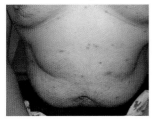
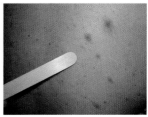

FIGURE 03-297. Pruritic papules and vesicles developed on this man's trunk and spread to his arms and face. He had been caring for his mother, who had shingles.

FIGURE 03-298. The classic varicella lesion is described as a "dew drop on rose petal" because it appears as a clear vesicle on an erythematous base.

General Comments

Definition

- Varicella is a common viral illness characterized by acute onset of generalized vesicular rash and fever.

Etiology

- Varicella zoster virus is a human herpesvirus 3 that can manifest with either varicella or herpes zoster (i.e., shingles, which is a reactivation of varicella).

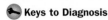
Keys to Diagnosis

Clinical Manifestation(s)

- Varicella is extremely contagious. More than 90% of unvaccinated contacts become infected.
- The incubation period ranges from 9 to 21 days.
- Peak incidence is in the springtime.
- The predominant age is 5 to 10 years.
- The infectious period begins 2 days before onset of clinical symptoms and lasts until all lesions have crusted.
- Most patients will have lifelong immunity following an attack of chickenpox; protection from chickenpox following varicella vaccine is approximately 6 years.
- Findings vary with the clinical course. Initial symptoms consist of fever, chills, backache, generalized malaise, and headache.
- Symptoms are generally more severe in adults.
- Intense pruritus generally accompanies initial lesions on the trunk.
- New lesion development generally ceases by the fourth day with subsequent crusting by the sixth day.
- Lesions generally spread to the face and the extremities (centrifugal spread).
- Patients generally present with lesions at different stages at the same time.
- Crusts generally fall off within 5 to 14 days.
- Fever is usually highest during the eruption of the vesicles; temperature generally returns to normal following disappearance of vesicles.
- Signs of potential complications (e.g., bacterial skin infections, neurologic complications, pneumonia, hepatitis) may be present on physical examination.
- Mild constitutional symptoms (e.g., anorexia, myalgias, headaches, restlessness) may be present (most common in adults).

Physical Examination

- Initial lesions generally occur on the trunk (centripetal distribution) and occasionally on the face; these lesions consist primarily of 3- to 4-mm red papules (**Fig. 03-297**) with an irregular outline and a clear vesicle on the surface (dew drops on a rose petal appearance; **Fig. 03-298**).
- Excoriations may be present if scratching is prominent.

Diagnostic Tests

- Laboratory evaluation is generally not necessary.
- CBC may reveal leukopenia and thrombocytopenia.
- Serum varicella titers (significant rise in serum varicella IgG antibody level), skin biopsy, or Tzanck smear are used only when diagnosis is in question.

DDx Differential Diagnosis

- Other viral infection
- Impetigo

- Scabies
- Drug rash
- Urticaria
- Dermatitis herpetiformis
- Smallpox (when suspecting bioterrorism)

Treatment

First Line
- Use antipruritic lotions for symptomatic relief.
- Avoid scratching to prevent excoriations and superficial skin infections.
- Use a mild soap for bathing; hands should be washed often.
- Use acetaminophen for fever and myalgias; aspirin should be avoided because of the increased risk of Reye's syndrome.
- Oral acyclovir (20 mg/kg QID for 5 days) initiated at the earliest sign (within 24 hours of illness) is useful in healthy, nonpregnant individuals 13 years of age or older to decrease the duration and severity of signs and symptoms. Immunocompromised hosts should be treated with intravenous acyclovir 500 mg/m^2 or 10 mg/kg Q8H IV for 7 to 10 days.
- Varicella is most contagious from 2 days before to a few days after the onset of the rash. Varicella vaccine is available for children and adults; protection lasts at least 6 years. Healthy, nonimmune adults and children exposed to varicella zoster virus should receive prophylaxis with live attenuated varicella vaccine (Varivax). Patients with HIV or other immunocompromised patients should not receive the live attenuated vaccine.
- Exposed patients with contraindications to varicella vaccine can be treated with varicella zoster immunoglobulin. It is effective in preventing varicella in susceptible individuals. It must be administered as early as possible after presumed exposure (within 4 days). If it cannot be obtained and administered within 4 days, providers should consider the use of IVIG within 4 days of exposure.
- Pruritus from chickenpox can be controlled with antihistamines (e.g., hydroxyzine 25 mg Q6H) and oral antipruritic lotions (e.g., calamine).

Second Line
- Foscarnet

Clinical Pearl(s)

- Infants who develop chickenpox are incapable of controlling the infection and should be given varicella zoster immunoglobulin (VZIG) or gamma globulin if VZIG is not available.

158. VARICOSE VEINS

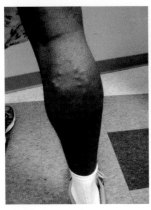

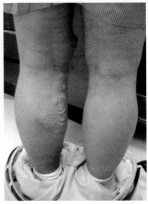

FIGURE 03-299. Right calf varicosities in this 40-year-old male are more pronounced on standing, secondary to incompetent venous valves.

FIGURE 03-300. Marked, tortuous varicosities on the left calf of this 50-year-old male, resulting in chronic edema.

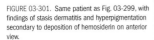

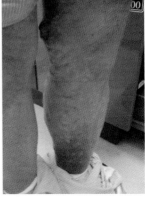

FIGURE 03-301. Same patient as Fig. 03-299, with findings of stasis dermatitis and hyperpigmentation secondary to deposition of hemosiderin on anterior view.

General Comments

Definition
- Varicose veins are dilated networks of the subcutaneous venous system that result from valvular incompetence.

Etiology
- Varices are caused by systemic weakness in the vein wall
- Valvular incompetence (**Fig. 03-299**) in perforator veins of lower extremity leads to reverse flow of fluid from high-pressure deep venous system to low-pressure superficial venous system, resulting in dilation of superficial veins, leg edema, and pain
- Rarely associated with deep vein thrombophlebitis
- Exacerbated by:
  - Restrictive clothing
  - Advancing age
  - Prolonged standing
  - Pregnancy
  - Obesity
  - Use of oral contraceptives
  - Obstruction in the ILIAC VEIN

Keys to Diagnosis

Clinical Manifestation(s)
- Present in approximately 30% of adults, with increasing incidence with age
- Increased incidence during pregnancy, especially with advanced maternal age

Physical Examination
- Dilation of superficial veins, leg edema (**Fig. 03-300**).
- Stasis dermatitis and hyperpigmentation secondary to deposition of hemosiderin (**Fig. 03-301**)

Diagnostic Tests
- Duplex ultrasound: gold standard for evaluation of varicose veins; quantitation of flow through venous valves under direct visualization

Differential Diagnosis

Conditions that can lead to superficial venous stasis other than primary valvular insufficiency include the following:
- Arterial occlusive disease
- Diabetes
- Deep vein thrombophlebitis

- Peripheral neuropathies
- Unusual infections
- Carcinoma

Treatment

First Line

- Leg elevation and rest
- Graded compression stockings: used early in morning before edema accumulates and removed before going to bed
- Weight loss
- Avoidance of occlusive clothing
- For associated stasis dermatitis: topical corticosteroids
- Treatment of secondary infection with appropriate antibiotics

Second Line

- Compression sclerotherapy: injection of 1% to 3% solution of sodium tetradecyl sulfate or 5% ethanolamine oleate
- Surgery: indications include the following:
  - Persistent varicosities with conservative treatment
  - Failed sclerotherapy
  - Previous or impending bleeding from ulcerated varicosities
  - Disabling pain
  - Cosmetic concerns

Third Line

- Surgical methods include (must be combined with compressive therapy) the following:
  - Saphenous vein ligation
  - Ligation of incompetent perforating veins
  - Saphenous vein stripping with or without avulsion of varicosities
  - Ambulatory "miniphlebectomies": avulsion of superficial varicosities with saphenous vein stripping
  - New treatments: endovenous obliteration using radiofrequency (diathermy) or laser as an alternative to traditional stripping of the long saphenous vein and powered phlebectomy for avulsing calf varicosities

159. VENOUS LAKE

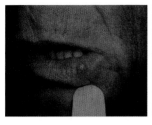

FIGURE 03-302. Venous lakes are often found on sun-exposed surfaces, which makes the vermilion border of the lower lip a common site.

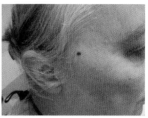

FIGURE 03-303. Benign dark purple papule containing venous blood that blanches under pressure.

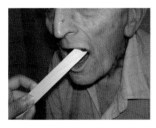

FIGURE 03-304. Large venous lake on the upper lip that blanched out under direct pressure. It can be confused with a nodular melanoma.

General Comments

Definition

■ A venous lake (varix) is a dilation of an endothelium-lined blood vessel with a very thin muscular wall.

Etiology

■ Unknown

Keys to Diagnosis

Clinical Manifestation(s)

■ They are found most often on the ventral surfaces of the tongue and on the lower lip (**Fig. 03-302**) and buccal mucosa and temporal area (**Fig. 03-303**), usually in older individuals.

Diagnostic Tests
- None necessary. Histology shows a dilated and congested vein in the superficial dermis. There is no evidence of vascular proliferation.

Physical Examination
- Lesions are sometimes multiple and can measure up to 1 cm in diameter.
- They are bluish-purple blebs that blanche upon pressure (**Fig. 03-304**) and may become firm if thrombosed

DDx Differential Diagnosis

- Hemangioma
- Melanoma
- Blue nevus
- Angiokeratoma
- Melanosis of buccal mucosa

R Treatment

First Line
- Cryosurgery

Second Line
- Laser ablation

Third Line
- Electrosurgery

Clinical Pearl(s)

- Lesions are often found over sun-exposed areas in middle age and older individuals.

160. VENOUS LEG ULCERS

General Comments

Definition
- Venous ulcers are shallow wounds with irregular borders that usually occur on the lower extremities above or over the malleoli. These ulcerations develop due to high venous pressures caused by incompetent valves or obstructed veins.

Etiology
- Venous stasis develops from valvular incompetence or obstruction, resulting in venous hypertension. Some authors propose that venous hypertension leads to malformation of capillaries causing leakage of fluid and reduced blood flow to

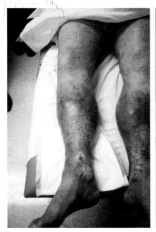

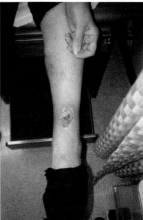

FIGURE 03-305. Severe venous leg ulcerations over the medial malleolus in this obese male with longstanding venous insufficiency, stasis dermatitis, pruritus, and marked hyperpigmentation from chronic scratching.

FIGURE 03-306. Punched-out recurrent venous ulcer with irregular border over the anterior shin, which occurred after minor trauma to this area chronically affected by stasis and recurrent cellulitis.

the skin. The resultant hypoxic tissue is prone to ulceration after minor trauma. The underlying vascular deficiency also impedes wound healing.

■ Risk factors include smoking, obesity, diabetes mellitus, phlebitis, increasing age, family history of varicose veins, history of DVT.

 Keys to Diagnosis

Clinical Manifestation(s)

■ Patients with venous stasis often have chronic skin changes on their lower limbs, including hyperpigmentation, hyperkeratosis, and dependent edema. Skin color changes are due to the extravasation of red blood cells and the resultant deposition of hemosiderin (**Fig. 03-305**).

■ Venous dermatitis or stasis dermatitis is common in these patients and is characterized by pruritic, red, and scaly eczematous changes.

■ Smooth white plaques of atrophic sclerosis are known as atrophie blanche and can be a clue that the patient has venous disease.

■ Patients often report a long history of dependent lower-extremity edema and aching pain in the legs that is often worse after standing for long periods.

Physical Examination

■ Venous ulcers are shallow, full-thickness ulcers, with irregular borders (**Fig. 03-306**) and areas of granulation tissue. Necrosis is extremely rare.

Diagnostic Tests

■ The majority of patients can be diagnosed clinically from the physical examination; however, up to 25% of patients have concomitant arterial disease. In these patients an ankle-brachial index test should be performed. Arterial insufficiency is suggested by an ankle-brachial index (ABI) of <1.0.
■ Patients with lower-extremity ulcers should also be evaluated for diabetes.
■ If vasculitis is suspected, a biopsy of the edge of the ulcer can confirm the diagnosis.
■ Any wound that is present for more than 3 months should be biopsied to rule out malignancy.

DDx Differential Diagnosis

■ Peripheral arterial disease (with ischemia and necrosis)
■ Diabetic ulceration (often secondary to neuropathy)
■ Decubitus ulceration (due to pressure over a bony prominence)
■ Vasculitis (with erythema and bullae)
■ Necrotic ulceration from infection
■ Basal cell carcinoma or squamous cell carcinoma

R Treatment

First Line

■ The goal of therapy is to improve venous return to the heart, thus decreasing edema, inflammation, and tissue ischemia.
■ First-line treatment includes compression bandages and elevation of the leg above the heart for at least 30 minutes three to four times a day. Bandages are used under compression stockings to provide a clean, moist environment to promote healing. Highly exudative wounds require absorbent dressings, whereas dry wounds may need a more occlusive dressing. There is no conclusive evidence that supports one type of dressing over another.
■ Smaller ulcers can be treated using compression stockings. Knee-high stockings with graded pressure providing at least 35 to 40 mm Hg of pressure at the ankle and 20 to 25 mm Hg at the knee are most effective.
■ Compression with either bandages or stockings is to be used only after arterial disease has been excluded as it can cause limb ischemia.
■ Underlying systemic hypertension and diabetes should be aggressively treated.

Second Line

■ Moist occlusive dressings and certain topical agents can aid in the healing of venous ulcers.

- Dressings can be nonadherent (Telfa), occlusive (Tegaderm, DuoDerm), or medicated like the Unna boot. Occlusive bandages have the advantage of reducing pain and can be changed by the patient every 5 to 7 days. These bandages do not increase the rate of wound infection if used appropriately.
- Daily aspirin (325 mg) is recommended to accelerate healing.
- Pentoxifylline may improve healing through its antithrombotic effects as well as fibrinolytic properties. Pentoxifylline 1200 mg/day has been shown to be an effective adjuvant to compression therapy.

Third Line
- Surgical intervention is not routine; however, options include sclerotherapy, replacement of venous valves, ligation, and stripping of veins. Skin grafts are also an option for nonhealing wounds.

Clinical Pearl(s)
- Overall prognosis is poor. Although 50% of ulcers will heal after 4 months, 20% are nonhealing after 2 years of treatment and 8% after 8 years. Recurrence is common.

161. VITILIGO

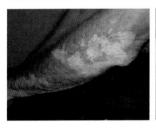

FIGURE 03-307. Sharply bordered area of vitiligo, which has been gradually progressive, on the left arm of this patient. This depigmented skin is vulnerable to sunburn (as depicted) and skin cancers.

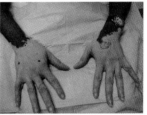

FIGURE 03-308. Nearly complete symmetric depigmentation of both hands with sharply defined borders, a common pattern in type A vitiligo.

General Comments
Definition
- Vitiligo is the acquired loss of epidermal pigmentation (**Fig. 03-307**) characterized histologically by the absence of epidermal melanocytes.

Etiology
- Three pathophysiologic theories suggest possible etiologies:
  Autoimmune theory (autoantibodies against melanocytes)
  Neural theory (neurochemical mediator selectively destroys melanocytes)
  Self-destructive process whereby melanocytes fail to protect themselves against
    cytotoxic melanin precursors
- Although vitiligo is considered to be an acquired disease, 25% to 30% is familial;
  the mode of transmission is unknown (polygenic or autosomal dominant with
  incomplete penetrance and variable expression).

Keys to Diagnosis

Clinical Manifestation(s)
- Initially the disease is limited, but the lesions tend to become more extensive over
  the years.

Physical Examination
- Hypopigmented and depigmented lesions favor sun-exposed regions,
  intertriginous areas, genitalia, and sites over bony prominences (type A vitiligo)
  (Fig. 03-308).
- Areas around body orifices are also commonly involved.
- The lesions tend to be symmetric.
- Occasionally the lesions are linear or pseudodermatomal (type B vitiligo).
- Vitiligo lesions may occur at trauma sites (*Koebner's phenomenon*).
- The hair in affected areas may be white.
- The margins of the lesions are usually well demarcated, and when a ring of
  hyperpigmentation is seen, the term *trichrome vitiligo* is used.
- The term *marginal inflammatory vitiligo* is used to describe lesions with
  raised borders.

Diagnostic Tests
- Physical examination
- Wood's light examination may enhance lesions in light-skinned
  individuals.

DDx Differential Diagnosis

Acquired
- Chemical induced
- Halo nevus
- Idiopathic guttate hypomelanosis
- Leprosy
- Leukoderma associated with melanoma
- Pityriasis alba
- Postinflammatory hypopigmentation

- Tinea versicolor
- Vogt-Koyanagi syndrome (vitiligo, uveitis, and deafness)

Congenital
- Albinism, partial (piebaldism)
- Albinism, total
- Nevus anemicus
- Nevus depigmentosus
- Tuberous sclerosis

Treatment

First Line
- Treatment is indicated primarily for cosmetic purposes when depigmentation causes emotional or social distress. Depigmentation is more noticeable in darker complexions.
- Cosmetic masking agents (Dermablend, Covermark) or stains (Dy-O-Derm, Vita-Dye)
- Sunless tanning lotions (dihydroxyacetone)
- Repigmentation (achieved by activation and migration of melanocytes from hair follicles; therefore, skin with little or no hair responds poorly to treatment)
- PUVA (psoralen phototherapy): oral or topical psoralen administration followed by phototherapy with UVA (150-200 treatments required over 1-2 years)
- Psoralens and sunlight (Puvasol)

Second Line
- Topical midpotency steroids (e.g., triamcinolone 0.1% or desonide 0.05% cream QD for 3-4 months).
- Total depigmentation (in cases of extensive vitiligo) with 20% monobenzyl ether or hydroquinone. This is a permanent procedure, and patients will require lifelong protection from sun exposure.
- Intralesional steroid injection.
- Systemic steroids (betamethasone 5 mg QD on 2 consecutive days per week for 2-4 months).

Third Line
- Topical immunomodulators (tacrolimus, pimecromilus) can also induce repigmentation of vitiliginous skin lesions. Their potential for systemic immunosuppression or increased risk of skin or other malignancies remains to be defined.
- Calcipotriol, a synthetic analogue of vitamin D_3, has also been used in combination with UV light or clobetasol, with limited results.

Clinical Pearl(s)

- Vitiligo may begin around pigmented nevi, producing a halo (*Sutton's nevus*); in such cases the central nevus often regresses and disappears over time.

162. WARTS (VERRUCAE)

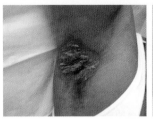

FIGURE 03-309. Large cluster of velvety warts occuring in the moist axilla of this AIDS patient.

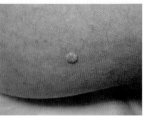

FIGURE 03-310. Solitary, persistent, keratotic wart on the leg of this patient on immunosuppressive medications.

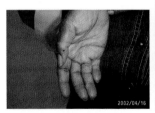

FIGURE 03-311. Broad-based, hyperkeratotic wart on the distal fourth digit with cylindric projections.

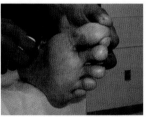

FIGURE 03-312. Several keratotic, callused, grouped plantar warts occurring over pressure points.

General Comments

Definition
■ Warts are benign epidermal neoplasms caused by human papillomavirus.

Etiology
■ Human papillomavirus infection; more than 60 types of viral DNA have been identified. Transmission of warts is by direct contact.
■ Genital warts are usually caused by HPV types 6 or 11.

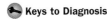 Keys to Diagnosis

Clinical Manifestation(s)

- Common warts occur most often in children and young adults.
- Anogenital warts are most common in young, sexually active patients. Genital warts are the most common viral sexually transmitted disease (STD) in the United States, with up to 24 million Americans carrying the virus that causes them.
- Common warts are longer lasting and more frequent in immunocompromised patients (e.g., lymphoma, AIDS, immunosuppressive drugs) (**Fig. 03-309**).
- Plantar warts occur most often at points of maximum pressure (over the heads of the metatarsal bones or on the heels).

Physical Examination

- Common warts (**Fig. 03-310**) have an initial appearance of a flesh-colored papule with a rough surface; they subsequently develop a hyperkeratotic appearance with black dots on the surface (thrombosed capillaries); they may be single or multiple and are most common on the hands.
- Warts obscure normal skin lines (important diagnostic feature). Cylindrical projections from the wart may become fused, forming a mosaic pattern.
- Flat warts generally are pink or light yellow, slightly elevated, and often found on the forehead, back of hands, mouth, and beard area; they often occur in lines corresponding to trauma (e.g., a scratch); are often misdiagnosed (particularly when present on the face); and are inappropriately treated with topical corticosteroids.
- Filiform warts (**Fig. 03-311**) have a fingerlike appearance with various projections; they are generally found near the mouth, beard, or periorbital and paranasal regions.
- Plantar warts (**Fig. 03-312**) are slightly raised and have a roughened surface; they may cause pain when walking; as they involute, small hemorrhages (caused by thrombosed capillaries) may be noted.
- Genital warts are generally pale pink with several projections and a broad base. They may coalesce in the perineal area to form masses with a cauliflower-like appearance.
- Genital warts on the cervical epithelium can produce subclinical changes that may be noted on Pap smear or colposcopy.

Diagnostic Tests

- Suspect lesions should be biopsied.
- Colposcopy with biopsy of genital warts should be performed in patients with cervical squamous cell changes.

DDx Differential Diagnosis

- Molluscum contagiosum
- Condyloma latum
- Acrochordon (skin tags) or seborrheic keratosis

- Epidermal nevi
- Hypertrophic actinic keratosis
- Squamous cell carcinomas
- Acquired digital fibrokeratoma
- Varicella zoster virus in patients with AIDS
- Recurrent infantile digital fibroma
- Plantar corns (may be mistaken for plantar warts)

℞ Treatment

- Watchful waiting is an acceptable option in the treatment of warts because many warts will disappear without intervention over time.
- Plantar warts that are not painful do not need treatment.
- Treatment for common warts is as follows:
  - Application of topical salicylic acid 17%. Soak area for 5 minutes in warm water and dry. Apply thin layer once or twice daily for up to 12 weeks, avoiding normal skin. Bandage.
  - Liquid nitrogen, electrocautery are also common methods of removal.
  - Blunt dissection can be used in large lesions or resistant lesions.
  - Duct tape occlusion is also effective for treating common warts. It is cut to cover warts and left in place for 6 days. It is removed after 6 days and the warts are soaked in water and then filed with pumice stones. New tape is applied 12 hours later. This treatment can be repeated until warts resolve.
- Filiform warts: Surgical removal is necessary.
- Flat warts are generally more difficult to treat.
  - Tretinoin cream applied at bedtime over the involved area for several weeks may be effective.
  - Liquid nitrogen can be applied.
  - Electrocautery can be performed.
  - 5-Fluorouracil cream applied once or twice a day for 3 to 5 weeks is also effective. Persistent hyperpigmentation may occur following Efudex use.
- Treatment for plantar warts is as follows:
  - Salicylic acid therapy (e.g., Occlusal-HP) can be effective. Soak wart in warm water for 5 minutes, remove loose tissue, and dry. Apply to area, allow to dry, then reapply. Use once or twice daily for a maximum of 12 weeks. Use of 40% salicylic acid plasters (Mediplast) is also a safe, nonscarring treatment; it is particularly useful in treating mosaic warts covering a large area.
  - Blunt dissection is also a fast and effective treatment modality.
  - Laser therapy can be used for plantar warts and recurrent warts; however, it leaves open wounds that require 4 to 6 weeks to fill with granulation tissue.
  - Interlesional bleomycin is also effective but generally used when all other treatments fail.
- Treatment for genital warts is as follows:
  - Genital warts can be effectively treated with 20% podophyllin resin in compound tincture of benzoin applied with a cotton-tipped applicator by

the treating physician and allowed to air dry. The treatment can be repeated weekly if necessary.
- Podofilox (Condylox 0.5% gel) is now available for application by the patient. Local adverse effects include pain, burning, and inflammation at the site.
- Cryosurgery with liquid nitrogen delivered with a probe or as a spray is effective for treating smaller genital warts.
- Carbon dioxide laser can also be used for treating primary or recurrent genital warts (cure rate > 90%).
- Imiquimod cream 5% is a patient-applied immune response modifier effective in the treatment of external genital and perianal warts (complete clearing of genital warts in >70% of females and >30% of males in 4-16 weeks). Sexual contact should be avoided while the cream is on the skin. It is applied three times per week before normal sleeping hours and is left on the skin for 6 to 10 hours.
- Sinecatechins (Veregen), a botanical drug product, is also effective for treatment of external genital and perianal warts. Formulation is a 15% ointment applied to the affected area TID for up to 16 weeks.
- Application of trichloroacetic acid (TCA) or bichloracetic acid (BCA) 80% to 90% is also effective for external genital warts. A small amount should be applied only to warts and allowed to dry, at which time a white "frosting" develops. This treatment can be repeated weekly if necessary.

Clinical Pearl(s)
- The importance of condom use in males and vaccination of females with quadrivalent HPV vaccine from age 9 to 26 to reduce transmission of genital warts should be emphasized.

163. XANTHOMA
General Comments
Definition
- Xanthoma is an abnormal deposition of lipids in the skin and subcutaneous tissues.

Etiology
- Hyperlipidemia due to hereditary factors and/or lifestyle
- Contributing factors may be endocrine or metabolic disorders (e.g., hypothyroidism, nephritic syndrome, diabetes)

Keys to Diagnosis
Clinical Manifestation(s)
- Onset can be asymptomatic and insidious or sudden with development of pruritic multiple yellow-red papules (**Fig. 03-313**) on buttocks, shoulders, or extremities (eruptive xanthomas).

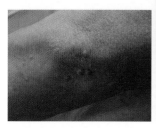

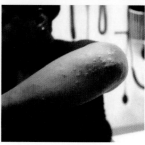

FIGURE 03-313. Dome-shaped, discrete yellow papules that appeared suddenly in a patient with uncontrolled diabetes.

FIGURE 03-314. This shower of eruptive xanthomas appearing from elbow to forearm occurred suddenly in this diabetic patient who ran out of her insulin.

Physical Examination
- Flat yellow lesions on eyelids (xanthelasma)
- Firm yellow nodules on the elbows (**Fig. 03-314**) and knees (tuberous xanthomas)
- Slowly enlarging subcutaneous nodules on the hands, ankles and over extensor tendons (tendon xanthomas)
- Yellow palmar creases (plane xanthomas)

Diagnostic Tests
- Lipid panel

Differential Diagnosis
- Necrobiosis lipoidica
- Rheumatoid nodules
- Neurofibromas
- Nodular elastoidosis
- Granuloma annulare
- Giant tumor of tendon sheath
- Erythema elevatum diutinum
- Histiocytoses

℞ Treatment
First Line
- Treatment of hyperlipidemia (statins, fenofibrates, dietary restrictions)

Second Line
■ Laser, electrocautery, excision or trichloroacetic acid can be used for xanthelasmas.

 Clinical Pearl(s)

■ Xanthelasma may or may not be associated with hyperlipidemia.
■ Eruptive xanthomas are associated with very high triglyceride levels.

164. XEROSIS

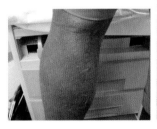

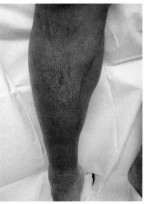

FIGURE 03-315. Chronically scaly, xerotic skin, worse during the fall and winter months because of dry, indoor heat and low humidity.

FIGURE 03-316. Dry, markedly pruritic, hyperpigmented skin with fissuring and bleeding secondary to scratching. Medial linear scar is from the harvesting of a donor graft for prior CABG surgery.

 General Comments

Definition
■ Xerosis is dry, rough-appearing scaly skin.

Etiology
■ Aging
■ Systemic illness (e.g. renal failure, diabetes, hypothyroidism, malnutrition, anorexia nervosa, carcinomatosis, HIV infection)
■ Medication induced (e.g., oral retinoids, diuretics, nicotinic acid, lithium)

- Congenital disorder of keratinization
- Atopic dermatitis
- Persistently low ambient humidity, infrequent use of emollients
- Use of harsh soaps and degreasing agents

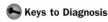 Keys to Diagnosis

Clinical Manifestation(s)
- Found most commonly in older individuals in the winter months (**Fig. 03-315**).
- Pruritus may be present.
- Dry skin on the shins (area of low density of sebaceous glands) (**Fig. 03-316**) is common in diabetics in winter months.

Physical Examination
- Dry, scaly skin
- Eczematous changes may accompany dry skin

Diagnostic Tests
- None usually necessary
- TSH, BUN, serum creatinine if clinically indicated

DDx Differential Diagnosis

- Ichthyosis
- Stasis dermatitis
- Asteatotic eczema
- Nummular eczema
- Eczema craquele

R Treatment

- Elimination of contributing factors: avoidance of soaps and detergents, decreased frequency of showering and bathing, use of humidifiers in winter months
- Frequent (4-6 times/day) use of emollients (moisturizers) to build a lipid layer to prevent transepidermal water loss; emollients containing urea, alpha hydroxyl acid, or ammonium lactate are very effective
- Use of soap substitutes

Clinical Pearl(s)

- Bathing in tepid water instead of hot water and patting dry rather than vigorous toweling is very helpful.

APPENDIX 1: TOPICAL STEROIDS

Super High Potency* Trade Name Clobex, Cormax, Olux, Olux-E, Temovate, Temovate-E	Generic Name Clobetasol propionate (0.05%): cream, ointment, solution, foam
Cordran	Flurandrenolide: tape 4 μg/sq cm
Vanos	Fluocinonide (0.1%): cream
Ultravate	Halobetasol proprionate (0.05%): cream, ointment
High Potency	
Cyclocort	Amcinonide (0.1%): ointment, cream, lotion
Halog	Halcinonide (0.1%): cream, ointment, soln
Diprolene, Diprolene AF	Betamethasone dipropionate augmented (0.05%): ointment, gel
Topicort	Desoximetasone (0.25%): cream, ointment
Topicort	Desoximetasone (0.05%): gel
Psorcone	Diflorasone diacetate (0.05%): cream, ointment
Aristocort A, Kenalog	Triamcinolone acetonide (0.5%): cream
Lidex, Lidex-E	Fluticinonide (0.05 %): cream
Intermediate Potency	
Cutivate	Fluticasone propionate (0.005%): ointment
Cutivate	Fluticasone propionate (0.05%): cream, lotion
Derma-Smoothe, Capex	Fluocinolone acetonide (0.01%): oil, shampoo
Aristocort A, Kenalog	Triamcinolone acetonide (0.1%): cream, ointment, lotion
Dermatop	Prednicarbate (0.1%): emollient, cream, ointment
Elocon	Mometasone furoate (0.1%): cream, lotion, ointment
Kenalog	Triamcinolone acetonide (0.2%): aerosol
Synalar	Fluocinolone acetonide (0.025%): cream, ointment
Luxiq	Betamethasone valerate (0.12%): foam
Cloderm	Clocortolone pivalate (0.1%): cream
Desonate, DesOwen, Verdoso	Desonide (0.05%): gel, cream, lotion, ointment, foam
Topicort-LP	Desoximatasone (0.05%): emollient cream
Cordran, Cordran SP	Flurandrenolide (0.025%): cream, ointment

*Potency varies with the product, its concentration, and the delivery mechanism.

(Continued)

Cordran, Cordran SP	Flurandrenolide (0.05%): cream, ointment, lotion
Locoid	Hydrocortisone butyrate (0.1%): cream, solution, ointment
Westcort	Hydrocortisone valerate (0.2%): cream, ointment
Low Potency	
Aristocort A, Kenalog	Triamcinolone acetonide (0.025%): cream, ointment, lotion
Aclovate	Alclometasone dipropionate (0.05%): cream, ointment
Synalar	Fluocinolone acetonide (0.01%): solution
Hytone	Hydrocortisone base or acetate (2.5%): cream, ointment
Hytone, Vytone, Cortisporin, U-cort	Hydrocortisone base or acetate (1%): cream, ointment
Cortisporin	Hydrocortisone base or acetate (0.5 %): cream

APPENDIX 2: CUTANEOUS MANIFESTATIONS OF INTERNAL DISEASE

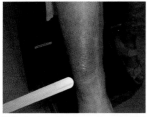

Flesh-colored, nonpitting, brawny plaque of pretibial myxedema found on both shins of this patient with Graves disease.

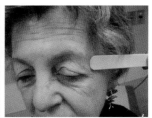

Puffy periorbital tissue, sallow, dry skin and loss of lateral third of the eyebrow (Queen Anne's sign) in this patient with hypothyroidism.

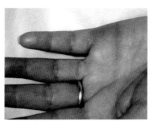

Red, hemorrhagic, painless macular lesion on the palm at the base of the fifth finger.

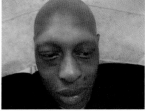

Global loss of scalp and body hair, beard, eyebrows, and eyelashes in this patient with associated autoimmune diseases (Graves disease and type 1 diabetes mellitus).

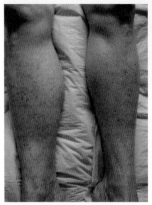

Numerous red, very small (pinhead size), flat petechiae that do not blanch on palpation and are located over both shins of this patient with idiopathic thrombocytopenic purpura (ITP).

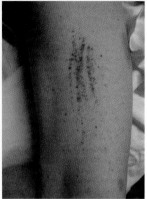

Petechiae can be distributed over lines of minor trauma, known as vibices, as on the arm of this patient with ITP following scratching.

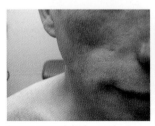

Gaunt appearance of HIV-infected adult patient caused by atrophy of the fat pad of Bichat following 1 year of treatment with protease inhibitors.

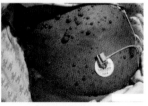

Numerous hyperpigmented, soft, pedunculated nodules or neurofibromas and several larger than 1 cm café-au-lait macules located on the abdomen of this patient with longstanding neurofibromatosis.

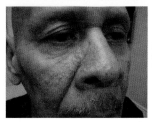

Multiple papules with a dome configuration known as adenoma sebaceum have been present on the cheeks of this patient since his early 20s.

APPENDIX 3: NAIL DISEASES

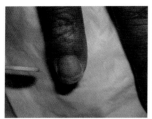

Transverse, parallel, paired white bands known as Muehrcke's sign, caused by hypoalbuminemia from nephrotic syndrome in this case, which results in localized edema of the nail bed.

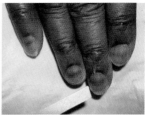

Hyperpigmented transverse bands (melanonychia), a drug-induced nail change, occurring in all nails of this patient following a course of hydroxyurea for thrombocytosis.

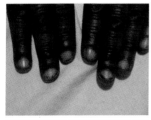

Multiple longitudinal collections of blood or splinter hemorrhages in distal nail beds of all fingers, caused by vasculitis secondary to cocaine.

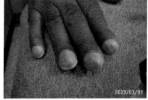

Typical bulbous shape of tips of fingers with hyperplasia of the vascular tissue at the nail base, causing a rocking sensation of the nail when the area is pressed. Note also the increased curvature of the distal nail.

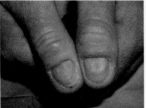

Deep, transverse, central grooves on the thumbnails of both hands caused by habitually "digging" (tic habit) and traumatizing proximal cuticle.

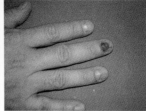

Subungual hematoma caused by proximal nail plate trauma producing pain and causing a slight elevation of the nail plate.

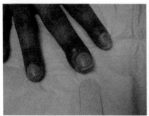

Painful acute paronychia that developed over 24 hours with erythema, edema, and accumulation of purulent material at the cuticle and lateral nail fold.

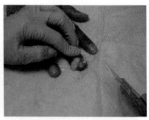

Successful drainage of an acute paronychia following the insertion of a scalpel under the proximal nail fold just above the nail.

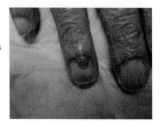

Flesh-colored, nodular growth, often referred to as Koenen tumors, protruding from the proximal nail fold in this patient with tuberous sclerosis.

APPENDIX 4: STINGS AND BITES

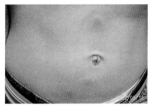

Pruritic, erythematous, raised hivelike fleabites, often referred to as papular urticaria, appearing on the abdomen in a previously sensitized individual.

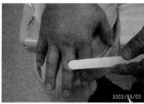

Intense, firm, edematous, erythematous reaction consistent with angioedema occurring several hours following a honeybee sting.

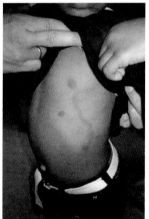

Cutaneous larva migrans appears on the lateral chest of this child as a thin, linear, serpiginous, raised tunnel-like lesion. When palpated, it has the consistency of an underlying thin string.

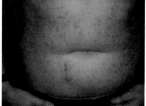

Erythematous pruritic papules consistent with seabather's eruption developed on the torso of this female swimmer following a swim in the Caribbean. The lesions are caused by a reaction to the stings of cnidarian larvae, which inflict their stings after a freshwater shower and are limited to the areas covered by swimwear.

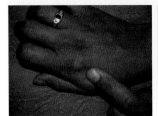

Papular, urticarial lesion on the dorsum of the hand following a mosquito bite.

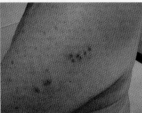

Bedbug bites occurring in a typical array of several red, intensely pruritic, hivelike papules distributed in a row on the upper arm.

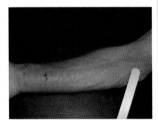

Deep puncture marks caused by a cat bite on the wrist of this patient with secondary lymphangitis extending up medial forearm. No fragments of cat teeth were identified on x-ray examination. The patient improved following wound irrigation and empiric therapy for *Pastuerella* organisms with amoxicillin-clavulanate.

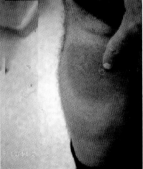

Erythema migrans presenting in the more common pattern of a slowly expanding, diffusely homogenous lesion occurring in 59% of cases. Note the central punctum from the preceding bite of the deer tick, *Ixodes scapularis,* which is seen in only 30% of the cases.

M